The Essence of Homeopathy Materia Medica

OrangeBooks Publication

1st Floor, Rajhans Arcade, Mall Road, Kohka, Bhilai, Chhattisgarh - 490020

Website:**www.orangebooks.in**

© Copyright, 2024, Author

All rights reserved. No part of this book may be reproduced, stored in a retrieval system, or transmitted, in any form by any means, electronic, mechanical, magnetic, optical, chemical, manual, photocopying, recording or otherwise, without the prior written consent of its writer.

First Edition, 2024

THE ESSENCE OF HOMEOPATHY MATERIA MEDICA

DR. MAHENDRA PRASAD MAHAPATRA

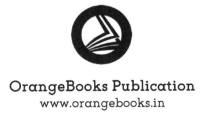

OrangeBooks Publication
www.orangebooks.in

Foreword

The Essence of Homeopathy Materia Medica by Dr. Mahendra Prasad Mahapatra represents the author's dedication to the art and science of Homeopathy. In his meticulous pursuit of each remedy he studied, he relied on the works of past masters, collecting the jewels of knowledge from various masters and reproducing the important key symptoms under each remedy. His hard work is making the student's studies much easier by placing in one book all that the student needs to study the important remedies of the Materia medica. I hope his book will be on the work desks of students and homeopathic practitioners as an invaluable reference to be read and reread.

Dato Dr Suriyakhatun Osman
MBBCh, MFHom
Bangi, Selangor, Malaysia

Foreword

The "Essence of Homeopathy Materia Medica" by Dr. Mahendra Prasad Mahapatra is one of the fine Homeopathy Books. Each remedy is described in detail. Dr. Mahendra Prasad Mahapatra has done a marvelous job. He was a great philosopher.

Thank you I am looking forward to this artistic job.

Dr. Satnam Singh S. Mehmi
BHMS, Pune

Acknowledgment

Dr Mahendra Prasad Mahapatra was a. noble, kind-hearted, and legendary homeopathic doctor in the middle and later part of the 20th century. He was fully dedicated to his profession and his patients. He was listening to the problems and symptoms of his patients carefully and thoroughly, following which he was recommending the treatment. Surprisingly, he was successful in almost all cases. He earned a good name in the Kidderpore area in Calcutta. Unlike other medical faculties, the philosophy of homeopathy is completely different. Here, the physician listens to the symptoms very carefully, and without an investigation, they diagnose the disease and treat the patient correctly. Today, in Allopathy and other medical branches, a patient has to spend lakhs of rupees in various investigations before the treatment. Besides, there are a lot of side effects in both Allopathy and Ayurvedic medicines. Today, I feel proud of the publication of the homeopathy book titled "The Essence of Homeopathy Materia Medica" and wish a grand success in circulation among the readers.

Dr. Kamalakanta Nayak. MS.
Senior Consultant Surgery
Odisha

Contents

A
Alphabet

Abrotanum	1
Acetic Acid	5
Acetaea Racemosa	6
Actea Spicata	9
Adonis Vernalis	9
Aesculus Hippocastanum	9
Aethusa Cynapium	11
Agaricus Muscarius	11
Ailanthus Glandulosa	13
Allium Cepa	14
Aloe Socotrina	15
Alumen	15
Alumina	16
Ambra Grisea	17
Ammonium Carb	18
Ammonium Mur	19
Artemisia Vulgaris	19
Amylenum Nitrosum	20
Anacardium Orientale	20
Angustura Vera	21
Antimonium Crudum	22
Antim Tart	23
Apis Mellifica	25
Apocyanum Cannabinum	26
Aralia Racemosa	27
Aranea Diadema	27
Argentum Metallicum	28
Argentum Nitricum	29

Arnica Montana 30
Arsenicum Album 32
Arsenic Iod 37
Artemisia Vulgaris 37
Asafoetida 38
Asarum Europaeum 39
Asclepias Tuberosa 39
Aurum Met. 39
Aurum Muriaticum 40
Aurum Muriaticum Natronatum 41
Argentum Metallicum 41
Argentum Nitricum 42
Azadirachta Indica 44
Apoplexy 44

B
Alphabet

Badiaga 46
Baryta-Mur. 48
Belladonna 48
Bellis Perennis 50
Benzoic Acid 50
Berberis Vulgaris 51
Blatta Orientalis 53
Borax 53
Bovista 54
Bromium 54
Bryonia Alba 56
Belladonna 57
Bufo 58

C
Alphabet

Cactus Grandiflorus 60
Cadmium Sulph 62
Cainca 63

Cajuputum	63
Caladium	64
Calcarea Arsenica	64
Calcarea Carb	64
Calcarea Carb	65
Calcarea Phosphorica	67
Calendula Officinalis	70
Camphora	70
Cannabis Indica	71
Cannabis Sativa	72
Cantharides	72
Capsicum	73
Carbo Animalis	75
Comparison between Hepar sulph and Calcarea sulph	76
Carbo Vegetabilis	77
(Acid Carbolis) Carbolic Acid	80
Cardus Marianus	81
Castor Equorum	82
Castoreum	82
Caulophyllum	83
Causticum	83
Ceanothus Americanus	86
Cedron	87
Chamomilla	87
Chelidonium Majus	89
Chenopodium - Anthelminticum	90
Chenopodium- Glaucum	90
Chimaphila Umbellata	90
China	91
China-Ars	91
China Sulph	92
Chionanthus Virginica	92
Chlorum	92
Cicuta Virosa	92
Cimea	94
Cina	95
Cinchona	95

Cinnabaris	97
Cistus Canadensis	98
Cobaltum	100
Coccinella	100
Cocculus Indicus	100
Coccus Cacti	103
Coffea Cruda	104
Cubeba Officinalis	105
Cucurbita Pepo	105
Cuprum Metallicum	106
Curare	110
Cyclamen	110
Cypripedium Pubescens	112

D
Alphabet

Daphne Indica	114
Digitalis Purpurea	114
Dolichos	116
Doryphora	116
Drosera Rotundifolia	116
Drosera	118
Dulcamara	119

E
Alphabet

Elaps Corallinus	122
Elaterium	122
Epigea Repens	123
Epiphegus Virginiana	123
Erigeron Canadensis	123
Eucalyptus Globulus	124
Eugenia Jambos	125
Eupatorium Perfoliatum	125
Eupatorium Purpurum	126
Euphorbium	126

Euphrasia Officinalis 127

F
Alphabet

Ferrum Arsenicum 128
Ferrum Iodatum 128
Ferrum Metallicum 128
Ferrum Phosphoricum 130
Ferrum Picricum 131
Ferrum Tauri 132
Fluoric Acid 132

G
Alphabet

Gallicum Acidum 136
Gambogia 136
Gelsemium 137
Ginseng 139
Glonoine 139
Gnaphalium 142
Gnaphalium Polycephalum 143
Gossypium-Herbaceum 143
Graphites 144
Gratiola Officinalis 147
Grindelia-Robusta 148
Guaiacum 149
Guarea Trichilioides 150
Gymnocladus-Canadensis 151

H
Alphabet

Hamamelis Virginica 152
Helleborus Niger 152
Helonius Dioica 154
Hepar Sulph 155

Hippomanes 158
Homarus 158
Hydrastis Canadensis 158
Hydrocyanic Acid 160
Hyoscyamus Niger 161
Hypericum Perforatum 165

I
Alphabet

Iberis Amara 168
Ignatia 168
Indigo 171
Indium Metallicum 172
Idoformum 172
Iodium 172
Ipecacuanha 175
Iris Versicolor 179

J
Alphabet

Jaborandi 181
Jalapa 181
Jatropha Curcas 182
Juglans Regia 182
Juglans Cinerea 182

K
Alphabet

Kali Bichromicum 184
Kali Bromatum 187
Kali Carb 189
Kali Chloratum 194
Kali Cyanatum 195
Kali Iod 195
Kali Nitricum 198

Kali Phos 198
Kali Sulph 201
Kalmia Latifolia 202
Kreosotum 203

L
Alphabet

Lachesis 205
Lac Caninum 208
Lac Dedloratum 209
Lac-Felinium 210
Lachnanthes 211
Lactic Acid 211
Lactuca Virasa 212
Lauroccrasus 213
Ledum Pal 213
Lilium Tigri 214
Lithium Carb 216
Lycopodium 217
Lycopus-Virginicus 222

M
Alphabet

Magnesium Carbonate 225
Magnesium Muriaticum 227
Magnesium Phosphoricum 229
Magnesium Sulphurica 231
Malandrinum 231
Magnum Opus 232
Mancinella 236
Medorrhium 236
Melilotus 239
Mentha Piperita 239
Menyanthes Trifoliata 240
Mephities 241
Mercurius 241

Merc-Sol (Mercurius solubilis) 243
Mercurius Corrosivus 245
Mezereum 246
Mitchella Repens 248
Morphinum Muriaticum 249
Moschus 249
Millefolium 251
Murex Purpurea 251
Muriatic Acid 252
Myrica Cerifera 253
Myrtus Communis 254

N
Alphabet

Naja Tripudians 255
Natrum Carbonicum 257
Natrum Muriaticum 259
Natrum Phosphoricum 263
Natrum Salicylicum 265
Natrum Sulphuricum 265
Niccolum Metalicum 268
Nitric Acid 268
Nux Moschata 270
Nuphar Luteum 272
Nux Vomica 273

O
Alphabet

Ocimum Canum 277
Oenanthe-Crocata 278
Oleander. 278
Oleum Animale 279
Oleum Jecoris 279
Onosmodium 280
Opium 281
Oxalic Acid 283

P
Alphabet

Paeonia Officinalis	286
Palladium	286
Pareira Brava	287
Paris Qudrifolia	287
Passiflora-In	288
Petroleum	289
Petroselinum Sativum	291
Phellandrium Aquaticum	291
Phosphoric Acid	292
Phosphorous	296
Phytolacca	300
Picric Acid	302
Platinum	303
Plantago-Major	304
Plumbum Met	305
Psorinum	308
Prunas Spinosa	311
Ptelea-Trifoliate	312
Pulsatilla	313
Pyrogen	319

R
Alphabeth

Radium Bromatum	322
Ratanhia	323
Ranunculus Bulbosus	323
Raphanus Sativus	325
Rheum	326
Rhododendron	327
Rhus Aromatica	328
Rhus Glabra	328
Ricinus Communis	329
Robinia Pseudacacia	330
Rumex	331

Ruta Graveolens 333

S
Alphabet

Sabina 335
Sabadilla 337
Salicylic Acid 338
Sanguinaria Canadensis 339
Sanicula 342
Santoninum 344
Sarsaparilla 344
Secale Cor 346
Selenium 348
Sepia 350
Senecio Aureus 354
Senega 355
Silicea 357
Sinapsis Alba 361
Sinapsis Nigra 361
Solanum Nigrum 362
Spigelia 362
Spongia Tosta 364
Squilla Maritima 366
Stannum 367
Staphisagria 369
Stramonium 371
Sticta-Pulmonaria 373
Stilliangia-Sylvatica 375
Strophanthus Hispidus 375
Strontiiana Carb 376
Strychinium 377
Sulphur 377
Sulphuric Acid 383
Syphilinum 385

T
Alphabet

Tabacum 388
Taraxacum Officinale 389
Tarentula Hispanica 389
Tarentula Hispanica & Tarentula Cubensis 391
Tarentula Cubensis 392
Tellurium 393
Terebinthinae Oleum 394
Teucrium Marum 395
Theridion 395
Tilia Europaea 396
Trombidium 397
Thuja Occidentalis 399
Tuberculinum 403

U
Alphabet

Uranium Nitricum 406
Urtica Urens 406
Ustilago 407
Urva-Ursi 409

V
Alphabet

Valeriana 410
Veratrum-Alb 411
Veratrum Viride 413
Viburnum Opulus 414
Vinca Minor 416
Viola Odorata 416
Viola Tricolor 417
Vipera-Torva 417
Viscum Album 418

X
Alphabet

Xanthoxylum 419

Y
Alphabet

Yucca Fillamentosa 420

Z
Alphabet

Zincum Metallicum 421
Zingiber Off.. 424
Zincum Metallicum- Baby (Borland)... 425

Alphabet

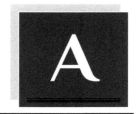

Abrotanum
Chilly Anti-psoric

Dr. Kent
- Rheumatic condition with heart irritation, epistaxis, Bloody urine anxiety and trembling. When there has been a history of diarrhoea. Metastasis is a marked feature. Inflammation of the parotid changing to testes or mammae is generally cured by Carbo veg or Puls but Abrotanum has cured when these remedies have failed.
- Susceptible to cold, complaints during constipation, injury.
- In boys it cures hydrocele bleeding from navel.
- Sharp pains here and there, especially ovaries and joints.
- Diarrhoea and constipation alternatively. The patient feels better any way during diarrhoea.

Dr. Tyler
It has many symptoms common with Aethusa.
- Too weak to hold up the head.
- Aethusa: Inability to hold the neck.
- Abrotanum craves bread boiled in milk.
- **Aethusa:** Idiocy irritable inhumane and even does all sorts of crack things.

- - Great weakness and prostration with a kind of prior hectic fever with children after influenza.
- Sensation as if stomach were hanging or swimming in water with Peculiar feeling of coldness and dryness to all orifices.
- Destroys worms especially ascaris.
- Boils with rheumatism or gout especially of the ankle and wrist joint.

Choudhary

In marasmus it can compare with the following remedies:

- **Aethusa:** Cynapium (see above Dr. Tyler)
- **Antimonium Crudum (Antim crud):** Vomiting of food and drink, diarrhoea and constipation alternatively. Ugliness and peevishness of children. does not want to be looked at or touched. Lack of mind rest. Thick white coating tongue.

Baryta Carb

- Dwarfish mind versus body large abdomen Chilli patient enlarge tonsil, tendency to enlarge cervical glands Offensive spicy susceptible to cold.
- **Calcarea Carb:** The emancipation is more marked in tissues than adipose. The muscles and bones suffer before the tissues are affected. 3F Chilly. Sweat on the head, wetting the pillow far around. Cold feet. Fat without fitness. Bones without strength. Sweat without heat. Tissues of plus and minus. Craving for egg, open fontanelle suture.
- Irritable, itching of the nose and rectum. Canine hunger or loss of appetite. Refused mother's milk. Touchy patient. Presence of worms in the stool. The beastly temper. picking of the nose. Wetting the bed. Child gets > by rocking.
  - **Iodium:** Hot patient, susceptible to cold. Voracious appetite. Can only quiet after eating. Swelling and irritation of the

glands < ascending, usually diarrhoeic in nature with diarrhoea.

- **Natrum Mur:** Suppress of intermittent. Marasmus of the children especially of neck, constipation, extra craving for salt. Aversion to bread. Mapped tongue. Herpes labialis, sadness, consolation < palpitation.

From Hahnemannian gleanings January 72: By F K Beilokossy M.D (Colorado).

- In Cryptorchismus (Undescended Testes) and dystrophia-adipose-genetalis (short penis and testis) It is almost specific.
- This translucent skin on his forehead temples and the veins shining through consider Natrum Mur thirty. If you see a lady with scrawny, wrinkled atrophic neck, covered with small of back or brown warts do not ask question, give Nat Mur thirty. Do not expect a cure before a year and repeat very seldom rising the potency each time, crust, black spots on the atrophic skin of the scalp, face or leg respond to the remedy.

Sanicula

- Marasmus of the children with marked emaciation of the neck, profuse sweat in head and extremities. The skin is wrinkled and hanging down in folds, dirty greasy skin. Unhealthy complexion. Subject to eruption, eczemas, ulcers and skin trouble of all kinds. Scaly dandruff over the scalp, eyebrows and other hairy parts. The face is full of pimples and acne, fishy brine smell of discharges, changeability of symptoms especially stools. Hot patient does not want to be covered, dread of downward motion. Tongue- Large, flabby, burning must protrude tongue to keep it cool.
- Ringworm on tongue, drinks little and often, constipation.
- Stool partially coming and partially receding. Burning feet must keep them out of bed.

Silicea

- Marasmus not due to food is lacking in quality and quantity but due to tampered assimilation.

- Unsurmountable fear is the greatest indication.

- Child weeps to keep its arm around the neck of her mother.

- Nervous, irritable, timid children. Large head and abdomen, open fontanelle suture, weak ankles. Aversion to mother's milk. Does not learn and play. Rough and yellow nails. He is an awful boy for knocking bits off of himself for falling and scratching his knees, every little scratch and hurt festers and ulcerates. They would never heal. And is very sore and getting sticking and burning pains. Such a patient has boils all over the body, which comes one after another. The child is very cold and chilly.

- Cold up to his knees. He cannot sleep for cold feet. Very tired. Always wants to lie down. At night he is terrorizing or others feels as if he was as sore on the side.

- He has constipation.

- The stool partly recedes and partly coming. Profuse sweat on head and extremities.

Calcarea Phos

- Almost like Calc carb but the difference is diarrhoeic in nature sunken abdomen.

- Sweat of head may or may not be present. Somewhat dark complexion.

- Growing pains in muscles. Thin and weak neck, too weak to hold the head.

- Stomach ache on every attempt to it. The stool is not watery. sputtering and offensive, and greenish. Diarrhoea with hydrocephalus usually, the child has tonsils and adenoids.

Petroleum

- Marasmus of the child subject to peculiar diarrhoea harassing all day long but mostly absent at night. The other prominent symptoms are marked garlic on breath and faeces of the patient.

- Aversion to fresh air, marked tendency to skin disease < during winter.

- Sarsaparilla. Marasmus of the children with syphilitic or Sycotic origin.

- The skin hangs in folds. The face becomes shrivelled, eruptions are prone to appear on the tongue and roof of the mouth. Offensive sweat about genitals restlessness before passing urine, passing of great quantity of salts in urine. Obstinate, constipation and attempt to pass tool is accompanied by an intense desire to urine.

Acetic Acid
Dr. Kent

- Persons having inherited Phthisis, and emaciation. weakness. Anaemia, loss of appetite, burning thirst and copious pale urine are a combination calling for Acidic acid. It is a good medicine for the bad effects of chloroform. It is a good medicine for nephritis acute scanty urine, oedema, and great weakness. It is a thirst. Apis IJH. 72-45.

- Eucalyptus nephritis after influenza.

- Koch's Lymph. 200. In nephritis, when indicated medicine fails, and there is history of family. Tuberculosis.

- Methylene blue: nephritis after measles.

Acetaea Racemosa

Chilly patient

Sensitive to cold

Dr. Kent

The patient is always Chilly.

- Sensitive to cold and damp weather which rouses rheumatic state and develops a state of rheumatism not only in the muscles and joints all over the body but also along the course of the nerves.
- All the symptoms are aggravated by cold except head which is ameliorated by cold.
- When questioned perhaps break into tears or Express in various ways the overwhelming sadness.
- Changeable symptoms are well marked in this medicine.
- Example the rheumatism will change in a day into chorea or again the choreic movements will keep on with soreness throughout the muscles of the body.
- Mental state following the disappearance of rheumatism is a strong feature of this remedy.
- Sometimes the rheumatism disappears in a short order and mind is not disturbed but then it is because a diarrhoea has come on with great soreness and aching of the bowels and because of flow from the uterus has given relief.
- Trembling in membranes and joints of the muscles with inability to exercise.
- The will over the muscles of the body jerking of the muscles is noted in state of emotion from becoming chilled any part of the body pressed upon.
- Soreness of abdomen with diarrhoea and coryza.
- Passion alternatively, alternation of diarrhoea and physical symptoms.

- Many symptoms during pregnancy.
- Every time the patient complaints a new group of symptoms.
- When vomiting not ceased in a pregnant woman with a previous history of rheumatism or chorea.
- During labour the patient screams out and grasps her hip.
- Chorea at puberty when menstruation was late.

Dr. Chowdhury
- There is a great abundance of sighing as an Ignatia.
- She is suffering from a great fear as if everybody around her would conspire and kill her.
- She get so suspicious to everybody and everything that she would not take medicines if she knew she was taking it.
- Stiffness in joints experienced in the morning as if he was wacked hard the day before.

Dr. Tyler
- In regard to diaphragmatic pain.
- The pain has its center in the chest.
- It was as if a person were pressing with his fist firmly on the sternum and forcing it inwards towards the spine.
- Aggravated by walking.
- When severe it would spread up the oesophagus and pharynx causing a peculiar tingling at the back of the throat which extended to shoulder and throat and down the arms to the fingertips.

Comparison
- **Caulophyllum in uterine affection:** Both are chilly patient but Actea very sensitive to cold damp weather.
- All its complaints aggravated during cold Damp weather.

- **Actea:** Rheumatic type of dysmenorrhoea with more the flow more the pain.
- **Caulophyllum:** Congestive type of dysmenorrhoea with severe spasmodic pain with first two days of menstruation.
- **Actea:** Darting shooting pains especially from hip to hip and left Infra mammary pains.
- Caulophyllum intermittent paroxysmal and spasmodic pain flying in different direction.
- **Actea:** amenorrhea or profuse dark coagulated. All the rheumatic and choreic symptoms aggravated during menstruation.
- **Caulophyllum:** scanty flow preceded by pain in the small of back great weakness and internal trembling are present.
- Leucorrhoea of little girls with moth spot on forehead.
- Heaviness of eyes and great weakness.

In Rheumatism

- **Actea:** Usually large joints are affected.
- Caulophyllum small joints are affected with erratic pain. It is good medicine when Rheumatism occurs in small joints (Rheumatism) at menopausal period.
- **Pulsatilla:** Both are weeping when questioned. changeable symptoms are marked in both the medicine but in Pulsatilla hot patient wants cold things and cold air and getting chills only during pain more severe the pain more severe the chill Pulsatilla gets ameliorated lying on left or painful side.
- Actea aggravated lying on side because pressure causing jerking of the parts.

Actea Spicata
Dr. Chowdhury
- It is a rheumatic remedy and it has special affinity for smaller joints particularly wrist.
- The patient goes out feeling well but after a slight exercise the joints start aching and swelling.
- Extreme tenderness of the affected parts aggravated by Touch movement and night.
- It bears great resemblance to Viola, Caulo, Sabina, Colo, Sticta.

Adonis Vernalis
Dr. Chowdhury
- It is meant for endocarditis valvitis and other heart conditions.
- Secondary to Bright's.
- Rapid and feeble action of the heart. irregular and intermittent pulse with oedema of the legs ascites and dyspnoea.

Aesculus Hippocastanum
Dr. Kent
- The conditions of Aesculus hip are aggravated during sleep hence symptoms are observed on waking. He wakes up with confusion of mind looks all around room in confusion, bewildered. Does not know the people wonders where he is and what is the meaning of the things he sees.
- It is especially useful in children that rouses up in sleep frightened and confusion like Lycopodium.
- Persons who suffer from palpitation when the pulsation extends to the extremities and the throbbing of the heart in sleep can be heard.

- It is the nature of this remedy to have flying pains all over the body. Dull Frontal headache from right to left, the pains usually felt in the back of the head as if the head would be crushed.

- Formication, tickling, shooting and itching all over the body and scalp. It is a good medicine for haemorrhoidal eyes and large blood vessels great redness of the eyes with lachrymation, burning eye boils and vascular appearance.

- Medicines having many troubles with the veins are often disturbed by hot bathing.

- The superficial pains are emulated by heat but deeper affections are ameliorated by cold.

- It has the tendency to produce varicose veins and ulceration and round about these we have marked duskiness.

- **Stomach:** Eructation sour, greasy, bitter, desire to vomit. Heartburn and gulping of food after eating.

- It has a great disturbance of stomach as soon as the patient takes food or a little while after it becomes sour and he eructates it till the stomach emptied.

- Such is the state of Phosphorus, Ferrum, and Arsenic.

- It has also congestion and ulceration of the stomach. Constant distress and burning in the stomach inclined to vomit. Such a state is present in the ulceration of the stomach.

- It has most troublesome haemorrhoids with fullness of the right hypochondriac region.

- The liver is full of suffering. After eating there is distress in bowels and stomach.

- Constant dull backache aggravated on attempting to rise from sitting, makes many painful efforts before he finally succeeds.

- Leucorrhoea with lameness of the back across sacroiliac articulation.

- After eye troubles have been cured varicose vein remain in the eye.
- **Digestive system:** Usually the older patient dull heavy rather depressed.
- Good deal of heartburn with acid eructation.
- Fullness and discomfort immediately after a meal sometimes amounting to a actual pain usually of burning character. Usually they have hepatic disorder with good deal of backache.
- They have considerable amount of thirst aggravated clothing in abdomen and morning.
- Sensitive to hot stuffy atmosphere.
- It can be differentiated from Lachesis with mental symptoms.

Aethusa Cynapium

Dr. Tyler
Inability to think or fix the attention before the class.

Agaricus Muscarius

Dr. Chowdhury
Chilly patient Antipsoric

- In locomotor ataxia there is a terrible pain in the heels as if they have been bitten.
- The pain as if touch or pierced by needle of ice.

Dr. Kent
- All the symptoms are aggravated after sexual intercourse especially in the symptoms of the spinal cord.
- Hysterical fainting after coition.
- Children are late in learning to walk and talk.

- It is due to mental defect a slowly developing mind children with twitching and early fainting nerves.
- Girls prior to puberty who have convulsion being scolded from excitement and shock.
- Late in mental development children who cannot remember, makes mistakes in writing and spelling.
- Twitching, trembling jerking and crawling are the characteristic of this medicine.
- Clumsy motion of the finger and nails in handling things she drops them (Apis, Bovista).
- All his symptoms are aggravated in the morning till noon and ameliorated towards evening.
- During sleep itching of the whole body without eruption.
- There is a sensation of ice coldness of the parts after scratching.
- Twitching and jerking of the eyes (Cicuta, Arsenic, Pulsatilla, Sulphur).
- Red nose as if frost bitten. It is as good as Ledum and Lachesis for the red tipped nose in old discharge.
- Aggravated from stimulants (liquor) Zincum.
- Tympanitic condition of the abdomen with rumbling and gurgling.
- Horribly foetid discharge and trembling and jerking of the muscles are present in typhoid.
- Diarrhoea morning hot flatus (Aloe) burning in the rectum soft stool great tenesmus violent urging to stool involuntary straining before during and after stool and pain in loin to leg continuing after stool.
- The urine feels cold on passing.
- Urine passes slowly in stream or drops, has to press to promote the flow. All the urinary disturbances are almost present in this

medicine. Urine becomes scanty and headache comes on goes many days and is constipated and headache ameliorated by stool.

- In Fluoric acid, headache comes on if he is not answer the call of urine.
- Metastasis especially if milk ceases and complaints come on.
- In male burning of the urethra comes on during coition or a sense of hotness of seminal fluid while being ejected.
- Violent sexual desire before and during but at the time of ejaculation the organism is wanting.
- It is a passive and pleasure less ejaculation.
- In old gleety discharge where there is a continual itching and tickling in the urethra and the last drop will continue discharging for a long time.
- Heart symptoms and prolapsus aggravated at the close of menstruation.
- Violent cough in isolated attack ending in sneezing.
- Sensation as if cold air were spreading along the back like aura epileptica.
- In heart disease when pain is prominent and the patient would not answer question.
- Cough ending in sneezing (Agar) cough ending in expulsion of casts of bronchial tubes (Cal acid).

Ailanthus Glandulosa

Dr. Chowdhury

- Malignant sore throat accompanying scorlatina, measles with other eruptive diseases.
- The fever is very high and the patient is in a stuporous delirium.
- The whole body is covered with a sort of dark miliary Rash.

- The tongue is cracked dry and parched from the nostril their flows a thin ichorous discharge.

Dr. Kent
- The medicine is suitable in the forms of sickness such as we find in diphtheria Scarlett fever measles and typhoid.
- The regular rash does not come out but in its place red spots, roseola like make their appearance and it is characterized by capillary congestion in spots and mottled spots.
- A continuous dreamy State of Mind throughout the week child cries all the time. Sees animals like rats running around feels rat or something small crawling up to the limb. There seems to be constant loss of memory.
- Throat much swollen dark red almost purple colour diphtheria with extreme prostration. throat livid swollen, tonsils prominent and studded with deep ulcer. The throat and tonsil very often appear as if they would pit upon pressure and some of these thymotic states diarrhoea sets in as a reactive method.
- Breathing hurried irregular, burning in palms and source hunts a cold place to put them.
- When the Scarlet fever Rash or the measles rash does not come out in its uniform fashion but in patches little circles here and there and it's dark irregular patchy livid eruption disappearing on pressure and returning very slowly, interspreads with small vesicles aggravated in forehead neck and chest.

Allium Cepa

Dr. Kent
- Rattles in larynx and throat and extends to the chest.
- On going to bed in evening all its complaints come on.
- Among the earlier symptoms will be sneezing.
- Complaints begin in the left and go to right.

- In coryza inflammation soon spreads for ears throat and larynx. jerking pain from throat towards ear.

- It is a good medicine for earache (Pulsatilla, Chamomilla).

- Cough of children with indigestion vomiting and Flatulency, will pass offensive flatus and will be doubled up with colic.

Aloe Socotrina

Dr. Kent
Hot patient

- With its diarrhoea the abdomen is distended with gas causing a feeling of fullness and tightness and he must often go for stool.

- Aloes patient is extremely irritable when under the influence of pain and the pains are generally in the abdomen. he hates people and repels everyone.

- Constant heat on the surface of the body with dry temperature hot patient burning extremities.

- Congestion of the head during bowel complaints.

- Bleeding are common in this medicine. Bleeding from nose, bowels and bladder.

- Growling in abdomen soon after supper. there are colicky pains in bowels from eating and drinking, when there is no diarrhoea even when there is a state of constipation.

- It is not a deep acting remedy think of Sulphur. Sulphur-ac, Kali bi and Sepia to treat the chronic liver diseases provided symptoms are present.

Alumen

- The stool is hard and knotty like stones come once or twice in a week.

- These hard lumps, as they pass, leave the rectum sore, tender and it pains for a long time after.

- Haemorrhage of large mass of putrid coagulated blood (in typhoid).

- Susceptible to cold aggravated during sleep and turning to the right side.

- It is particularly indicated in chronic sore throat and pharyngitis. The relaxed and ulcerated condition of throat and spasmodic constriction in throat makes swallowing very difficult. The voice is entirely lost.

- It has a tendency to induration. The tonsil becomes indurated. Every cold settles on the throat and tonsils become more indurated. Here it complements with Baryta carb in the medicine the induration is so prominent or the ulcers indurate under it.

- Its headache is very peculiar. The indications are there is pain with burning on top of the head. Pressure on the head, but ameliorated from pressure like Cactus. The patient frequently wants to change a cold cloth on the head to get ameliorated.

- Thirst for ice cold water. it has action on the spinal cord.

- Sense of coldness in the back.

Alumina

Involuntary spasmodic twitching of the lower jaw due to great exhaustion. The upper lip covered with numerous little blisters and its dry and cracked.

Dr. Tyler

- Gets a sore throat from taking onions.

- Seeing blood on a knife has horrid ideas of killing herself.

- Can only pass stool when standing.

- Persons taking their food and drink through aluminium vessels a prone to create skin disease. The symptoms are itching of eyelids and constipation with straining even for soft stool (I J H 61-20).

Dr. Kent
- Catarrhal headache every time he gets cold the thick discharge becomes thin and he gets headache.
- Difficult in swallowing. Granules form on the soft palate, tonsils and pharynx.
- A long dry cough in the morning.
- When blowing the nose tearing through the eyes.
- It can complements with Argentum metallicum in sore throat of singers (when the patient starts song there is accumulation of mucus in the throat and gets ameliorated after the mucus comes out. Phosphorus).
- When he gets aggravated from beginning of song and ameliorated from continuous singing PT.
- Myelitis burning of the spinal cord sensation as if a hot iron band or hoop around the waist. Numbness of the leg with softness of the soles.
- They have a gray appearance. They feel worse in the morning and gradually pick up towards the evening. Sensation as if everything is going in a wrong manner.

Ambra Grisea

Dr. Chowdhury
- During menses the legs become quite blue from distended varices and also painful.
- It is a very shy patient. Always likes to sit on the last bench especially girls in school or college.
- Discharge of blood between periods at every little exertion- a long walk, lifting something, bleeding starts and becomes a nuisance for them. Bleeding whenever she went for shopping.

Dr. Kent
Premature old age

- Great depression alternate with vehemence.
- Morning Aggravation
- Company
- Embarrassment in company
- Conversation
- Warm Drinks
- All gone sensation in stomach after normal stool.

Ammonium Carb

- Sensation of Oppressive fullness near the bridge of the nose as if everything inside would burst.
- All the head troubles usually located in this region. The headache may be pulsating, beating but it is always located in the forehead.
- It is extensively used in whitlow and panaritium. The finger is extremely inflamed and deep seated periosteal pain is felt & red streaks run up to the axilla from the inflamed areas. He also has inflammation and pain. The ball of great toe which looks red and swollen.

Dr. Tyler
Unconquerable desire to eat sugar.

- Pain in the wrist joint where sprained long ago. Warts, burning, stitches and tearing corns.
- Drowsy by day, sleepless by night. Heat on hand with cold feet.
- Complaints caused by Charcoal fumes.
- It's fluids are all acrid, the acrid saliva excoriates the lips so that they crack in corner and middle and becomes very dry and scabby.

- In diphtheria and chest troubles < after sleep.
- Cough that may be left by influenza which should yield to Bryonia but may fail to do so (Amm carb phos).
    o Asthma at new moon and before menses with cough.
    o On lying down.
    o Nose obstructed during night (Ammonium carb, Lycopodium, Nux Vomica).
    o It is a good medicine in old age.
    o Obesity is symptoms of Ammonium carb but it is not found in Dr. Kent.

Ammonium Mur
Dr. Chowdhury
- In the mouth and throat we find accumulation of viscid saliva which is difficult throughout.
- The cough of this remedy is Peculiar in as much as the cough excites the salivary glands and while coughing the mouth fills up with saliva.
- After amputation of foot when there are tearing, stitching pains aggravated in bed ameliorated from massage.
- Much sneezing, watery burning discharge, yet stoppage of nose, coryza with burning of larynx.

Artemisia Vulgaris
IJH April June 1988
- Irritable and excitable before the attack of epilepsy.
- Attacks accompanied by profuse sweat of offensive or garlicky odour.
- Somnambulism gets up at night and works remembers nothing in next morning KP.

- Petit Mal epilepsy without aura.
- History may show tendency of stealing.
- Usually the head turn towards the left during the attack.
- Chewing motion of jaw, grinding of teeth.
- Looking up coloured lights produces dizziness.
- Eyes turn up before attack.

Amylenum Nitrosum
Dr. Chowdhury
- Smacking of lips as if in the act of tasting and a constant movement of the lower jaw as if chewing.
- The surging of blood to chest face and head are found both in Belladonna and Amyle but in Belladonna aggravated from laying and Amyle ameliorated from laying.

Anacardium Orientale
Dr. Chowdhury
Ineffectual urge to stool find both in Nux and Anacardium. In Nux it is due to irregular peristaltic movement of the rectum but in Anacardium it is due to paralytic condition of rectum with a sense of purging.

- It produces eruptions which are umbilicated in nature.
- In spinal affections, its symptoms are as follows a great tired feeling of all the limbs, incomplete palsy of voluntary muscles, trembling cramps in calves when walking, stiffness and lassitude in knees as if paralyzed and sensation of bandage in the legs.
- **Digestive System:** Irritable bad tempered, unable to curse and swear but cowardly. They have a blunting sensation. Blunting in hearing and smell. Sometimes they have a nasty odour of nose and mouth.

- Any excitement brings on abdominal pain. They are liable to get sudden attack of profuse salivation. They are moderately thirsty but cold or drink cold drink brings on acute pain. Very often they complain of feelings of nausea in the morning. They also complain of good deal of gurgling in the abdomen rather than actual distension. They are aggravated chill and ameliorated from exposure to sun.

- They have an urgent desire to stool yet there is difficulty in passing stool and the stool is soft.

- Usually the patient is a mental worker - a student, a teacher, a retired scholar. He stumbles over the door - sill or evidence some other form of clumsiness His furrowed forehead indicates a headache which is confirmed by intorvation.

Angustura Vera

Dr. Chowdhury

Its action is confined principally on motor nerves and mucus membrane hence it makes admirable remedy in rheumatic affections and paralytic complaints.

Fatigue of the arms on movement boarding almost on paralysis and cracking in joints are some of the symptoms to indicate it in the above complaints and therefore it should be studied in close comparison with Bryonia.

- Craving for coffee and warm things. Aversion to meat especially pork.

- Oversensitive the slightest offence and mere trifles irritate him.

- It resembles Ruta G in its action over the muscles and bones. It has sore bruised feeling like Ruta.

- It has a special affinity for the long bones such as humerus Tibia and fibula. Carious affection of the bones with coming out chips of dead bone from the affected bone. It also causes necrosis of the lower jaw.

- It is meant for tetanus either traumatic or otherwise when there is twitching and jerking of the muscles aggravated by Touch.

- Like Ambra grisea it's cough is followed by hiccup and belching.

- Stiffness of the elbow joints and paralytic heaviness in arms after holding the arm for a long time upward.

Antimonium Crudum

Dr. Chowdhury
Protrusion of rectum with loose bowels.

Dr. Tyler
Rush of blood to head, troublesome itching on head with falling off of hair.

- Gnawing pain in carious teeth after every meal.

- Severe continual itching on chest the whole day.

- Decided disposition to shoot himself, to know other kind of suicide. This forced him to leave his bed otherwise he was unable to get rid of it.

- Stool first natural then several loose evacuation then a small but hard evacuation with straining.

- It is complementary of Graphites as regards the skin symptoms as well as Silicea of Petroleum and Thuja even sometimes of Sulphur. It should be used in lower potency. (See H G November 70).

- Calcarea carb is often a ground remedy of Antim crud in warty condition.

- When complaints come after taking the refrigerated items. (HG 755).

Dr. Kent

- Diarrhoea ending in dysentery. stool liquid mixed with lump Aloe.
- A person takes bath at night but gets hoarseness in the morning.
- When a patient get cold it's coryza suppressed and he gets headache and vomiting starts. Metastasis from cold to stomach.
- Gout with abdominal symptoms.
- Pustular Rash surrounded by red areola.
- Cough after chickenpox Antim crud.
- Cough after smallpox Calcarea carb.

Antim Tart

Chilly patient anti psoric anti Sycotic.

Dr. Tyler

- It is almost specific for impetigo contagiosa use CM potency.
- It is equally acts in pustular eruption of small pox like Cicuta, Rhustox, Thuja and Variolinum.
- On waking up from sleep the child seems stupid and is so excessively irritable that he howls if one simply looks at him.
- In children the cough is provoked when ever the child gets angry, eating brings on the cough which culminates in vomiting of mucus and food.
- A nursing infant suddenly lets go of the nipples and price as if out of breath and seems better when held upright and carried about. Now this is the beginning of capillary Bronchitis.
- In threatening paralysis of the lungs it can be compared with following medicines.
- Lachesis aggravated from rising from sleep.

- Kali iod pulmonary oedema with great of rattling of mucus in the chest. Raising of greenish and frothy sputum looks like soap suds.

- **Moschus:** when there is loud rattling of mucus and the patient is restless especially after Typhoid fever. The pulse goes less and less strong and finally the patient goes into syncope.

- **Justiesa:** Constipation, thirst yellow sputum rattling of mucus, unable to raise it out.

- Drowsiness usually occurs after whooping cough.

- It is a good medicine for heart diseases where ECG shows elevation of STP QR.

- The symptoms are coldness of the body, drowsiness, irregular and slow pulse.

- Do not give Digitalis in this case. It is a good medicine for coronary thrombosis, myocardial infarction. (All India Homeopathic Journal.)

- It's difference with Veratrum alb as follows and antim tart more drowsiness.

- Veratrum album more cold sweat on the forehead.

- In pneumonia both Antim tart and Opium have great sleepiness but the difference is Opium the face is dark red or purple or there maybe sighing or strenuous breathing and the face is always pale or cyanotic with no redness and the breathing is not strenuous.

Dr. Chowdhury

- The cough is provoked by crying, eating, drinking and becomes angry.

- In gastric trouble its vomiting is just like Ipecac. Its vomiting is associated with precordial anxiety. Cold sweat on forehead and faintness after vomiting. Distension of the hypochondriac region and drowsiness.

- In cholera there is sharp cutting colic before stool. Burning in rectum after each stool during after loose stool drowsiness and, profuse perspiration leading into collapsed thread like pulse white coated tongue with red papillae and the edges are characterized by red.
- In smallpox were after one batch drying up fresh makes it appearance and some get dry others mature.
- It is psychotic remedy. We have warts behind the glans penis. It is also used in secondary orchitis the effect of checked gonorrhoea and as such can be compared with Pulsatilla.
- Antim tart has more vomiting and retching while Ipecac has more nausea.

Apis Mellifica

In Apis case when Rhus tox is given by mistake give a dose of Sulphur which acts as a intermediate deterrent after Rhus tox and before Apis (H G 75 December - 540).

Dr. Chowdhury

Hot patient

- It has quite a lot of congestion to head and face in consequence of which a general aching of the brain is complained of. This violent congestion may lead into meningitis or meningeal irritation.
- The gradual increase in torpor, the sudden shrill cries, squeaking grinding of teeth boring of the head in pillow warn us for the indication of terrible attack.
- The other indications are twitching of the one side of body and semi paralysis of other. Scantiness of urine, turning up of big toe, offensive odour from mouth, thirstlessness or extreme thirst.
- It is a good medicine for fever of cerebral and suppression of eruption.

- The brain as a result of such suppression soon becomes cloudy. Delirium not of an active type soon appears violence is not a feature of these patients. They are in a state of stupor and they mutter constantly.

- Their tongue is ulcerated, cracked and blistered and trembles as soon as it is the protruded. The prostration is so great that they frequently slide down in bed. Tenderness and bloated condition of abdomen with foul smelling diarrhoea scanty urine moist cough pale waxy colour of skin great sleepiness with piercing shrill crying are few more important symptoms.

- In meningitis it can be compared with Helleborus.

- **Helleborus:** the wrinkled forehead, dilated pupils, drooping of the lower jaw, automatic motion of one leg and one arm, suppression of urine, chewing motion of the mouth, dark snooty nostril, constant picking of nose lips and bed clothes.

- Uneven distribution of heat is good indication of Apis. One portion is heat and the other portion is cold.

Dr. Kent
Severe mental shock ending in right sided paralysis.

Apocyanum Cannabinum

Dr. Kent
- Dropsy followed hemorrhage. Chilly, thirst for cold water but cold water disagrees ameliorated from warm water.

- Chest troubles ameliorated from laying down (Apis) this is due to hydrothorax.

Aralia Racemosa

- It is a good medicine for asthma cough and other respiratory troubles.
- The cough occurs at about 11:00 p.m. generally after a short sleep with tickling of the throat. The respiration is dry wheezing and aggravated from laying down on back.
- There is a sense of constriction in chest it feels as if foreign body were in the throat.
- The patient is extremely susceptible to the least current of air which causes frequently sneezing with copious excoriating nasal discharge.
- The patient perspires profusely while asleep.
- Asthma aggravated in spring season.

Aranea Diadema

- Aggravation of all complaints and symptoms by exposure to cold and them emulated by bright and sunny days.
- Unvaried and unchanging periodicity.
- Complaints appear with great regularity and precisely the same over everyday every other day every week or every month as the case maybe.
- The symptoms are clock like.
- The spleen is often enlarged.
- Fever with chilliness without heat and sweat.
- Headache emulated by smoking ameliorated by open air.
- The patient often wakes up from sleep with a peculiar sensation of some part of the limb's feeling enlarged and augmented.
- Colic with rumbling bowels liquid stools numbness of the arms and legs at 4 o'clock in the morning everyday.

Argentum Metallicum

- In arthritic rheumatism when swollen profusely bruised on pressure. The pains are tearing in nature. There are sometimes electric light shock in joints and limbs.

- The muscular systems are affected and cramps like pains are the special feature of it. The parts feel stiff and numb, calf muscles feels too short when going downstairs.

- Epilepsy of hysterical women and men who have lost a good deal of the seminal fluid. The attack is followed by delirious rage. The patient jumps and striking those nearby.

- Headache of Businessmen. The pain increases slowly and when at its height ceases suddenly.

- Diabetes with swelling of the ankles.

Dr. Kent

- Every time the patient goes to sleep, a electric like shock running through the body.

- Itching of the ears scratches till it bleeds.

- Headache pressive pain ameliorated from pressure and application of external warmth.

Ghatak

Chilly patient

- Loss of intellectual power memory and recollection.

- Nervous debility.

- Great weakness with pain in the lower extremities.

- All its symptoms are aggravated from rest and ameliorated from Motion. The patient walks all the time in spite of his troubles.

- Its mental symptoms are aggravated after sleep.

- Palpitation with vertigo or pain in the head aggravated lying on back.

Argentum Nitricum

Dr. Chowdhury
- The patient is subject to frequent errors of perception while walking through the street she dreads the corners as they seem to her to be projecting out and she feels afraid she will be bumping against them.
- The structures on the side of the street seem to her as if about to stumble down and crush her.
- All this is due to imperfect coordination of the ocular muscles.
- In epilepsy the dilatation of pupil for days or hours before the attack, great restlessness following the attack and trembling of the hands.

Dr. Tyler
- It is one of the most flatulent remedy. He is distended to bursting, gets scarcely any relief from passing flatus or eructation.
- A slight colic wakes him from uneasy slumbers (light sleep) and he has 16 evacuations of greenish very foetid mucus with quantity of noisy flatus.
- It has Claustrophobia (apprehension being in a closed room).
- Numbness in the fore arms at night. The wristband of the night dress has to be cut, everything pulled away from arms.

Pierce
- Argent nitricum patient is worrier and seems to like it at any rate she will not allow the mind to be diverted. Her ailments are naturally a source from which she can exert a good deal of trouble and she anticipates all sorts of dreadful things as the possible outcome. She will not consult a physician for fear that he will tell her she has Cancer, Heart disease, Bright's disease, Cerebro-spinal meningitis or any other complaints that she has heard reports in the newspaper and she is finally induced to see

the doctor will not believe what he says because she knows that he is keeping things from her.

- Yellow diarrhoea turning green after standing (Argentum Nitricum, Rheum, Sanicula).

- Bluish stool changing to green on standing (Phosphorus).

- Diarrhoea as soon as one drinks Argent nitricum.

- Diarrhea as soon as one eat Trombodium.

- Argentum nitricum is to abuse of cauterization what Mag phos is to after effect of catheterism.

- **Digestive System** - Development of headache coming on usually at the end of a day's work ameliorated from very dilute alcohol.

- Cold food and drink seems to ameliorate the abdominal pain but ice cream aggravates.

- Craving for strong tasting pungent food.

- The pain starts right in the middle of the epigastrium and tends to spread towards the left side of the abdomen under the left ribs.

- In acute gastritis and gastric ulcer they do get a good deal of vomiting and the vomit maybe blood streaked or coffee ground.

- Though sour drink ameliorates the nausea yet the gas the gas aggravated from sour drink (HG June 82).

Arnica Montana

- It is a good medicine for dyspepsia, tympanic condition of the abdomen with sense of full and bursting.

- Belching is loud and continuous. He is a great subject to obstinate constipation. Rectum is loaded with faeces but they are not expelled easily, when they do come out after excessive straining, they look flat and ribbon like.

- This is due either to enlargement of prostate or to retroverted uterus. The stool and flatus are extremely offensive. The stool contains undigested food particles with violent belly ache.

- In dysentery there is discharge of profuse dark venous blood at long intervals which ameliorates the symptoms. It is usually associated with tenesmus of the neck of the bladder and bruised sensation in the anus. Sometimes a painful prolapse of the rectum is present.

- It is an admirable remedy in nephritis violent chills followed by extreme nephritic pain with nausea and vomiting. The pain extending from right hypochondriac region to groin. It almost feels knife plugging into the kidney. It is accompanied by frequent desire for urination but has to wait a long time to pass the urine. Very often urine is full of blood and pus.

- Great coldness of the nose is a great indication of the remedy.

Dr. Tyler

- It can bring out a very nasty dermatitis when used externally too long or too strong even. Sometimes a cellulitis is formed.

- It is a good medicine for wasp stings apply Arnica Q.

- Urtica urens is said to be for bee stings.

- Cantharis 200 for gnat bites.

- Intracranial hemorrhage (due to injury) with unconsciousness with dilated pupil on one side and cannot bear the light think of Arnica and Cicuta.

- To antidote the coal for drugs such as Anacin, Aspirin, Saridon think of Arnica, Carbo Veg, Lachesis, Mag phos according to indication.

- Fever with enlarged and tender spleen and with tetor from mouth.

Dr. Kent

- The patient wakes frequently at night with frightful and dreadful dreams. There is great distress in the heart. He keeps his hands on the heart and says I will not survive.

- Arnica patient is morose, wants to be alone.

- Indisposed to speak and approached.

- Its fear comes only during night but in opium fears remain day and night.

- Mental symptoms alternate with uterine symptoms.

- **Aristolochia: Clematis:** First traumatic blisters, caused by rubbing, Arnica Fear of approach.

- Bryonia fear of poverty.

Arsenicum Album

Dr. Chowdhury

- It has been said that persons handling Ars get ulceration of the scrotum and penis.

- The burning pain of Arsenic is really due to destruction of tissues either progressing or impending.

- It is a good medicine for vertigo or dizziness from Malaria. Complaints of great heaviness in the head and Humming in the ears. It goes of in the open air and returns as soon as enters the room.

- Arsenic patient can only see the lower part of his field of vision, so that he lifts his head high and throws it somewhat backward. when looking at a distant object sometimes the whole vision is dim and objects look as if he has been looking through white gauge.

    1) Everything looks black Capsicum.

    2) Everything looks blue Actea spicata.

3) Everything looks bright and glistening (Can).

4) Red spots before his eyes (Hyoscyamus).

5) Candle light seems surrounded by red halo (Rutag).

6) Everything looks yellow (Cina).

7) It is useful in mumps especially metastasis to the testicles.

8) Toothache is mostly first lower tricuspid. It is very severe and is excited by cold weather and is aggravated by the sound of other talking. There is also other condition is when to take his associated with dysmenorrhoea and also when toothache precedes menses.

9) **During Apyrexia:** the patient desires for refreshing drinks such as wine, coffee, lemonade.

10) In typhoid fever, there is the circumscribed redness of the cheeks.

11) In angina pectoris the patient gets aggravated from sitting either bend forward or head thrown back.

12) In asthma very often there is coexistence of emphysema and Cardiac affection. aggravated by lying down and midnight.

- Ferrum met has midnight aggravation but the patient gets ameliorated by sitting and moving slowly. He keeps his chest uncovered to get relief. These patients flush easily and subject to epistaxis.

- **Graphites:** He gets hungry during this time and told relief it's men indications are anxiety restlessness prostration burning and category cold rated by cold madam anxiety when anything expected to him.

- Arsenic main indications are Anxiety, restlessness, prostration burning and cadeveric odour.

- Burning ameliorated by heat Arsenic.

- Cold ameliorated by cold Ledum.

- Arsenic alb great agitation and anxiety with whole body burn like fire (Radium).

- Arsenic has black colour stool.

- Bromium black colour stool. These patients are prone to painful blind varices and we find them very averse to the application of warm or cold water because it aggravates the complaints. The patient only get ameliorated by application of his own saliva.

- **Leptendra:** The stools are jet black, almost like a tar and the patient complaints of severe aching burning sensation in the region of the liver especially behind the liver (Farrington).

- There is cutting pain and distress near the umbilicals and epigastrium. It is a good medicine in infantile liver and cholera.

- Psorinum black stool with offensive odour.

- Silicia black offensive and frothy stool.

- **Stramonium:** Black and fluid stool usually when it appears in typhoid.

- Good medicine for suppression of urine.

- It is a good medicine in retention of urine due to atony of bladder after parturition.

- The patient feels no desire whatsoever to pass water, give this medicine without thinking and when it feels think of Causticum, Hyoscyamus.

- In bronchial asthma after Arsenic think of Kali bichrome Kali carb, Thuja, NS (Homeopathic Glenings June 1973).

- Bronchial asthma and its treatment.

- It is a good medicine for Scorpion bite give a single dose of 200 potency (Hahnemanian Gleanings August).

- The patient is very particular about the accuracy of the information he gives.

- **Curious Arsenic Symptoms:** Homeopathic Gleanings November 75 (552).

- Any kind of pain after drinking cold water aggravated from sitting and lying down ameliorated from standing.

- In fever when there is midnight aggregation and if Arsenic fails it should be suspected as a hidden focus or TB condition and the medicine is usually Pyrogen or Bacilinum.

- When these medicines fail the background is Syphilitic and Syphilinum should be tried.

- The patient was in the habit of wetting his lips with his tongue.

- The patient is fastidious, sensitive fond of sour and cold things. suppose there is an abrasion or wound then secondary infection takes place because the damage tissues are putrefying.

- Arsenic can be employed as an antiseptic. Ars useful for bad effects of vaccination. Skin disease appears after shoe bite.

- When there is a history of taking Arsenic (crude) give HS or K I according to modalities.

- Abdominal colic with coldness of palms and soles. in abdominal trouble when indicated medicine fails and if there is history of malaria give Arsenic. Vomiting and diarrhoea takes place simultaneously.

- It is a good medicine for black spot all over the body especially nose.

- In skin diseases when indicated medicine fails and if there is history of Malaria give Arsenic give Arsenic 6 or 30.

- In London hospital Doctor Andrew Kellner a cardiologist handling 60% of the heart cases which were not under Allopathy with Arsenic low potency. He opines that in the high BP patient is one who crosses the bridges before he comes to them. They think of tomorrow's problems today and try to find out solution today. Pain hollow of knees rising from a seat (Ars- hy).

- In filarial attacks during the attack Streptococcin is good. In chronic cases Ars alb and Hydrocotyle.
- In congestive cardiac failure with all the indications of Arsenic when it fails give Strych-Ars.
- When Arsenic seems indicated but does not fit in give RT.
- Arsenic counter acts in effects of penicillin (Sulphur).
- Dysentery has a specific effect on pyloros and claims effect in pyloric spasm. (William Grigs).
- In asthma when Arsenic is indicated but fails sycotic complaints yield the case it has also 3:00 a.m. aggravation in asthma.
- Whatever indicated medicine might be given give one or two doses of Arnea diadema for sound sleep during night.
- Asthma in children when Ars N.S. fails give Morgan 200 to CM (IJH 73-103).
- Dr. Kent discharge ameliorated inveterate catarrh of the nose always enquire about the suppression of some discharges is otorrhoea, leucorrhoea and ulcer (Arsenic, Calcaria sulph).
- Usually the patient feels better when discharge in the nose is thick but when he gets cold the discharge becomes thin and he gets headache, chilliness of fever etc.
- This condition remains for a few days and again the discharge becomes thick and the patient feels better.
- It's fever is like China but there is no thirst during Chilly the patient wants only little quantity of hot water during hot stage, he wants cold water.
- It's fever has no time it may come at any time.
- Itching without eruption (Alu, Dol, NS).
- Its itching are alternate with burning.
- Headache alternate with rheumatism.

Arsenic Iod

Dr. Chowdhury
Its discharge is profuse greenish yellow and pus like and a persistently excoriating.

Ghatak
- TB this remedy presents almost all the symptoms of active TB. Profound prostration Rapid and irritable pulse fever off and on, easy and debilitating sweats, emaciations, frequent diarrhoea.
- It is both chilly and hot patient. The patient wants to open the doors and windows and after sometime wants to close it again. He cannot stand open air if it is cold.

Dr. Kent
- Bathing aggravates.
- Aggravated lying on painful side.
- When Ars iod did not promptly ameliorate the acrid coryza Stillingia 30 is the remedy.

Artemisia Vulgaris

IJH April June 1988
- Irritable and excitable before the attack of epilepsy.
- Attacks accompanied by profuse sweat of offensive or garlicky odour.
- Somnambulism gets up at night and works remembers nothing in next morning KP.
- Petit Mal epilepsy without aura.
- History may show tendency of stealing.
- Usually the head turn towards the left during the attack.
- Chewing motion of jaw, grinding of teeth.
- Looking up coloured lights produces dizziness.

- Eyes turn up before attack.

Asafoetida

Dr. Chowdhury

- It is a good medicine for the hysteria in women.

- Reverse peristaltic movements. Globus hystericus. Distension of the abdomen with loud belching which.

- Hysteria from suppression of habitual discharge such as sudden checking of long standing expectoration of a chronic diarrhoea or menses.

- Very sensitive to external impression especially to excitement and noise together with great distension of the abdomen with flatulence which pass upward.

- Supra orbital neuralgia < night.

- Pulsation at the pit of the stomach with an empty all gone feeling at about 11AM.

Dr. Kent

- The face becomes puffy, dark-red, dusky (Carbo an, _,Aurum, Puls) It indicates some cardiac disorder mainly venous stasis of the heart.

- Fatty, flabby, purple patient extremely nervous with extreme sensitive to pain. Hysterical women fainting easily.

- It has deep flate ulcer, on the periosteum and bones, discharging watery, ichorous, offensive discharge. Ulcer surrounded by varicose veins.

- Milk in the breast of non-pregnant women. Milk ceases ten days after delivery.

Ghatak
Left of Patient

- Left Sided.
- Fainting Easily.
- Suppression of Discharge.
- Hypersensitive to touch.
- All its discharges are offensive.
- Difference between Lachesis and Asafoetida are:

Lachesis: Aggravated after Sleep Asafoetida:- Ameliorated after Sleep.

Asarum Europaeum

- Chilli patients sensitive to cold it is a nervous chilliness and not ameliorated by warmth or covering dysentery with long yellow twisted string of in odorous mucus.

Asclepias Tuberosa

- Its cough and pains + modalities are like Bryonia Alba but it is also aggravated in damp and cold weather but lacks in constipation dryness of mouth and thirst which is prominent in Bryonia.
- It is useful in pneumonia of Sub acute type with pain especially at the base of the left lung which shoots downwards ameliorated from bending forward.

Aurum Met

Dr. Chowdhury

- The discharge in this remedy is very offensive.
- The pain of Aurum Met is burning in character and > by application of cold water.
- In prolapse of uterus, a kind of bruised pain – generally < after lifting a heavy load associated with constant, profuse corroding

leucorrhoea and backache indicate it in these affections of the uterus.

Dr. Tyler: Loss of Gold has driven many to suicide. Potentised gold has brought many back to life and hope.

- The person goes on questioning and does not wait to get his answers. He may go on thinking of suicide, but you may not be able to know this, because he will not tell you.
- A person wants to do too many things at the same time. (Sec/ J.H. N. 166)
- Heart stops for one or two beats and suddenly starts.
- Bony growths of osteoarthritis, leads to habitual abortion.
- Dr P Sankaran of Bombay said In High BP I found that most of the patients had history of grief, shock, disappointment or some such background. So I thought of Aur Mur which is known to cover the effects of grief and has a specific action on the heart and blood vessels. Many of these patients also have much anxiety and restlessness and such other symptoms of Arsenicum Album. So I selected Aur Ars as the likely remedy. Many patients have high BP and have internal tension. And they are not consciously nervous. They are worried but they do not admit it. Arsenic is for expressed worry situation. In this case give Aur Sulph.
- Adrenalin is a good medicine for high BP. All these medicines should be used low potency. (IJH 92.114)
- Sensation as if ball moving in the abdomen (Aur-sulph).

Aurum Muriaticum

Dr. Chowdhury
- Great Sycotic remedy causes suppressed discharge to appear.
- Depressed now.
- Indicated in all sorts of Heart disease.

- It affects on the bones and periosteum causing caries and erosion.
- Swelling and induration of glands characterised by heat, hardness and tension.
- Lips, nose, lungs, uterus, liver, spleen shows signs of induration.
- It is a good medicine for haemorrhage of the climacteric period in Sycotic constitution.

Aurum Muriaticum Natronatum

- It is indicated in Uterine Fibroid, big tumour commonly associated with arteriosclerosis and high BP.
- Kali Iod is also a good medicine for uterine fibroid (IJH 71-22).
- For Undescended testis both Aur Mur and Aur Mur Nit are highly indicated. (H G Feb 76-84).

Argentum Metallicum

- In arthritic rheumatism when swollen profusely bruised on pressure. The pains are tearing in nature. There are sometimes electric light shock in joints and limbs.
- The muscular systems are affected and cramps like pains are the special feature of it. The parts feel stiff and numb, calf muscles feels too short when going downstairs.
- Epilepsy of hysterical women and men who have lost a good deal of the seminal fluid. The attack is followed by delirious rage. The patient jumps and striking those nearby.
- Headache of Businessmen. The pain increases slowly and when at its height ceases suddenly.
- Diabetes with swelling of the ankles.

Dr. Kent
- Every time the patient goes to sleep, a electric like shock running through the body.
- Itching of the ears scratches till it bleeds.
- Headache pressive pain ameliorated from pressure and application of external warmth.

Ghatak
Chilly patient

- Loss of intellectual power memory and recollection.
- Nervous debility.
- Great weakness with pain in the lower extremities.
- All its symptoms are aggravated from rest and ameliorated from Motion. The patient walks all the time in spite of his troubles.
- Its mental symptoms are aggravated after sleep.
- Palpitation with vertigo or pain in the head aggravated lying on back.

Argentum Nitricum

Dr. Chowdhury
- The patient is subject to frequent errors of perception while walking through the street she dreads the corners as they seem to her to be projecting out and she feels afraid she will be bumping against them.
- The structures on the side of the street seem to her as if about to stumble down and crush her.
- All this is due to imperfect coordination of the ocular muscles.
- In epilepsy the dilatation of pupil for days or hours before the attack, great restlessness following the attack and trembling of the hands.

Dr. Tyler

- It is one of the most flatulent remedy. He is distended to bursting, gets scarcely any relief from passing flatus or eructation.
- A slight colic wakes him from uneasy slumbers (light sleep) and he has 16 evacuations of greenish very foetid mucus with quantity of noisy flatus.
- It has Claustrophobia (apprehension being in a closed room).
- Numbness in the fore arms at night. The wristband of the night dress has to be cut, everything pulled away from arms.

Pierce

- Argent nitricum patient is worrier and seems to like it at any rate she will not allow the mind to be diverted. Her ailments are naturally a source from which she can exert a good deal of trouble and she anticipates all sorts of dreadful things as the possible outcome. She will not consult a physician for fear that he will tell her she has Cancer, Heart disease, Bright's disease, Cerebro-spinal meningitis or any other complaints that she has heard reports in the newspaper and she is finally induced to see the doctor will not believe what he says because she knows that he is keeping things from her.
- Yellow diarrhoea turning green after standing (Argentum Nitricum, Rheum, Sanicula).
- Bluish stool changing to green on standing (Phosphorus).
- Diarrhoea as soon as one drinks Argent nitricum.
- Diarrhea as soon as one eat Trombodium.
- Argentum nitricum is to abuse of cauterization what Mag phos is to after effect of catheterism.
- **Digestive System:** Development of headache coming on usually at the end of a day's work ameliorated from very dilute alcohol.

- Cold food and drink seems to ameliorate the abdominal pain but ice cream aggravates.

- Craving for strong tasting pungent food.

- The pain starts right in the middle of the epigastrium and tends to spread towards the left side of the abdomen under the left ribs.

- In acute gastritis and gastric ulcer they do get a good deal of vomiting and the vomit maybe blood streaked or coffee ground.

- Though sour drink ameliorates the nausea yet the gas the gas aggravated from sour drink (HG June 82).

Azadirachta Indica

Afternoon fever starting at from about 3:00 to 4:30 p.m. To 7:30 p.m. With slide chilliness glowing heat in ice face and palms and so on.

Apoplexy

- **Stromo:** Expiration of breath, great difficulty, spasmodic drowning of head to either side > In full light. Passes head frequently from the pillow, eyes wide open. Pupils dilated, hands constantly kept.on genitals, urine suppressed.

- **Gels:** The condition is preceded by headache, nausea, giddiness, and staggering eyelids. And limbs heavy. Speech-heavy complaints due to nervous exhaustion. Dark red face.

- **Zinc:** Stupid great frustration loss of all reflexes. Complete comatose condition in sensibility.

- **Opium:** Love of liquor with worry and sleep. And sleepless nights. Exciting dreams of head congestion, preceding the attack. There is much Vertigo and, a heavy head. The sensory attack. Sensorium not clear, Hard of hearing heavy speech untidy gait with the attack, snoring respiration.stony look purple face, visible pulsation in temporal artery. Twitching of facial muscles.

- **Phosphorous:** Suddenly falls unconscious. Life looks extinct. Pulse and respiration lost face red, body cold to touch, mouth drawn to the left, hyperemia of the brain, hot head, irresponsive to all stimuli, laying on the left side.

- **Lachesis:** Purple puffy face with convulsive movements, blowing respiration, paralysis on the left side, throbbing and burning of the head cannot bear touch on the throat or anything near the mouth.

- **Aurum Met:** Heart pulse depressed move high BP paralysis left side (apoplexy has developed mainly on syphilitic background.)

- Cerebral thrombosis has also developed from a Syphilitic background and the possible medicines are. (Phosphorus., Plumbum, Arsenic Iod) (I.J.H.M. 71-100).

Alphabet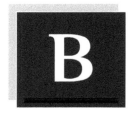

Badiaga

1) Soreness and induration are the characteristics of this remedy.
2) The part affected are sore to touch.
3) Good medicine for syphilitic condition - with the above symptoms.
4) Headache associated with inflammation of the eyes > at night but < after sleep and motion.
5) When the patient coughs, there is flying out of mucus from the mouth. It shows the spasmodic nature of cough and followed by sneezing.
6) On the skin we notice quite a lot of freckles and rhagades.

Streptococcin: any kind of disease may be cured by this medicine depending upon the following history.

History of recurrent sore throat, tonsillectomy, Appendectomy, series of inoculation.

In skin diseases when Sulphur fails with the above history. It is – for arthritis with the above history.

When the adject glands are affected due to primary legion apply this medicine.

Baryta carb

Spasm of the esophagus difficulty in swallowing. Bolus of the food goes down a little and then causes spasm and he gags and chokes. This symptom more strong in mer.cor. Paralysis extending from above downwards (Baryta, Merc sol) paralysis extending from below upwards (Conium, Magnesium).

Person suffering from severe attack of pneumonia, when called the attention that their lungs are not right they are full of smoke and they get the smell of pine smoke give Baryta-carb high. if he complains paper burning-caffeine.

Persons suffering from severe attack of Pneumonia, when call the attention that their lungs are not right. They are full of smoke.

Baryta - Carb

1) Mania during pregnancy.
2) There is a sort of loquacity but there is any coherence in her speech.
3) Great tendency to go out of the house.
4) They can hardly make up their mind to do any thing.

Doctor- Talcott

1) Patient thinks his legs are cutoff and that he is walking in his knees.
2) Unhealthiness of the skin thrush not surmount to felicia.
3) Moist eruption on the head and behind ears are common. These lead to falling off of hair. Tumors of scalp. Of tension on whole face as if white of egg had dried on it.

Streptococcin

It is an excellent remedy for sequel of tonsillectomy and impetigo (IJH 63.29 229).

Usually Baryta cases are followed by SYPH, especially in mental idiocy, SYPH and Baryta C. again idiocy in children.

Baryta-Mur

- It has a particular action on the cardiac orifice of the stomach where it causes induration and narrowing as well as narrowing. The result is great epigastric tenderness as well as over sensitiveness of the stomach.

- It causes induration of pancreas with profuse flow of saliva like-. It is great help in abdominal aneurysm. The patient rules in agony with attack of anxious dyspnoea.

- Mania due to increase sexual passion.

- Acts upon the multiple sclerosis of the brain and cord and there is entirely loss of voluntary muscular power.

- In hypertension of old people headache with less pain and more heaviness, noises in the ears, vertigo, high systolic pressure and comparatively low diastolic pressure. The patient may have bronchial affection with great accumulation of mucus in the chest with difficult expectoration. Increase of uric acid and decrease of chlorides in the urine (See 1970 - hypertension).

- It is good medicine for lipoma. It has Baryta like mind and Natrum like cravings (IJH-71.22).

- Baryta carb is a very good drug for multiple lipomas over the body and for multiple neurofibromata (IJH Dr. Kent) desires cold air but cannot bear it.

- It is a natural complement of "Conium" in glandular affection but it is deeper. Sneezing is sleep without waking.

Belladonna

Belladonna lies with his feet crossed and cannot uncross them.

Theridon - sits with them crossed and is powerless to uncross (The H recorder December 1931) when the cows draw up the milk, when they are milked give Belladonna 3X an hour before being milked.

Bells + Dona = beautiful lady

1) In mania he calls for his food and when gets it instead of making good use of it he bites its spoon into two then grabs at his dish and snarls and barks like a dog, he then tries to throttle himself and those around him to kill him. Usually these symptoms are found in hydrophobia.
2) He tastes and smells everything more acutely. The sense of sight and hearing is keener.
3) **In epilepsy** - when it occurs recently the aura feels like running over and extremity or as if fear is rising from the stomach. The convulsions commence in upper extremities and extend to the mouth. There is also a clutching sensation in the throat.
4) It is a good medicine for cough. The child cries before coughing and this is a good drug of pain before coughing. Tickling sensation in the throat. Cough frequently ending in sneezing.
5) It is a good medicine for dysentery. The stools are thin greenish bloody or Papescent white. They are small in quantity, frequent and involuntary. Some times during summer complains of babies and during dentition. It is a good medicine when Chamomilla and Podophyllum fails. Greenish diarrhoea of children during dentition having following symptoms.
    1) Tymphanitic abdomen < after each meal and the irritability of the temperament was great. Seems to suffer from abnormal appetite give Bell-200.
    2) In pregnancy when pain comes intermittently give Bell 6.
    3) Dr. Kent: The patient is over sensitive to touch, sound, light, talking of others, motion, jar especially jar of bed.
    4) Usually the patient is thirsty, and its thirst is like arsenic. Craving for lemon and lemon juice during fever.

5) Dryness prevails throughout its mucus membrane.
6) Metastasis from taking cold in the head to other organ.
7) In head pain, bending head backwards >.
8) All it complains < from motion except neuralgic pain of the legs which > from motion.
9) The patient wants to be wrapped and > open.
10) It is highly indicated in gallstone colic and appendicitis.
11) Menstrual flow is bright red with clots.
12) It is indicated in right sided pleurisy. Great pain, extreme soreness of the parts. Cannot lie on it, < from Jar of the bed.
13) Its mental symptoms are > from taking light food.

Sweat on cover part (Bell) Sweat on uncovered part (Thuja).

Bearing down sensation & gt; than standing (Bell). Bearing down sensation & lt; lying. Hypertension during pregnancy (Bell, Glonoinum).

Bellis Perennis

Dr. Tyler
- Complains due to drinking cold drinks, when the body is heated, ill effects of sudden chill from wet.
- Cold when one is hot.
- Eruption on the face or any other part of the body from application of cold water or ice after being.
- Heated.
- Feeling of discomfort or bruised in a pregnant woman due to mechanical defects of the faetus.

Benzoic Acid

1) **Diarrhoea:** The stools are profuse, exhausting and entirely watery, running right through the diaper in Podophyllum. The smell resembles of burnt gunpowder. This brownish watery

stools contain little pieces of faecal matter that look like tiny portions of sponge.
2) Rheumatism from Sycotic or syphilitic origin. It is a good medicine for the ganglion of the wrist.
3) In arthritis, cracking of the joints indicates that the bones are involved & > from movement, though < at beginning is an indication that not the bones but the ligament and muscles are involved <; by movement and to desire to keep the parts rest, indicates that all the parts of the joints are actively inflamed (IJH 73-100).

Dr. Kent
1) Its metastasis takes in different way. Profuse urine alternates with scanty urine. The patient gets all the trouble during scanty urine and > from profuse urination.
2) Dwells upon unpleasant things. Profound sleep alternates with sleepless nights.
3) The urine becomes scanty and redevelops swelling of the tongue, sore throat, < from profuse urination.(MERC SOL).
4) Metastasis from rheumatism to stomach. Nausea and vomiting stops. (MAG CARB).

Berberis Vulgaris

Chowdhary
- Biliary calculi when jaundice follows in violent stitching pains are felt in the hypochondriac region these cause him to hold his breath. The stool becomes grey coloured. It is sometimes complicated with fistula in anus and persistent troublesome cough.

- Bubbling feeling as if water were coming through the skin. Similar bubbling sensations are felt in the joints and other parts of the body.

- Sensation of a tight cap pressing on the whole scalp.

Gleanings November 1975 (520)

- The patient is apt to sit with both hands clasping the head.

- Symptoms are apt to alternate rapidly in a thirsty feverish condition can change quickly into thirstless frustration. A voracious appetite can suddenly give away to complete anorexia.

- Acute polyuria can alternate with oliguria.

- Stitches occur in the region of the liver, acute pains coming on suddenly and with instant Intensity increases both by movement and pressure. The left lobe may be especially affected.

- Burning stinging tearing, stitching, pains occur in joints indicating early sign of multiple arthritis. Neuralgic pains are felt deep to the fingernails associated with swelling of the digital joints.

In discoloration left by eczema after the eczema has been cured, think of Berberis (IJH 72-66).

Dr. Kent

- If pains are stitching, tearing, shooting, darting and wandering in character. It may travel in any direction. Usually, the pains starts in a particular organ and radiate in different direction.

- Stitching, tearing pain before, during and after stool.

- Fowl and bitter taste in the mouth with rush of blood.

- Chest, Liver, Kidney and other troubles after fistula operation.

Blatta Orientalis
Chowdhary
- It is better in acute cases with fussy persons or corpulent constitution.
- It has saved many cases from threatened suffocation due to excess of mucus in the bronchi.
- Oppression of breathing, restlessness, profuse perspiration increases from lying down of some of the symptoms increases in new moon and full moon.

Borax
Dr. Chowdhury
- Dirty and unclean sort of patient, a patient whose hair is constantly tangled and knotted, whose eyelids are loaded with gummy exudation, whose nostril are always crusty and inflamed from flowing of an excoriating coryza, whose mouth is full of apthous sores that prevent eating and whose tongue is cracked and dry.
- Every little injury suppurates (Hepar, Silicea, Calendula, Petrol).
- Red nose of young women.
- Great irritability and fretfulness of mind before the almost natural afternoon.
- **Stool:** becomes cheerful after the stools, restlessness through the afternoon. She find it difficult to settle down to any definite work, she changes from one work to another and roams about this indefinitely this restlessness cannot be accounted anyway.
- Discharges more frequent during afternoon and evening.
- The patient says that the urine is hot like boiling water when passing.
- Eczema of the tip of the fingers, Hering gives Fever medicine as Borax, Nat.C. Nat.M, SKP.

Dr. Kent
- Anxious, restlessness, fidges found in this medicine.
- All its complaints are ceased after 11 pm and after Stool.
- Small vesicles appear around the mouth and forehead of children, (Natrum mur).
- Nausea when engage with a work.

Bovista

Dr. Chowdhury
- The patients are somewhat bloated, they are more or less puffy and the integument about them is somewhat velvety.
- Sense of enlargement-feeling hugeness. The ovaries feel too large, the uterus seems enormous.
- Haemorrhage from nose, especially in the morning after awaking, or during night.
- Menorrhagia during night (Mag Carb, Natrum mur).
- Flow takes place in the morning (Sepia).
- Flow takes place in the evening (Phosphorous).
- In Diabetes Mellitus it is an excellent remedy where the urine is yellow green or turbid like lime water and desire to urinate is frequent.
- In abdominal colic, the pain is increased than by pressure and eating and is associated with red urine white line on scratching the skin, permanent mark left on scratching.

Bromium

Dr. Chowdhury
- It has been used in stitching in testicles after separation of gonorrhea and goiter.

- It has a peculiar vertigo It has a sensation feet deep in the brain as if vertigo or apoplexy would come. The giddiness is always < on looking at running water and hence the patient is unwilling to go over the bridge. The vertigo > by nose bleed showing the congestive nature of its giddiness.

- In Pneumonia the lower lobe of the right lung is affected. Great oppression of breathing is experienced and although the rattling shows great accumulation of mucus very little is expectorated. (stomach troubles after eating either diarrhea or vomiting)

Dr. Tyler

- Chronic stomach ulcer with vomiting or diarrhea < after eating. , black faecal stool, must go to stool after eating.

- Acids, oysters, tobacco smokes, warm things, hot drinks, hot tea. Membranous stool, black fecal stools, must go to stool after eating.

- Hemorrhoids diarrheic > by application of saliva.

Dr. Kent

- It is a hot remedy and its complaints come in hot weather especially summer, sudden appearance of cough in hot weather.

- Its glands are stony hard and rarely suppurate.

- Hardness of the glands with inflammation.

- Cough and sneezing when handling the old books in racks.

- Hoarseness from overheated, usually it is a left sided medicine.

Bromium Baby: Borland

- Fair hair, fair skin, happy, friendly cheerful, nervous, usually their nervousness increases in the evening, darkness, sensation as if some persons were coming behind him, fatty, crops of boils on or acne on face or shoulder increases warm or rest decreases after eating.

Bryonia Alba

- Eating much at a time (arsenic).

- Great soreness of chest with dry cough (Bryonia).

- Great soreness of chest with loose cough (NATRUM Sulph).

- It appears to be related somewhat to Causticum in the laryngeal rattles which it cause to Bryonia in muscular pain and painfulness to cough and pulse in the yellow or yellowish green (Dr. SG Stearns).

- Constipation is always a guiding symptom of Bryonia it is invariably present with the headache.

- In fever he picks off his dry and parched lips and makes them bleed.

- In diarrhea we have soft pasty and mushy stool, the stool causes soreness and boring pain in the rectum. The smell is putrid like that of old cheese. It may also be involuntary. Distinction in abdomen, rumbling, tenderness are present.

- It is indicated in fluent coryza beginning with violent and frequent sneezing and associated with stitching headaches and hoarseness. It generally follows arsenic.

- It is useful in synovitis. The affected joint is red but not that vermilion red of Belladonna nor the rosy, red of Apis.

- In separation or slow development of rash or eruption, and whenever we find the child getting drowsy and the fever more persistent and the disappearing of rash we should think of Bryonia it can be compared with following medicine.

- Apis mel - It is usually used after Belladonna and Bryonia.

- When the congestive space is having being super ceded by cerebral symptoms, the result of much effusing. The eruption what little is left oedematose.

Antim Tart:
- Indicated in suppressed eruptions particularly of the type of variola. It is characterized by great drowsiness and distinct involvement of the lung tissue with bluish appearance of the face and a rattling breathing.

Belladonna
- Comes in the first stage of the disease, when in spite of great febrile excitement the rash doesn't appear. It throws off the fever still higher.

Cuprum met
- Cerebral symptoms show themselves .Convulsion with screaming, clutching of the head into the palms of the hand boring of the head into the pillow and spasm of the abdomen or the muscles are chief indication.

Gelsemium
- When due to defective reaction the rash doesn't appear and chill becomes dull or listless.

Helleborus
- Great stupor, the dark sooty nostril, the suppression of urine. The constant chewing motion of the mouth, the ever present Cephalic cry the wrinkled forehead, dilated pupils and dropping of the lower jaw are the conditions.

Zincum Met
- Cerebral exhaustion, defective vitality, impending paralysis of brain. Constant fidgeting of the lower extremities . Rolling the head from side to side.

Dr. Tyler
- Aggravation at 3 am on; delirium, profuse night sweats, toothache, 9 pm is also the bed hours of Bryonia, profuse urination 6 to 7 pm, the symptoms < in the morning, some symptoms aggravates in evening.

- In Natrum mur patient when headache ensues, do not give it directly. Its best to give few doses of Bryonia till the acute phase is over then give NATRUM Mur.
- Headache from stooping as if everything will fall out at the forehead, as if everything will press out of the forehead.
- Very much inclined to yawn. Frequent yawning all day.
- Profuse nocturnal stitches from 3 am.
- Ask the patient do not take (Bryonia, Lyco and Petroleum is the remedy) Cabbage.

Dr. Kent
- Its complains come slowly. After exposure or overheated. The patient feel uneasiness in the morning.
- Most of it's troubles are associated with headaches.
- Generally the patient gets < from heat, warm room, closed room from cold.
- All its troubles are > from cold except stomach > from heat. The patient desires to take cold water but it < than the stomach troubles > from hot drinks.
- Eye troubles after disappearance of rheumatism or gout.
- All troubles > from sweat.
- It has only day diarrhea.
- It affects the upper extremities.

Bufo

Dr. Chowdhury
- It produces imbecility, impotence, and great tendency towards masturbation.
- In epilepsy, fits occur during coition or worse at times of menses and during sleep.

- These symptoms are almost always preceded by great irritability of mind. The convulsions are usually followed by profound sleep (Blister in hand which recurred annually.)
- The least pressure on the right hypogastric region causes violent fits, strong craving for alcohol.
- Involvement of the lymphatic system after injury, its good medicine for septic lymphangitis. Complains > putting the feet in hot water.

Dr. Kent

- Its mental symptoms like Baryta carb.
- Imbecility childlike behavior, titters at everything.
- Becomes angry if misunderstood. this is the indication of approaching insanity.
- When there is history of inherited epilepsy. Their offspring exhibit it in different ways, one will be an imbecile, another insane, another will die of cancer, and another will be epileptic. It has the physical constitution, when the epilepsy has been turned aside by strong drugs, phthisical constitution when discharges' have been suppressed by closing fistulous openings or by stimulating ointments.
- In the epilepsy the aura felt in the abdomen.
- Music is unbearable.
- Mouth wide open before attack.
- Inclination to carry the hand constantly to the gentile organ.
- Milk is mixed with blood.

Alphabet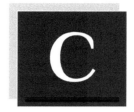

Cactus Grandiflorus

Dr. Chowdhury

An excess of any of the body fluids.

- Constricted aching pain around the heart (Diaphragm).
- Constrictive pain < during menstrual period with palpitation accompanied by sadness, anxiety and sighing.
- Arsenic, Calcarea carb, - constriction while bending. In calcarea carb the constriction is > by throwing his shoulder back.
- **Cuprum:** Constriction after anger and from driving.
- **Moch:** Constriction with trembling of the heart.
- Phos constriction while the patient is coughing.
- Mental symptoms fear of death, despondence about cure,
- A great apprehension about some impending calamity.
- Sadness taciturnity And an irresistible desire to cry.
- Sometimes the pain starting from the apex of the heart shoots down along the left arm to the end of the fingers. Oedema Cyanosis, feeble intermittent pulse and palpitation of the heart are frequent symptoms. The slightest mental or physical exertion aggravates the complaints.it is frequently associated with vertigo. Loss of consciousness and Dyspnoea.It is generally worse while walking at night And laying on left side.

- Ambra grisea, Staphysagria: palpitation from music and Antim tart, sulphur palpitation from having stool.

- **Conium:** Palpitation after stool.

- **Crotalus, Lachesis:** Palpitation during menopause.

- **Digitalis Sepia:** Palpitation after coition.

- **Digitalis, Opium:** palpitation from grief and after fright.

- Kali carb the troubles are due to distorted cardiac wall due to deposits heart action is weak and has feeling as if the heart over hanging tightly drawn hands.

- Phosphorus palpation where the patient is unable to have sexual intercourse as each attempt on question brings on most dire results. We also used it in palpitation of old maids who are generally so nervous that even the entrance of an unexpected visitor into the room brings on palpitation of the heart.

- **Natrum mur:** Bad effects of quinine. Enlarged spleen with hypertrophy of the heart. The heart pulsation shakes the whole body. feeling of coldness about the Heart.

- Palpitation aggravated by mental exertion and laying on left side.

- Palpitation aggravated before menses Spongia, Cactus, Natrum mur, Sepia.

- **Spongia:** palpitation before menses unable to lie on back with head low which brings on a spell of suffocation she is often raised from sleep as if something is stirring and sits up with anxiety dread and fears death pressing pain in pericardial region.

- Pneumonic complication such as constant violent grasping breath etc are frequently present.

- Sulphur palpitation when going upstairs or when climbing a hill there is violent orgasm of blood in the chest and a sort of sensation of boiling in that religion and a great tremor on his right arm.

- A great craving for fresh air is present during deep inspiration and from leaning forward of the chest.
- Dyspnoea is Marked in every change of position. the pains are very sharp shooting through hand to back or radiating from heart down the arm or over the chest.
- Herring used it in pneumonia with the patient expectorated of blood every 4, 6, 7, 8 hours.

Dr. Kent
- Its chief symptoms are constriction contraction and congestion of the affected parts.
- It mainly affects the circular fibres.
- Irregular distribution of circulation some part is hot and another is cold.
- Congestion of the head hot head with cold extremities Bryonia Arnica.
- Irresistible inclination to weep.
- Dreams of falling.
- Vertigo aggravated from physical exertion turning in bed stooping rising from a recumbent position and deep inspiration.
- Weight on vertex by pressure aggravated from sounds hearing, falling and strong light.
- Heat on the head from mental exertion.

Cadmium Sulph

Dr. Kent
- Sore eyes rousing up with every cold paralysis of the lids, ptosis.
- It commonly affects one side of face and one eye.
- After an apopleptic attack when the patient recovers but weakness of one arm and leg remains it competes with Phosphorus.

- Formication of skin and deeper tissues.
- Crawling in paralyzed parts.
- Violent thirst every time he takes cold water which he craves.
- Goose flesh comes out, a creeping or horripitation like Capsicum.
- The nausea is distressing, nauseated all the way down to the abdomen (CP, Antim tart, Ars) irritation of the stomach after tedious sickness like cerebrospinal meningitis, typhoid, yellow fever.
- The patient vomits everything.

Cancer with burning prostration and vomiting it gives >.

Cainca
Dr.Chowdhury
- Severe pain in the region of the Kidneys in the morning.
- The pain is so intense that the patient is unable to change his position.
- It is usually described as a sort of stiffness of the back.
- Urine is passed copiously and often day and night aggravated by travelling.

Cajuputum
- Stricture of the Oesophagus (Ars, Baptisia, Bryonia, Natrum).
- Feeling of Enlargement. Head feels as cone as bushel.
- Sense of persistent choking as in hysteria.
- Constant inclination to spit.
- Urine smells like cat's urine.

Caladium

For bad effects of Tobacco.

Dr. Kent

- Forgetful, feeble minded.
- Hot Patient.
- All it's symptoms are < from warm except stomach which > from warm drink and the patient desires for warm drinks. Eats without hunger and drinks without thirst.

Calcarea Arsenica

- Left sided medicine.
- Hypertension due to chronic nephritis.
- Nephritis with tenderness on back of it in the Kidney area.
- It is indicated in chronic nephritis.
- Sense of lightness of the body as a floating in air convulsion.
- Its head pain if moves from the side lain on and goes to the side not Lain on > from mental exertion.
- Loss of desire for food but thirst for cold water.

Calcarea Carb

Dr. Chowdhury

- The skin is unhealthy and least scratch suppurate.
- It is a great remedy for fibroid tumours.
- Desires for egg raw potatoes and flour.
- Great burning is felt in the vulva.
- It is a well-known remedy for cataracts and chronic dilation of the pupils.
- The stools are of varying character.

Although white stool with a sour smell Is the prominent symptom of it. prolapsus ani are frequent occurrence.

- The constipation is associated with haemorrhoidal affection and it is mostly mucus haemorrhoid.

- Bad effects of emission, onamism, lascivious fancies excite desire but the organ has become too frail for an erection. And emission takes place too soon. with consequent weakness of limbs and Excitement of nerves.

- Warty growth on sexual organs smelling like ____ and herring Brine.

- Swelling of the breast before menstruation leucorrhoea occurring before puberty and in infants.

- When conception does not take place in spite of normal condition.

- Cramps in toes and soles of feet during pregnancy.

- It is a good medicine for scantiness of milk after child birth. Child averse to take mother's milk. Nauseating, a few doses of calcarea carb given to the mother will rectify it.

- In Phthisis the sputum is yellow lumpy sweetish and when thrown into water it resembles of falling star.

- Complaints come on after working in mud and clay Standing On The Water.

- Epilepsy with a sensation of something running in arms or from pit of stomach down through abdomen into feet. vexation fright onanism and suppression of chronic are principal cause.

Calcarea Carb

Dr. Tyler
- Picture of teething cough and bronchitis.
- Picture of Rickets during teething.

- Picture of anaemia.
- Picture of tuberculosis.
- Picture of mental deficiency, and decay.
- Fatness without fitness.
- Sweating without heat.
- Bones without strength,
- Tissues of plus quantity and minus quality.
- Desires eggs, eats lime, slate pencils, chalk, clay sweets ice cream. Aversion coffee, meat milk.
- White stools (calc, mag mur, chelodonium, cardus marinus, Ammonium muriarticum and sanicula) Watery or sheep dung stool also indicates bad liver Thumb sucking- the most important remedy is Ipecac. The potency should be not less than 1M. Sometimes Calc carb is also a medicine.
- In Calcarea Exertion brings on so many complaints.
- In walking a furlong. He gets a rise of temperature.
- It shows a tubercular diathesis.
- Every time the child exerts, It goes down with tonsilitis or fever.
- Sometimes we give Bryonia, Rhus tox, Bell but fail.
- It can postpone the menstrual period by 3 or 4 days if possible. Give this medicine 10M before the ovulation. 4 doses a day for 2 days.
- It is a good medicine for sterility.
- It can be given as an intermittent remedy or straight repeating.
- Epilepsy of young girls, regular fits in sleep. Regular fits in sleep between age 20 to 35. Bufo is another remedy for epilepsy. Where colossal sweat is present when the patient is in a very bad fit and the whole body is moist with sweat. (IJH 79-55)

- 50% of the Calcarea Children are not flabby and fatty, rather, they are emaciated (See Dr. Kent stomach appetite).
- Sometimes the Calcarea patients are very hot. Like sulphur with burning palms and souls. The greatest aspect is that Calcarea has got craving for open air. Especially because he perspires so much, but they are averse to and aggravated by Cold both like Sulphur.
- It has the internal feeling of heat with external coldness. In a Calcarea, carb patient gives Calcarea iod 6 when reducing of weight is desired.
- Drenching in wet or working in clay when Rhus tox Fails, gives Calcarea. It is a good medicine for renal colic, but Calcarea renalis is more suitable.
- Urticaria > from open air is cured by Calcarea. After Apis fails, it follows well when the pupils are dilated.

Calcarea Phosphorica

Dr. Chowdhury

- The girl maybe having pain from the first or second period itself especially when nearing the period she writes the period cancel area for 10 M you may straight away give this remedy first.
- The neck is so thin and weak it cannot support the head.
- **Diarrhoea:** the stools are green slimy undigested hot watery spluttering and extremely offensive.
- Sleep is restless yet the child is Drowsy all day.
- It is better indicated in those cases of chronic diarrhoea in children where constant continuous and persistent purging has led on to hydrocephaloid condition.
- It is a preventive in hydrocephalus.

- It has been recommended as a prenatal remedy in women during pregnancy to women who have given birth to hydrocephalic children.
- Sexual Desire is increased in both sexes.
- Erection is painful, it occurs even when riding in a carriage.
- In women we find nymphomania particularly before catamenia.
- She feels pulsation in the parts with increase sexual desire even urination brings erection on clitoris. There is creamy like leucorrhoea.
- Desires salt smoke meat bacon.
- The tongue is white furred with disgusting bitter taste in the morning.
- When waking up hunger is more felt At Special hour 4:00 p.m.
- It is a good remedy in diabetes mellitus where lung is implicated.

Dr.Tyler
- Instead of SF the Calcarea phos is typically anaemic and dark complexioned.
- Dark hair and Eyes. thin and spare instead of fat children.
- Emaciated unable to stand, slow in learning to walk.
- Sunken flabby abdomen, growing pains in muscles, adenoids.
- Eye strain produces headache we should give Natrum mur headache before 1:00 p.m. lunch hour in morning session of school or Calcarea phos headache in afternoon session of school these being given only high in frequently (IJH 69 - 154).
- If a child refuses to eat even after taking vitamins tonics appetizers etc think of Calc especially Calc phos (Arthur and Roberts).

- Pain all over the body like electric shocks and at other times like tricking of cold water also pain severe at night with creeping sensation numbness and coldness.
- It prevents hydrocephalus and TB children given to mother in high potency during pregnancy 2 /3 doses.
- **Calc sulph:** repeated daily, prevents cleft palate, hare lip and other deformities where even one child has been born like that.

Dr. Kent

- Convulsions of children but the remedy must be given when not in convulsion to secure the best results.
- The child grasps the head with hand and screams.
- Fluent coryza in a cold room and stopped in a warm room.
- Every cold settle in the tonsils (Bryonia, Arnica) Infants want to nurse all the time.
- Diarrhoea aggravation from least food.
- Colic followed by diarrhoea.
- The woman has no better friend than Calcarea phos her suffering at puberty when she is slow in maturity often met by this medicine.
- From taking cold at first menstrual period often comes a painful menstruation that lasts during menstrual life.
- Child refuses mother's milk.
- It may be given to a woman who has brought fourth one or two children that may be considered Calcarea phos babies.
- It's pains are more marked in this lower extremities.
- Sleepy day time and evening.
- Sleepless after going to bed till midnight. very sleepy in the morning.

Calendula Officinalis

Intense pain in the right shoulder joint after throwing stone or some heavy thing > by hot application.

Camphora

Dr. Chowdhury

- It is an important remedy in Mania with melancholy violent rage.
- The patients scratches bites and tears her clothes and foams at the mouth.
- Great precaution is necessary or else she would throw herself out of window.
- Incessant fits of crying which the patient is hardly able to explain.
- Feels better in anyway as soon as the patient stops to think.

Dr.Tyler

Mental Symptoms:

- Pericardial anxiety.
- Great anxiety and restlessness.
- Suffocative dyspnoea I am dead no I am not dead yes I must be dead.
- Attacks of terror by night and solitude.
- Afraid to go to sleep at night.

Dr. Kent

- The patient wants to be covered and suddenly wants to be uncovered.
- This is a very serious condition this occurs with opisthotonous convulsion,
- Inflammation of the brain liver kidney bladder comes from violent shock and cold with great exhaustion.

- In acute complaints there is violent thirst but in chronic troubles it is thirstless during heat and when the pains are on he wants to be covered.

- The coldness is > by cold he wants more cold.

Ghatak

- Changeable condition both mentally and physically hyper sensitive to cold.

- It's fever comes suddenly with excessive chilliness but the patient wants to be uncovered during chill and wants to be covered during warm.

- Wants more warm during warm and more cold during cold.

Cannabis Indica

Dr. Tyler

- All perceptions and conceptions all sensations and emotions are exaggerated to utmost degree.

- Distance seems infinite and time endless.

- Very excited dancing about a room laughing talking nonsense knew it but could not stop without effort which he did not care to make shouts leaps into the air claps hands for joy sings extemporises (speaks without thinking) words and music on becoming conscious finds himself dancing laughing and singing before a looking glass.

- Incoherent talking tendency to blaspheme (speaks of God in terms of irreverence).

- Accents the last syllable in all words and laughs immoderately.

- Said he had been transported to hear in and his language usually common place becomes quite enthusiastic.

- Despair fear of being eternally lost on hearing the name of god cried "stop! that name is terrible I cannot bear it. I am lying".

Dr. Kent
- The Limbs and parts same enlarged mental symptoms > by walking in the open air.
- It is useful in chordee during gonorrhoea.

Cannabis Sativa
- Things seem strange and uneasy.
- When he speaks it seems that someone else were speaking.
- Sensation of enlargement of the nose.

Cantharides
Spanish flies

Dr. Chowdhury
- It increases the sexual Desire so much that the night sleep is disturbed and there is painful and persistent erections often brings on cutting pain along the spermatic cord to the testicles which feel as if drawn up.
- On the skin the vesicles filled up with yellowish white serum. it look so large that the parts look blunt or scalded.
- We use it in psoriasis, Pemphigus, Eczema and variola when the vesicles are numerous and affected parts look burnt as if from fire.
- It is particularly useful in erysipelas when the vasications begin on the nose and then spread out the cheeks and other parts.
- it is useful in Mania and delirium when we have violent paroxysms of rage, tearing of clothes and biting and kicking. They bark like dogs aggravated from bright dazzling objects and touch.

Dr. Kent
- Violent delirious state intermingled with sexual ideas and talk.
- Eruption burn when touched.
- Thirsty but with aversion to drink water because a little drink brings much pain in bladder.

Capsicum

Dr.Chowdhury
- It affects principally the mucus membrane of the body where it produces a sensation of constriction it also affects bones particularly the bones of the face.
- Its burning pain is like the application of Red Pepper on the skin and aggravated from cold application and slightest drought of cold air.
- It resembles Cantharis in the simultaneous presence of tenensmus of the bladder and rectum but it locks in other keynote symptoms of congestion.
- Dysentery usually associated with backache.
- It is expressed as a drawing pain in the back.
- Regarding its action on the urinary organ burning in the bladder.
- Burning In the whole channel and the orifice of the urethra. the patient suffers from frequent unsuccessful desire to urinate.
- When passed the urine scalds and smarts.
- It is useful in second stage of gonorrhoea when the discharge assumes creamy appearance and when the chordee is so violent that the patient is compelled to Seek relief by emerging the parts in cold water.
- It is a good medicine for intermittent fever but the thirst commences long before the chill like Natrum Mur and Eupatorium but lacking in bones pain.

Dr. Tyler
- Needle like stitches in forepart of urethra when not urinating.
- Stitches on suffering parts with cough.
- Violent pulsation of arteries of abdomen clacking, rapid pulsation in some of the larger arteries.
- Chilliness between scapulae cold water dropping down back.
- Abdomen as if it would burst & yawning by day and sleeplessness by night. Sensation as if falling from a height during sleep (Thuja).
- Eructation of Red Pepper feel and taste.
- Sensation of cold water in stomach.
- Symptoms generally left side for lightheaded people.
- Tendency to get fat lacks muscles bloated skin fat flabby red face children.

Ghatak
- Fat flabby dirty chilly indolent.
- Burning not > from heat.

Children: Borland
- Fatty dirty indolent clumsy backward slow in learning in school.
- Flushing usually with red cheeks with their acute fever.
- They get sore throat, high temperature, flushing face, irritable, sleeplessness, thirst + + but get shivering after drinking.
- Very often they get acute urinary irritation burning during micturition.

Carbo Animalis

Dr. Kent
- It's complaints come insidiously the parts affected are hard indurated and purple.
- Bubos sluggish in nature become enlarged hard purple and Burn.
- Ulcers and fistulous opening where the walls become hard and Burn and the discharge becomes acrid.
- All gone sensation in the pit of the stomach while the child put on breast.
- It has yellow Brown saddle over the bridge of the nose (Sepia).

Ghatak
- Excessive Chilly with great prostration.
- No tendency to suppuration.
- Usually, it's pains are burning and stinging in character with slight tenderness.

Dr.Chowdhury
- The glands affected are hard and indurated and there is dirty bluish and lose appearance of the skin.
- Old maltreated Syphilitic bubous that in spite of surgical operation and cauterization refuse to heal and keep on secreting offensive discharge.
- It is used in last stage of pneumonia and phthisis. pulmonalis when huge cavities have taken place due to extensive destruction of lung tissues. suffocative hoarse cough that shakes the entire brain with expectoration of green purulent offensive mucus and pus.
- It is used in far sightedness while walking along the streets. the objects seen to be far off.
- Sensation of looseness feel in various parts.

Ghatak Tuberculosis

- The patient is normally exhausted weakened quite disproportionate to the amount of discharge of any type.
- This peculiarity is a sign during diathesis and must guided against otherwise full-fledged.
- This is to be expected. It usually found amongst the child bearing female and the active stage is found to start from a delivery.
- It's discharge is slightly offensive and sanides.
- Night sweat of offensive nature is found in this remedy. Greatly exhausting the patient.
- Carbo veg is near sighted what the Carbo animalis is far sighted.

Comparison between Hepar sulph and Calcarea sulph
Dr.Tyler

- Both are sensitive to drought and touch but Hepar Sulph is very sensitive to dry cold and better in damp weather.
- Calcarea sulph aggravated in Damp cold weather Hepar sulph sensitive mentally angry at the least trifles and almost murderous in its rage.
- Both have unhealthy skin that will not Heal while with Hepar sulph every little hurt festers.
- **Hepar Sulph:** cold foot sweats.
- **Calcarea Sulph:** Burning soles.
- Hepar Sulph wants to cover.
- **Calcarea sulph:** Throws away covering.
- **Hepar Sulph:** splinter like pain.
- **Calcarea Sulph:** not present.
- According to Nash it is a good medicine for Bright's disease where pus is present in the urine with great pain in the Kidneys day and night use Calc sulph 12.

Calcarea Sulph
- It is very useful for acne and summer boils and abscesses will point with a small pus head discharge a little pus and then the remaining big indurated portion will resolve by itself whereas in Silicea there is a small opening which will keep on discharging.

Carbo Vegetabilis

Numbness of the limbs. Dreams of fire, burglars, fearful of horrible things.

Fever: He wants cold water during chill and no thirst during fever.

Choudhary:
- Great weakness renders him for vertigo. When he wants to move, he has to hold on something or else he will fall.
- Tenderness of the epigastric region with sensation of rawness of the stomach, extending all the way along the oesophagus to the middle of the chest. Great acidity of the stomach is complained of and with this goes frequent eructation of wind. Tension is felt in the region of the ribs which too is sensitive and painful. Feels offended with grumbling. The result of flatulence is equally troublesome. Passing of hot and offensive flatus. Fatty food disagrees. Milk causes flatulence. They are frequently victim of hemorrhoids and the haemorrhoidal knobs are blue and they frequently suppurate. The piles become more active each time they go on spruce (engaged with liquor).

Difference between Carbo Veg and Lachesis in abdominal complaints:
- Both have complaints come on due to various habits.
- Milk disagrees in both the medicines but in Lachesis inspite of this intolerance to milk there is strong craving for it.
- Carbo Veg: fullness, heaviness and sleepiness after eating mostly to flatulence.

- **Lachesis:** It is more a sensation of pressure than fullness. It feels like a load, as if stone were suspended in the intestinal region. Sensation of constriction is very marked in Lachesis whereas it is a bit less in Carbo Veg.
- **Lachesis:** the weakness is due to Cardiac debility.
- **Carbo Veg:** It is due to loss of some important fluid.
- **Lachesis:** Strong desire for liquor.
- **Carbo Veg:** No desire for liquor.

Nux Vomica and Carbo Veg:
The same fullness and sensitiveness to pressure are to be found in both medicines.

- Pyrosis, acid eructation. bobory of this are same in both remedies but in Carbo Veg intensity of distension is much marked.
- In Nux, though it has lymphanitis but lacking in bursting sensation of Carbo Veg.
- Nux patient suffers more or less ineffectual vomiting with violent retching and excessive Irritability.

Carbo veg and Pulsatilla

- In both the complaints come after taking food, rich and greasy food, flatulence, bitter or sour eructations are common in both but Pulsatilla has a sensation of lump at mid sternum. In Pulsatilla it has more or less slow digestion as evidenced by the bringing up of food partaken several days ahead of the vomiting.
- The temperament and thirstlessness of Pulsatilla are always guiding.

Dr.Tyler:

- According to Dr. Kent: sluggishness, laziness and turgescence are the guiding symptoms. Everything about the economy is sluggish, lazy, full, distended, swollen and puffed. The limbs feel full, so the patient longs to put the feet up to the leg so the blood run out.

- Flatulence night after night and still needs to do it again and again. Night after night if it is not a Carbo veg case where no other drug, perhaps Argentum Nitricum.

  Guernsey says: complaints from obstructed flatulency (may be pains in the head, around the heart, or anywhere which have > by the discharge of flatus.

- Ch. Post influenza states: exhaustion of mind and body, apathy, depression and hopelessness. Cadmium, Nux.

- Acute post influenza states: Carbo Veg.

Dr. Kent

- Sluggishness, laziness, coldness, burning and fullness in different parts are the five salient features. The sluggishness is so prominent that the patient cannot realize anything. He is quiet indifferent.

- Inability to perceive or feel the impression. His affection is practically bloated up. Herd everything without pleasantly or unpleasantly and without thinking about it. Nothing arouses him. He cannot bring himself realize whether a thing be so or not, or whether he loves his family or not or whether he hates his enemy or not.

- Sleep: the sleep is full of anxiety and is an awful one on going to sleep. There is anxiety, suffering, jerking and twitching and he has horrors, horrible visions, sees ghosts. He wakes up in anxiety and covered with cold sweat.

- Exhausted, unfresh after sleep. He does not want to sleep in dark.

- Its headache is mostly occipital. It becomes so heavy, he is unable to lift the head from the pillow (opium). the patient suffers from catarrh. He is at his best when there is free discharge. He cannot stand suppression of discharge.

- Every time he has suffering of stomach, he is likely to get coryza, every time he goes into an overhead room, he is likely to get coryza. He suffers from the heat of chilling by the cold.

- Every draft chills him. He breaks into copious sweat on forehead. If he becomes overheated and his head perspires and then a draft strike that sweating head, his catarrh will stop at once and headache will come on.

- Aversion to milk which causes flatulence.

- It is the greatest medicine at the beginning of whooping cough. Its cough has all the gagging, vomiting and redness of the face found in whooping cough. It is the best medicine when no indication is obtained. The patient coughs until the chest is sore as if it had been beaten all over the chest. He sleeps into a paroxysm of coughing (Lachesis). He rouses from sleep with coughing, gagging, sweating and suffocation. He has two or three paroxysms during night.

(Acid Carbolis) Carbolic Acid
Dr. Chowdhury

- In Diphtheria: it is characterized by absence of pain.

- The accumulation of deposits in the faeces emits a very offensive stench. Excessive prostration, violent fever and thirst are present but water returns through the nose.

- The urine is generally dark smoky and greenish and urination is accompanied by involuntary discharge of mucus from the anus. greenish urine (Camphor, Arsenic, Aurum, Colchicum).

- Nervous dyspepsia of painful character and in return and in drunkards has been cured by Acid carb. There is intense distress in stomach with deathly faintness and gross sensitiveness to smell. The transverse colon suffers particularly from soreness. diarrhoea and constipation alternatively.

- Offensive breath.

- Strong desire for stimulants and tobacco.

Cardus Marianus
Choudhary
- Tenderness is felt in the left hepatic lobe and pressure causes oppression and cough.
- The other symptoms to follow are depression of mind, vertigo, dull heavy pain in forehead, eyes and temples. Bitter taste, nausea and sour green vomiting.
- It acts like Nux vomica where symptoms arising after taking too much liquor.
- It is a very good medicine for gallstone. It has no power to expel the stone but it is considered it does not allow for the formation of new stones.
- At climacteric where other complaints associated with liver trouble.
- It is the remedy to help in alcoholics to give up drinking (card mar).

Dr. Kent
- Motions with all the complaints.
- Very sensitive to cold and subject to attack of bilious vomiting at regular or irregular intervals. Sick headache ending in bilious vomiting and the patient gets low.
- Dragging pain in right hypochondriac region when lying on left side(Arnica, Mag mur, Nat S).
- Liver symptoms when complicated with lung and heart symptoms with expectoration of blood.

Castor Equorum
Choudhary

Herings recommends it in very high terms of it in cataract and ulcerated nipples of the worst kind of nursing women. When the nipples turned into scar and sore from prolong sucking of infant. It resemblance Causticum, Asterin Phytolacca. Persons having thick skin with a tendency- to become chapped (Antim crud, Graph, Petroleum). it is used in chopped hands and chapped breasts. It is used for external use warts of chest, tongue and forehead.

Castoreum
Herring

- Weakness and prostration affect after typhoid or any other exhausting disease.

- Swelling of the fingers with rounded elevation in the center. The size of a pea surrounded by an angry suspicious looking base. It was extremely sensitive and the patient felt drawing sensation as if a string there pulling the center of the tongue towards the hyoid bone. This kind of change may turn into malignancy.

- The patient yawns while suffering from dominant colic. in diarrhoea yawning present. Throughout day even when he is sleeping, he is yawning constantly.

- In amenorrhoea and other uterine troubles the abdomen is distended with wind and the pain starting in the middle of thighs, extends over the limbs, blood leaves the uterus in drops with tenesmus like pain.

Caulophyllum

It is a good medicine for after pains.

1) Female patient belonging to dystocia (difficult child birth), dystonia (a state of of the small joints and or also present yellow brown pigmentation of skin of face or body).
2) Rheumatic girls who suffer from sterility or repeated abortion.
3) Versicolour or brown spots.
4) Pain in left lower abdomen flying in all directions. The pains are intermittent or paroxysmal. They are of crampy, drawing, shooting or bearing down types.

Actaea Racemosa

1) Dreams of impending evil.
2) Fear of riding in closed vehicles.
3) Opening and shutting in brain.
4) Sensation of cloud enveloping the head.

Causticum

Paralysis: right side (Cantharis, Graphites) paralysis left side (Lachesis, Nux Vomica).

Dr.Chowdhury

It is anti-psychotic, syphilitic and psoric. Chilly patient.

- It is guided to patients who are melancholic, low spirited and anxious most of the time particularly at the dread hour of the evening. He calls for light. When shadows grow larger and the vanishing light of the day mingles with the darkness of the night they are apprehensive about some impending calamity.

- Redness of the face during anxiety with a frequent desire to pass stools is most characteristic.

- Aggravation of complaints while thinking about them.

- He is a gross subject to vertigo which may be the precursor of a coming paralysis.

- There is a tendency to fall either forward or sideways on rising in morning and sometimes in the bed at night.

- In chorea, we have constant twitching of the muscles of the face. During sleep legs and arms are constantly jerked out. The patient lies down on stomach and keeps on making spasmodic jerks.

- Intense photophobia which obliged the patient to wink constantly with flickering sparks and black spots before the eyes. It is a good medicine for cataract. The patient feels as if he were looking through a gauze. This dimness of vision comes up when he blows his nose. Aggravation with existence of warts on eye brows is a common feature.

- The cough is induced by crawling sensation in the larynx and after talking.

- It cures itch when it occurs on tips or wings of nose.

- Large protruded warts occurring in various parts of the body and bleed easily.

Dr.Tyler

- Affects especially persons dark haired, dark eyed and of darkest mood and temper looks on the dark side.

- Feeling of empty space between brain and cranial bones.

- Children emaciated especially about the feet with large tumified abdomen with eruption on scalp and inflamed eyes after otorrhoea and the child stumbles when it attempts to walk.

- He thinks fairly well when he had the eruption but when it disappears his mind goes out.

- Fissure seems to form upon the least provocation. Fissures about the lips and wings of the nose, the corners of eyes, arms.

- Apprehension of impending danger with urging to stool. (gels, arsen).

- It is a good medicine of colic after failure of colocynth, amelioration by bending double at night.
- Hahnemann gives a curious mental symptoms what he have come to call spoonerism confound letters and syllables, for instance says cluent coryza instead of fluent coryza.
- The least things make the child cry.
- Pain on sound felt on drawing on cold air.
- Tongue coated white on both sides, red in the middle.
- Bread causes pressure on stomach.
- He urinates so easily that he is not sensible of the storms can scarcely believe in the dark that he is urinating till he makes sure with his hand.
- Marbled skin of thigh and legs.
- Neuralgia moving from occiput upwards and forwards over vertex.

Renal Colic
- Excruciating pain which radiates from kidneys to testicle.
- Attack comes on while sleeping, urine passed in drops.

Dr. Kent
- It is deep acting constitutional remedy and is needed in acute diseases too. Patient improves for a time then comes to a standstill position.
- The paralytic weakness is associated with the rheumatic diathesis. The patient himself can endure neither heat or cold. The pains are ameliorated from heat both in dry weather.
- If frightened, he is almost sure to have some form of convulsive condition. epilepsy from the age of puberty from fright. Epilepsy, chorea, paralysis, hysteria during menses.

- **Mentals:** Always anticipating some dreadful event. It is found in old broken down mental cases after prolonged anxiety, after a prolonged struggle of some sort. everything excites him. The more he thinks about his complaints, the worse they become. The suppression of eruption is apt to bring out most symptoms. Suppression of eruptions from zinc ointment. He was fairly well when he had the eruption. When these eruptions are suppressed in children, chorea is apt to follow.

- It produces copious, thick, tough, gluey discharges from the mucous membrane.

- It is indicated in post diphtheric paralysis. (Lachesis, Cocculus)

- Sits down to the table with hunger but on seeing the food his appetite vanishes. The thought, smell or sight of food takes away his appetite. (Kali bich empty all gone feeling in the stomach with aversion to food) (China- canine hunger but loathes the sight of food).

- Thirst after eating, thirst for cold drinks with aversion to water. (Lachesis)

- Trembling in the stomach. Bread causes a sensation of heaviness and pressure.

- The rectum is inactive and fill up with hard faeces and which passes unnoticed and involuntarily.

- A woman who is too greatly embarrassed to pass through a crowd of observing men to the closet at the end of the railroad, at the end of the journey finds that she is unable to pass the urine affecting to strain the bladder.

Ceanothus Americanus
Dr. Chowdhury
- It is a good medicine for spleen.

- Aggravated lying on left side.

Dr. Tyler
Pain in the left side

Pain high up under the clavicle.

- Pain a little lower than it - Sambucus.
- Still lower - Acid flour.
- Move to the right - Aurum met.
- Under the left breast - Cimicifuga.
- The real splenic sick requires - China, Chelidonium, Berberis, Calc sulph, Conium, Ceanothus.
- When given in low potency it causes diarrhoea.

Cedron
Dr. Chowdhury
- He notices a great aggravation after coition.
- She complains of pain over eyes, of languor, debility and lassitude after each act.

Chamomilla
- Face sweats after eating and drinking. It is antidote to coffee. It is palliative in membranous dysmenorrhoea. Chilly patient.
- Nervous child go into convulsion when punished.
- All complaints are ameliorated from heat except teeth which aggravate from heat and ameliorate from cold.
- When there is pain in the ear, child carries the hand to the ear. Complaints aggravated in the first part of the night. 9 am and 9 pm colic while urinating.
- Ask the patient do not take coffee when NV or Chamomilla is the remedy. Every time the child is put to breast cramp in the uterus, cramp in the back (Pulsatilla).

Dr. Chowdhury
- Hot sweat on the head and scalp.
- Pain associated with numbness (Aconite, Rhus Tox, Helonis, Platina, Graphites).
- Gastritis where it comes after anger, a sensation of fullness and distension of hypochondria, nausea, eructation of putrid gas, heat and sweat on face, bitter taste in the morning, yellowish white coating on the tongue, collection of saliva or a sweetish metallic taste in the mouth.
- In threatened abortion: the discharge of dark blood, frequent micturition, restlessness, yawning and shuddering.
- Fever: chill without thirst. Intermingling of chill through certain parts of the body extremely chilly and cold and other parts are hot. (Children irritable and difficult to please. (Cham, Cina and Nux Vomica).

Dr. Tyler
- Chamomilla cannot bear pain.
- Cannot bear himself.
- Cannot bear other people.
- Cannot bear things.
- If you see a baby having brilliant chills, warm and wet head, cries or howls, insists on being carried, the music starts afresh and the trouble is aggravated at night.

Nash
- An ugly patient who refuses to see you, first send a dose of Chamomilla.
- Wind, colic, abdomen distended like a drum. Wind passes in small quantities with only relief by applying warm cloth.

- Rash of crying to women and nursing infants caused by heat or errors in diet with watery greenish chopped diarrhoea corroding anus.
- Profuse on covered parts.

Dr. Dippe
- She feels as though she were walking around on the ends of the bones of her leg and did not have any feet.

Dr. Pyrrell
- When the husband complaints of the wife being cross and irritable and he cannot get along with her, give him a dose of Chamomilla.
- When teeth are extracted give Chamomilla on first day followed by arnica in subsequent days.

Chamomilla
- Colic during urination (Chamomilla).
- Colic during and passing stool (Rheum).

Chelidonium Majus

Dr. Chowdhury
- A great craving from hot drinks that brings untold relief. Unless boiling hot their stomach will not relieve.
- The patients are lethargic mentally and bodily. They are sleepy and yawn frequently but when they try to sleep unattainable.
- A great heaviness, stiffness and lameness of limbs are quiet characteristic so it becomes an important remedy in rheumatism. The coldness of the tips of fingers is an important indication. The pain is always worst from least touch and definitely helped by bathing the part with hot water.
- In cough, there is sensation of dust in the throat.

Dr. Tyler
- Chelidonium – swallows.
- Cranium feels too small.
- All complaints lessen after dinner.
- Burning sensation in eyes aggravated after sleep.
- Heaviness in stomach after drinking hot.
- Sweet things taste sour so much that even the homoeopathic medicines taste sour. When the patient comes and tells the medicine is tasting sour give Chelidonium.
- Dr Farrington differentiates between Lycopodium and Chelidonium by saying that Lycopodium has got sour taste and Chelidonium has bitter taste. (I J H M 71-76)

Dr. Kent
- In pneumonia, the patient sitting up in bed with high fever bending forward upon his elbows, holding himself perfectly still as motion aggravates.

Chenopodium - Anthelminticum
Dr. Chowdhury
Pain beneath the joint of the right shoulder blade with a sensation of giddiness in the forehead and ringing in the ears. (Chelidonium)

Chenopodium - Glaucum
1) Severe pain under the left shoulder blade.
2) Toothache ameliorated from general sweat.

Chimaphila Umbellata
Dr. Chowdhury
- It is one of the principal remedy in obstructive vesicle irritation due to catarrh of the bladder.

- The patient experiences pain both in the region of kidneys and bladder.

- The urine is thick dark coloured and full of copious sediments. It is also ropy, bloody and full of pus. It scalds and smarts during and after the passage of urine. This painful irritation is felt along the whole length of urethra and from the bladder to the meatus. He is unable to pass even a drop of urine without standing with his feet wide apart and body inclined forward. These symptoms usually found in prostatitis. A peculiar sense of swelling felt in the perineum and on sitting sensation as if a ball is pressing upwards.

- It is indicated in hypertrophy of breast of females with tumors (benign and malignant).

China

Dr. Kent

- Sensitive to odors of flowers, of cooking tobacco.
- Cannot ride on a carriage or anything that jolts.
- Food tastes bitter or too salty.
- Convulsion during haemorrhage.

China-Ars

Ghatak

- Great prostration or emaciation appear slowly.
- Copious sweat.
- Diarrhoeic tendency.
- Chilly patient.
- Sensitive to cold.

Hungry type of patient.

China Sulph

- It is generally adopted to persons of dark complexion and to persons in state of prostration due to excessive loss of blood.

- Great sensitiveness of the last cervical first dorsal vertebra pressure. During fever the entire length of spinal column becomes painful.

- The time of paroxyms is generally 10 or 11am or 3 and 10pm. The paroxysm anticipates about the heart each time. It starts with decided strong short chill of 3pm. During chills the patients' nails and lips turn blue with ringing in the ears. Thirst is present during chills but in China. Nux Vomica thirst during chill but its thirst is present in paroxysmal stage.

Chionanthus Virginica

- It is a good medicine for jaundice which returns annually. Its symptoms are like Chelidonium but lacking intrascapular pain.

- Any complain after jaundice especially headache since jaundice.

Chlorum

- Sudden loss of voice.

- Prolonged expiration.

- Incessant dry cough, fever and profound sweating.

Cicuta Virosa

Dr.Chowdhury

- It produces congestion of the base of the medulla oblongata.

- It is a convulsive remedy and the convulsions are violent in character.

- Ophisthotones is a leading feature of this remedy.

- The whole body becomes rigid. We notice spasms in the muscles of neck and chest. The rigidity is so great that neither the curved limbs can be straightened nor the straight one curved. The whole body in fact becomes hard as wood. The head is turned or twisted to one side it becomes difficult. Foaming at the mouth. Violent tremors. Twitching and the bluish appearance of the face are important symptoms.

- Chronic concussion of the brain after arnica has failed.
- It is good medicine for various kinds of skin diseases. The eruption as a rule starts in the corner of mouth or face and extends to the head. Its exudation generally dries into a hard lemon yellow scab.

Dr.Tyler

- Convergent strabismus in children if periodic or spasmodic or bound by convulsion- blow or fall.
- After swallowing a sharp piece of bone or other injuries to the oesophagus, the throat closes and there is sense of suffocation, inability to swallow.
- Complete powerlessness of limbs after spasmodic jerks.
- Wish to come near the warm stove.
- Vertigo- objects seem to move in circles to move hither and thither though they retain their right shape.
- Most she is more firmly because she sees nothing firm or steady about her. Thinks she is herself unsteady. Imagines she is swaying. Everything swings backwards and forwards like a pendulum. Objects seem to come near and then recurs again from her.
- Has cured epithelioma of lips after swallowing a fish bone.
- It is indicated when the following symptoms are present:
- Violence of the convulsion
- The pustular rash
- After effects of blows to the head.

- Convulsion from center to circumference (Secale).

Dr. Kent
- Great irritation of the whole nervous system so that a little touch or pressure causes convulsion. Convulsion extends from center to circumference. The head face and eyes are first affected. An aura in the stomach gives warning to the convulsion. Some complaints spread from the chest especially heart. The rigors and chills begin in the chest and there is sensation of coldness in the heart and from there it refers to other parts. Any irritation in the throat and oesophagus will become violent convulsion. Convulsion from severe pain in bowels. Convulsion from disorder of stomach, from chilled, from fear of other mental condition.

- Mentals: at times he knows no one. Becomes idiot. childish behaviour, everything looks strange, doesn't know where he is, wants to be alone, dislikes to society, singing, shouting, dancing like toys. Jumps about like a child. Child grasps off ones clothing in fright tensed manner. Between the convulsion the patient is mild, gentle and placid (reverse Nux vomica), over estimation of himself (Plat).

- Cramps of convulsion in different parts, when occur after head injury. Cerebrospinal meningitis with convulsion aggravated from touch. Hot head with cold extremities (Bryonia, Arnica) sweat on the scalp when sleeping, staring and fixed pupil with upturned eyes. (Cuprum) strabismus is the only spasm which comes periodically from cerebral irritation.

Cimea
Dr.Chowdhury
- It is considered a good medicine for intermittent fever. (China, Capsicum, Eupatorium, Nux Mosch)
- In the prodromal stage thirst becomes intensified.

- All his limbs, joints and tendons ache more violently during the stage of chills.
- The tendons feel as if they were contracted and they constantly yawn and stretch.
- Thirsty but when satisfies it aggravates cough and brings on violent headache.

Cina

- Big fat rosy scrofulous children.
- Irritable temper.
- Glutton's appetite (she who over eats).
- Grinding of teeth sleeping during.
- Abnormally cross and ill-humoured does not want to be touched, crossed (intervened) or carried.
- Desires many things and rejects everything.
- Desires to be carried with pressure on abdomen.

Cinchona

Dark complexion. Habitually silent. Biliary colic with fever. Ars sulph, flab 200 Black spots in different part of body. Usually cover by Ars. When fails give China.

Dr. Chowdhury

- Restlessness and unrefreshing sleep with lot of dreams.
- Fixed ideas where ever he goes or whatever he does, he feels that his enemies are of his heels trying to thrust him in every way.
- In delirium of insanity he displays a great dread of dogs to other animals specially at night.
- On being called loudly, the consciousness revives and the patient may even ask questions but soon his consciousness ebb away.

- There is a great tendency to congestion of head, usually occurs after haemorrhage and seeing enemies. This is evident from flushing of the face and throbbing of the carotid. Sensation as if skull would burst. Aggravation from draft of air, touch and exposure to sun.

- Intense photophobia, intolerance of noise and acuteness of smell are present.

- Slightest food taken in stomach causes pain. Voracious appetite. Longing for highly seasoned food, liquor, violent thirst for cold water, longing for dainties, pulsations in the stomach, rumbling and gurgling in the abdomen.

- Diarrhoea at night and after it comes in insidiously and gradually.

- **Fever:** prodromal thirst, it may begin at anytime of the day but rarely at night. Presence of thirst during chilly and heat is contraindicated.

- Asthma during-Aurum. Cold sensation in the abdomen during every inspiration.

Dr. Tyler

- Hahnemann says long and repeated doses of this medicine causes secondary injury effects.

- Three times soft stool with smarting burning pain in the anus with bellyache before and after each stool.

- Looseness of bowels like diarrhoea.

- Frequent diarrhoeic blackish stools.

- Severe purging.

- Diarrhoea of undigested faeces like kind of dysentery.

- Frequently says - diarrhoea very debilitating, stools acrid, undigested, watery, bilious black, involuntary, painless, putrid, profuse.

- The biliary calculi patient is usually fair, fat, and flabby. Obesity plays a role here, especially women.

Dr C Thayer states

- China is most certain to eradicate the tendency to gallstones. I usually give china 6x, six pills twice a day till ten doses are taken and so on till at length the dose is taken once a month. I have not failed to cure in a single instance, permanently, radically every patient with gall stone colic who has taken the remedy as directed.
- For preventing renal colic: Natrum phos 1x 4 times daily.
- Terebenthina 1m to be administered (1 J H 64-29).
- Dr. Ian Mackenzie gives a diagnostic tip. In cases stimulating intestinal obstruction. The possibility of gallstones ileus in a strong multiparous elderly woman who continues to have attack of severe upper abdominal pain should always be considered. (In gall stone colic when indicated when fails I always get good results by giving in dose of S P 1M).

Cinnabaris

Dr. Chowdhury

Hot patient, bleeds easily.

- There is great abundance of warty growth on the skin. These excrescences are specially for shaped and are very common on the prepuce. History of sycosis and syphilis. Face is red and swollen, different kind of eruption especially red on skin.
- Violent itching of the corona glandis with profuse secretion of pus, redness and swelling of prepuce. Syphilitic phymosis with foetid gangrenous odour, induration of testicles and warty excrescences of various parts of body.
- The bones of the skull and hair is very sensitive to touch and painful. A sensation of congestion over whole head but principally over forehead is constantly present.

- Pressing sensation on bridge of nose as if he has been putting on a pair of heavy spectacles. This sensation of heaviness often extends to temples and goes to ears.
- Like MS it has metallic taste in mouth and there is increased flow of saliva.
- It is a good medicine for syphilitic troubles provide the indication of a great dryness of throat during sleep is present. wave of heat starting in abdomen extending upwards to it.
- Nodes on shin bones, forcing pain legs below, knee areas, the neck and head aggravated at night, ameliorated from sitting in bed.
- When allergy appears after the application of Variolinium in women on head.

Cistus Canadensis
Dr. Chowdhury
- It is meant for gangrene, ulcers, and bites of mad dog, animals and poisoned wounds. As a local wash it is said to arrest foetid discharges from ear, throat and other parts of the body. It acts on the neurosyphilitic ulcer.
- It is a good medicine for scrofula. Different glands of the body are affected.
- Very sensitive to cold and every exposure ushers in new complaints. Cold feeling in different parts of the body is well marked.
- A spongy feeling in the throat is a characteristic symptom.
- A continuous feeling of dryness of heat feeling in the throat is complained of. The patient swallows constantly to get ameliorated. The least inhalation of air removes all sensation of heat in larynx and trachea and produces a sensation of coldness in those regions.
- It is useful in cones of mammae.

Dr. Tyler

- Aversion to fat, meat, salt. Great craving for cheese.

- Great dryness of heat in the throat aggravated after sleeping eating and drinking.

- As if ants were running through the whole body (after lying down) then anxious difficult breathing, obliged to get up and open windows, fresh air relieves, immediately on lying down the sensations return. Great chilly, great prostration, every cold brings on engorged glands. Wants more spices too.

- Besides cheese, longs for acid food and fruits which give pain and diarrhoea. Diarrhoea from coffee and also from cold weather.

Dr. Kent

- It runs very close to Calc and it has the same exhaustion from exertion dyspnoea, sweating and coldness that we find in cal.

- Chronic diarrhoea with enlarged glands.

- Dyspnoea on going upstairs.

- It has eruption, herpes, and scaly eruptions. Salt returns on the hands of ends of the finger with cracking and bleeding of the fingers in wind and from working in cold water.

- All its complaints are aggravated from meat and exertion. It is anti psoric, Sycotic and tubercular.

- Old discharges from ear date back to eruptive diseases.

- If he is compelled to fart, headache comes on. (Lycopodium)

- The parotid gland is so much enlarged that it pushes the head one side.

- In acute coryza, the nose fills up with thick yellow mucus and when it is blown away it leaves the nasal cavity empty and there is irritation, one will say it is dryness one will say it is coldness and another will observe it as burning. There is amelioration when the nose fills up with mucus again.

- Old deep seated oozing ulcers about the ankle and shin with copious acrid discharge.
- The glands of the neck are enlarged in lines like knotted rope.
- Burning bruised pain in coccyx aggravated touch (Carbo animalis).

Cobaltum
Choudhary
- Backache followed by seminal emission ameliorated from walking, lying down and rising up.
- Constant headache aggravated by bending forward.
- Weakness, trembling and foot sweats are some of the symptoms.

Coccinella
Dr. Chowdhury
- Usually the right side is affected. The patient is disturbed at night from the neuralgia of the teeth, gums and mouth. Accumulation of profuse saliva in the mouth.
- Aggravation of all symptoms at night and sight of bright objects.
- Its pains are throbbing in nature associated with ice coldness of the extremities.

Cocculus Indicus
Dr. Chowdhury
1) It acts on the cerebrospinal system, where it produces a kind of paralysis, depending on the disorders of the spinal column. It has a special affinity for the lumbar region of the spine. Hence he comes across many symptoms indicating weakness of the legs, thighs and the back. They cannot lift their eyes on waking but drag them along. Trembling of all limbs.

2) It effects of anger and grief. (Coccus, Graphitis, Staphy, Hyos, Platina). every anger settles down on the liver and causes pain.

3) Sensation of hollowness and emptiness present everywhere in the body. Headache with sensation of opening shutting of the scalp in the occipital region.

4) Its headaches are two types: nervous and gastric.
    - *Nervous:* as it is brought on by mental efforts.
    - *Gastric:* associated with nausea, vomiting and other disturbance of digestion.

5) It is a good medicine for dyspepsia originating either from the abuse of stimulants or from long studies. Confused feeling in the head after eating or drinking, nausea, vertigo, metallic taste in the mouth with a great tendency for salivation. Burning in oesophagus extending to bones. Aversion to food, violent abuses of gastralgia with cramping in stomach. Sensation of emptiness and hollowness. There is great accumulation of flatulence due to flatus but not due to decomposition of food as in Carbo veg. Tendency to diarrhoea only during day. (Petroleum). Certain amount of urgency is noticeable as he has caring any time to dress. Stool yellow and faecal, Prolapsus recti after stool are the features of this medicine.

Dr. Tyler

- Frightened look, little concern for his own health. Very anxious about others sickness. (Ars, Phos)
- Pain in bowels and sensation as if bowels would protrude of the left inguinal ring. (Cocculus has been found useful in left sided inguinal hernia.)

- It has cured a case of delirium at the onset of menses, the patient says "I always see something alive on walls, floors, chairs, or anywhere, always rolling and on roll on me."

- A hideous dream came over him as soon as he closed his eyes which made him get up again.

- The thought of food makes the patient gag.

- The thought of food or the smell of food in the other room or kitchen will nauseate the patient.

- Sensation as if a worm is crawling in the stomach.

- Flatulent colic about midnight, awakened by incessant accumulation of flatulence, which distended the abdomen causing oppressive pain here and there. Some has passed without remarkable relief. Bilious flatulence constantly collected for several hours. He was obliged to lie on one side for relief. Irresistible desire to sing even if he was engaged.

Dr. Kent

- All the nervous impressions are slow in reaching the center. If you pinch the patient on the great toe he waits a minute and then says "oh". in response to questions he answers slowly, wants plenty of time to turn the head cautiously to see things. Wants plenty of time to turn the head cautiously to see things. Wants plenty of time to move to think, to do everything. The whole economy is slowed down, inactive.

- Extreme irritability of the nervous center. The least noise or jar is unbearable.

- Limbs straightened out and held there for a while are painful when flexed.

- Any complain arising after loss of sleep.

- Time passes quickly. He cannot realize that it has been a whole night.

- Loathing of food every time the patient gags when food is mentioned.
- Copious menstrual flow. Too soon, too long. Gets menses two weeks before time. Woman prostrated from grief, anxiety and from prolonged loss of sleep. Headache, vertigo, nausea, violent cramping pain in bowels, clutching pain in uterus during menstruation.

Coccus Cacti
Dr. Chowdhury
- It is a good medicine in whooping cough. Tickling sensation in the larynx is the characteristic symptom of this remedy. This tickling sensation wakes him up at about 2:30 p.m. and make him cough incessantly ending in vomiting of profuse tough stringy tenacious white mucus. The cough is aggravated in the morning about 6 to 7 a.m. it does not cease until a quantity of tenacious mucus is raised.
- **Anacardium:** cough brought on by anger and vexation. It's remarkable feature is belching after each fit of coughing.
- **Ipecec:** there are spasms of the glottis before paroxysms. The child stiffens up during cough and becomes rigid and turns blue in face. There is also nose bleed, bleeding from the mouth and vomiting.
- **Mephitis:** the child passes both urine and stool and turns blue during the spell of coughing.
- **Natrum mur:** violent bursting pain in the forehead during coughing associated with involuntary micturition and sticks in the region of the liver.
- **Sanguinaria:** whooping cough associated with diarrhoea.

Dr. Kent

- It's cough comes at the beginning of cold weather and last till warm weather comes. The patient is cold and his complaints come in cold weather.

- It has a contrast modality example when he becomes sick from exposure to cold he is always aggravated in a warm room and ameliorated in cold air.

- There is a General hyperesthesia of the skin and mucus membrane and sensitive to the pressure of clothing. With the chest trouble there is much dyspnoea.

- He cannot walk without bringing on difficult breathing which is aggravated by ascending aggravated in the warm of the bed ameliorated from clearing out mucus by coughing, lying in cold room without much covering and drinking cold water.

- Aggravated after eating and waking.

Coffea Cruda

- Over sensitive to noise. Pains are aggravated with noise. Even the opening of the door and ringing of the bell produced great suffering pain in the extremities aggravation from noise is the greatest indication of the remedy.

- All it's complaints are aggravated from cold and cold air except pain in the mouth which is ameliorated from cold.

- Very sensitive to wine.

- Person addicted to coffee. There is no fever.

- Intense stinging burning pains in the skin with the redness and heat with course Rash coming on suddenly. The sensitive part is aggravated by cold air of any kind, from fanning from Motion yet aggravated by warmth, aggravated from anyone walking across the floor.

- It can be compared with belladonna, both have hot head red face and brilliant eyes but Belladonna is sluggish, stupid and sleepy but is Sleepless.

Cubeba Officinalis
Dr. Chowdhury
- It is an important remedy for Gonorrhoea especially after the violent inflammatory stage of the disease is over. The violent strangury and tenesmus as seen in Cantharis and NV are over but there still remains a thick, yellowish, greenish discharge which is by no means scanty. There is certain amount of scalding pain during micturition. It is a good medicine for gleet.

Cucurbita Pepo
Dr. Chowdhury
- It is a good medicine for tapeworms.
- The most important indication is nausea soon after eating.

Cuprum Ars
- It is a great remedy for certain conditions and complications attendant on cholera as neuralgia of the abdominal viscera and uremic convulsion resulting from edema of the brain nephritis etc. We would rarely think of prescribing this in cholera. unless there is violent colic associated with frequent vomiting. Passing of cold sweat. The patient in his agony squeezes his abdomen with both hands. Dr. Bhaduri mentions the icy coldness of the whole body with cramps and obstinate hiccups.
- It is indicated in diabetes, when the urine becomes dark red and emits a peculiar garlic odor. The high specific gravity and the presence of ketone and dia-acetic acid are further indications.

Cuprum Metallicum

- Violence is the characteristic of Cuprum Met: Violent spasm, violent cramps, violent cough and violent diarrhoea. They are pale rather depressed looking or they are bluish with blue lips and extreme distress. They often present with a lot of jerking, spasm and twitching.

- In a uraemic coma, when there is suppressed urine with high temperature and convulsion, constant protruding and retracting of the tongue give cuprum aceticum 1M every 2 hours instead of cuprum met (1 JHM 71-92) and that kind of things when feeling awful the patient chats quite incoherently never sure of what he is chatting about.

- It is a good medicine for Endrine poisoning. The symptoms are unconsciousness with severe spasm and jerking. Give cuprum met CM diluted in alcohol every 15 minutes. (JH-33-54)

- Bufo is also a good medicine for Snake bite.

- In uraemic coma, when there is suppressed urine with high temperature and convulsion, constantly protruding and retracting of the tongue give Cuprum aceticum 1M every 2 hours instead of Cuprum met (1 JHM 71-92) and that kind of things when feeling awful the patient chats quite incoherently never sure of what he is chatting about and it is difficult to stop him. if extremely ill however they become delirious they cannot remember who they are or where they are or anything about themselves. They are bored stiff if they are idle. Therefore they are always doing something. They are very fretful and either apt to burst into tears or else they are apt to be very amusing and show off with a sort of buffoonery. They prefer cold food and milk and get ameliorated from it. They get a lot of cramps with the abdominal colic with gushing of sudden stools. During the colic abdomen is very tender to touch.

Dr. Kent

- It is a conservative remedy and complaints come with great violence.

- In whooping cough the face becomes livid or blue, the finger nails become discoloured. The eyes are turned up, the child coughs until it loses it's breath and then lies in a state of insensibility for a long time ameliorated from drinking cold water.

- Spasmodic condition and constriction of the xiphoid sternum with cracking of voice. The patient thinks he would die if he would not get relief from it. Some say it feels as if a lump in that region and others as if much wind were collected in the stomach. This constriction and dyspnoea occur sometimes in Cholera Morbus and in painful menstruation.

- In old age and in premature old age it is useful for those cramps that come in the calves, the soles of the feet and the toes and the fingers at night in bed. When an old man who has been single a long time marries, his cramps will often prevent him performing the act of coition. He has cramps in the calves and soles as soon as he begins the act. It is also meant for premature old person when cramps prevent the sexual act but when cramps occur during the sexual act Graphites, Sulphur may also cure this stage.

- In epilepsy it is prevented by violent constriction in the lower part of the chest followed by sudden shriek and passing faeces and urine during the attack.

- In Puerperal State: before or after delivery, the case maybe of uremic character, no matter the urine is scanty and albuminous. During the progress of labour the patient suddenly becomes blind. All eyes seems to her to disappear and in the room, as the labour progresses, convulsion comes on commencing in fingers and toes.

- In Cholera Camphor, Cuprum and where it rum other three principle remedies and their difference is like this:

- Camphor: it is a cold remedy. coldness of the body without usual sweat. coldness comes on soon after a little evacuation. The patient does not want to go.

- Cuprum: it is a spasmodic remedy. He is full of cramps and its compelled to cry out with the pain from the contraction of the muscles.

- Veratrum album: has copious exhaustive discharge, copious sweat, vomiting diarrhoea, coldness of the Sweat ameliorated by hot drinks and application of hot bottles.

- Podophyllum: it is a good medicine for Cholera. It has copious offensive gushing discharge with cramps in the bowels and the diarrhoea is painless in character.

- Convulsion from repression or driving in of eruption, from suppressing discharges. It restabilises the suppressed discharges and stop the convulsions.

- Metastasis: The same thing may occur from suppressed discharge, eruption and a suppressed diarrhoea and goes to the brain, affects the mind and brings on insanity, a wild active maniacal delirium, cuprum is not passive in its business. violence is manifested everywhere.

- Convulsions with flexion and extension are common to Cuprum.

- Headache after epileptic attack paralysis of brain with symptoms of collapse. metastasis to the brain from other organs.

- About the face convulsion, jerking of the eyes, twitching of the lids, bruised pain in the eyes. Spasms of the muscles of the eyes so that the eyes jerk and twitch first from outside and then from inside.

Choudhary
- In the stomach and bowels periodical cramps. It has cured colic in the form of violent cramps coming every two weeks with perfect vigorosity. It has been in stomach and pain under the xiphoid. Appendix that seems as if it would take his life.

Dr. Chowdhury

- In epilepsy, eclampsia epileptic form and puerperal convulsions and other nervous convulsion, cuprum becomes indicated by the severity of its muscular spasms.

- There is generally great restlessness between the attacks either filling of the entire interval or only a part of the time. In epilepsy aura begins in the knees and ascends. The first attack generally coming on during night, arms and legs jerk, specially the legs are jerked convulsively as if by electric shock. Urine flows involuntary. Clenched thumb during the paroxysm.

- Mental Symptoms:

- Maliciousness is the predominant feature of the mental stage. They glow over other peoples Miss Fortune and the feel happy when they find themselves in distress. They bite and strike and do everything to annoy their nurse and companion. Great fear and become afraid of anybody approaching them. They shrink away and try to escape from anybody. Sometimes we find them bellowing like Coffea, at other times they seem to be in convulsive stage they constantly protrude and retract that tongue like a snake.

- Gastric symptoms constant nausea like if Ipecac. The patient brings up gushes of whey like fluid and truly bites ones mother and is only ameliorated by drink of cold water. great burning is complained of in epigastrium of Deathly feeling of constriction Beneath The sternum. Intense cutting pain in the umbilical region as from a knife associated with tenesmus or contraction of abdominal muscles should call for cuprum.

Guernsey

One of the strongest indications for the use of this remedy is a strong Metallic taste in the mouth (RT) never well since whooping cough (IJH 65-96).

Curare
Dr. Chowdhury
Palaces after epileptic attack

- It is a great remedy for paralysis of various kinds and various parts of the body. We have ptosis, facial and buccal paralysis, paralytic failure of power to swallow, paralysis of the deltoid muscles and the general paralysis of the motor system. A tired pain all over, weakness and heaviness of arms, weakness of hands and fingers and trembling of limbs which frequently gave away while walking are very prominent symptoms of this remedy.

- The patients are haggard looking, pale and nervous, the eyes are sunken and they complain of dark spots before their vision. Noises in the ears as of whistling, deep red cracked bleeding tongue, constant dryness of mouth are indications of a Grave condition.

- Farrington: vertigo when associated with weakness of the legs. Sometimes the giddiness is so prominent the patient falls down like fainting while standing or walking.

- It has great dyspnoea aggravated by falling asleep.

Cyclamen
Dr. Kent

- Aversion to motion yet motion ameliorates her pain of uneasiness.

- Aversion to open air yet open air ameliorates many complaints.

- Most symptoms are ameliorated by walking and motion.

- Very restless at night.

- Alteration of moods is a striking feature of mental state.

- Vertigo when walking in open air. Objects turn in a circle in a room and when sitting. Everything turns dark before the eyes and you fall as if fainting.

- Pains aggravated lying on painful side and back.
- Pressure in the vertex as if brain were over enveloped in a cloth. Headache with flickering before the eyes on the rising in the morning. Headache from disordered stomach and ameliorated by Cold application.
- Convergent strabismus dilated pupils, heat and burning swelling of upper legs dryness and itching of lids.
- Dullness of hearing Humming ringing and roaring in both the ears.
- Sense of smell diminished. Dry or frequent coryza worst in warm room ameliorated in open air.
- Pale sickly face, dark under the eyes in women, contracted forehead and frown.
- Taste is lost or perverted, flat, bad, putrid, rancid. All food taste too salty. Saliva increased.
- Loss of appetite and even our run to food. Thirstlessness except in the evening during fever.
- Desires lemonade (Nit ac), inedible things.
- Aversion to bread, butter, fatty things, meat satisfy after the first mouthful (Lycopodium).
- Colicky pain in the abdomen rumbling and gurgling in the evening ameliorated by moving about.
- Diarrhoea after coffee diarrhoea in chlorotic women subject to sick headache and menstrual irregularity haemorrhoids that bead drawing pressing pain about the anus as if a spot would suppurate.
- Menstrual flow when profuse the mental symptoms are better. Labour like pains in the menstrual period. Commencing as the smell of back and running down each side of the pubis. After menses milk in the mammae. Complaints after weaning (China).

Mammae swollen and very hard after menses. Mammae swollen and containing milk in non pregnant women.

- Cough comes on during sleep from dryness and constriction of trachea ameliorated in open air.

Dr. Chowdhury

- Burning in the region of heart, inflammatory action of the heart, great lassitude and a sensation of something alive running in the heart.
- Hiccups during pregnancy.

Dr. Tyler

- No thirst the whole day but it occurs in the evening when face and hands become warm.
- Fine sharp itching on the hairy skull which when he is scratches always re-commences on another spot.
- Immediately after a meal rumbling in the hypogastrium, this recurs every day.
- Sore pain in the heels. (Petro)
- Menstrual flow more profuse while at rest (Cyclamen).
- menstrual flow more profuse at walking.

Cypripedium Pubescens

Dr. Chowdhury

- It is a good remedy for sleeplessness when due to overcrowding of brain with all kinds of personal ideas.
- Little babies are often seen to wake up in the middle of the night and laugh and gamble in the bright light, if this continues night after night the parent should take warning as often such functional irritability and cerebral hyperesthesia end in convulsions.
- In Insomnia it may be compared with Coffea and Scuttelaria.

- Coffea: due to an ore excitement of body and mind the result of excessive Joy or agreeable surprise.
- Scuttelaria: due to nearest the patient wake up suddenly with some disturbing disagreeable dreams and finds it hard to fall asleep again.

Alphabet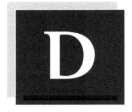

Daphne Indica
Dr. Chowdhury
- Sensation as if a part of the body being separated from the rest of the body.
- Offensive sweat, urine breath.
- The tongue is coated in one side only.

Digitalis Purpurea
Dr. Kent
- Slowness of the pulse rate is the principle feature of this medicine even the pulse rate may come down up to 40 or 32. It has irregular respiration with constant desire to take a deep breath.
- The liver becomes congested, tender and soreness. Bilious stool, jaundice with slow pulse rate.
- Sinking feeling in the pit of stomach not ameliorated by eating.
- Sleep is full of horrible dreams Nightmare bright dreams of falling that is very common with cardiac affections this is due to irregular supply of blood to the head for the irregular heart.
- At first it's pulse rate is slow but later it may be intermittent or irregular.

- When he goes to sleep the bread seems to fade away then he wake up with gasp (Lachesis, Phosphorus, Carbo veg) remedies that affect the cerebellum particularly producing a congestion to the cerebellum. When a patient goes to sleep the cerebrum says to cerebellum "now you carry on this breathing a little while I am getting tired" but the cerebellum is not equal to the occasion. It is congested and just as soon as the cerebrum begins to rest, the cerebellum goes to sleep too and let the patient suffer and in that way we get suffocation.

- Fear of suffocation at night. Likes mostly to lie flat on the back without a pillow.

- In enlarged prostate where there is constant teasing to pass urine in many instances where the catheter was being used for months or years because he is unable to pass urine in a natural way.

- It is capable of curing acute and chronic gonorrhoea. it has cured inflammation of that thing delicate membrane covering glans penis, dropsical swelling of the genitals.

- Loss of appetite and violent thirst.

- Constant nausea with cardiac trouble sometimes ameliorated by eating.

Chouwdhury

- It has vicarious menstruation like Bryonia and Phosphorus.

- Dropsy due to hepatic origin (Aurum met, Camphora, China, Lycopodium).

- Apocyanum is another great remedy for dropsy from heart disease. In this remedy too we find a great sinking feeling, a weak irregular intermittent and slow pulse, but the urine unlike that of digitalis copious and nearly involuntary from the relaxed sphincter. The skin is unusually dry.

Dolichos
Dr. Chowdhury
- Sensation of Splinter felt in the throat below the angle of right lower jaw.
- Violent itching without any eruptions aggravated by scratching.
- Jaundice with irritation of skin, distension of abdomen with flatulence.

Doryphora
- In Gonorrhoea it is indicated by intense itching and burning in glans penis which looks swollen and bluish and urination is associated with excruciating pain.
- Great trembling of extremities.
- It has been used in urethritis in children caused by local irritation.

Drosera Rotundifolia
Dr. Kent
Spasmodic cough is the characteristic symptom of this remedy.
- Lancinating in various parts of the body especially in head and much support the head with hands must support the chest when coughing.
- Corrosive itching in various parts of body with measles like eruptions.
- Ordinarily the face is Hot and Cold extremities, except during coughing of which time the face becomes red and congested.
- Putrid test in the mouth is common symptom in phthisical condition.
- Cough after eating and drinking cold thing.
- Colic after sour food.

- Sympathetic cough from spinal irritation.
- Spasmodic cough comes often during or after an attack of measles.
- Cold sweat on forehead and extremities.

Dr. Chowdhury
- The cough is attended with a sense of constriction in the chest with pain in hypochondria and the patient supports these parts with his hands during coughing.
- When Drosera is indicated but fails to act, think of Sulphur and Veratrum album.

Dr. Tyler
- It is a deep acting medicine and should not be repeated frequently.
- It is a good medicine for spinal caries, Scoliosis of TB glands and sinuses. Goitre where there is history of TB himself or inherited.
- It has power to dissolve the scar tissues of TB origin.
- It acts upon the rheumatoid arthritis of TB origin.
- Intestinal TB with diarrhoea and pain in the left side of the abdomen is cleared by it.
- A number of patients after months of steady treatment with other remedies and with waiting periods of Amelioration and relapse on getting Drosera, come back no more or only after periods of months to years of good health.
- Cough with yellow slimy expectoration and hoarseness of voice.
- Single cutting stitch in the middle of the anterior aspect of left eye recurring from time to time.
- A fine stage in right calf which comes while sitting and goes on walking.

- Tearing pain in right angle joint as if it were dislocated only when walking.

- Painful shooting pressure in the muscles of the upper and lower extremities of the same time in every position.

- All the Limbs are as if bruised or are also painful externally.

- Febrile rigor all over the body with heat on face but Ice cold hands without thirst.

Drosera

- Asthma aggravated from talking - Meph

- Asthma aggravated from cold weather - HS, Aconite, Causticum

- Asthma aggravated from rainy season - Ars album, Dulcamara, NS.

- The Drosera Mentally is paranoid the suspicious in character. Great aversion for Sour food.

- It is a great remedy for asthma when there is a history of TB in the family and TB from baci. give severe reaction. The patient is extremely restless, cannot stick one subject or one place for long time. Full of great anxiety and mistrust. He thinks he is surrounded by more but false people. Anxiety as if extremities would not leave him in peace and they are persecuting him. Anything may inflame his wrath of anger. Slightest contraindication throws him into rage.

- He shows and stamps his feet on ground. He thinks he posses the qualities of a Superhuman being, Supreme magician, a great Dictator. in the middle of night he wakes up in conversation, shrieks, shakes with fear shuttering, confused and unintelligent phrase. Wanders restlessly to and fro. He wants light everywhere. He is afraid of everything, of everybody. He is well protected or other guarded wherever he goes for fear of attacks on his persons. Adults suffering from laryngeal TB and hoarseness of voice.

Dulcamara

It is a good medicine for fungus growth inside the ear. There may be pain and fever. The appearance of the fungus is black and white like the ones we see on a piece of bread on a wet day. it is more applicable when wax is suspected trickle into the ear and causes fungus growth. (IJH 67-151)

Dr. Kent

- The Dulcamara patient is disturbed by every change of weather from warm to cold, from dry to moist and from sudden cooling in the body while perspiring. He is ameliorated in dry weather, aggravated by cold and damp weather, evening, night and rest.

- Diarrhoea and the close of summer, hot days and cold Nights, with changeable stool. Diarrhoea of Infants, yellow slimy stools, yellow green stools and quite a mass of Slime, showing a marked catarrhal state. It is sometimes ameliorated by Pulsatilla and Arnica but in Dulcamara every time the child gets cold the diarrhoea or dysentery sets in.

- The patient who has been out in the heat of Sun and catches the cold draft at night, which means hot days and cold night.

- Rheumatism from suppressed perspiration from sudden change of weather, aggravated rest and night.

- Every cold settles on the eyes, on the whole it has a tendency to bring back the old troubles when exposes to cold.

- Stuffing of the nose and the patient sleeps with his mouth open during cold damp weather.

- Affections of the mucus membrane, skin first becoming vasculated and then breaking open and oozing. It is specially related to very sensitive bleeding ulcer with false granulations, phagedenic ulcers. Ars.alb leads all the other medicines for ulcers that are phagedenic ulcers. Arsenic is a typical remedy for spreading sores, For spreading ulcers and especially those that come from a bubo that has opened and not Healed.

- In Bronchial asthma think of NS.

- Asthma with headache after the disappearance of tetters on the face.

- It is eruptive medicine producing vesicles, Crusts, dry brown crusts, keloids, Crusts, herpes. It's eruptions are just like impetigo multiple little boils like eruptions. it produces little boils and the boils spread eruptions upon the scalp that look so much like crusto-lactae. Extreme soreness, itching, and the itching is not ameliorated by scratching and the scratching goes on until bleeding and redness takes place. Children only few weeks old break out with the scalp eruptions. (Sepia, Graphites, Arsenic, Petroleum, Syphilinum). It has ringworm and herpes circinatus. It comes sometimes on face and scalp. Children sometimes have ringworm on the scalp. Dulcamara will always cure these ringworms in the ear.

- It has rheumatic and catarrhal headache and it is conducted in two ways. in some patients whenever he takes cold, from the cold, damp weather, he commences to sneeze, and to get coryza and soon comes a copious take yellow flow from the nose. On the other hand it has dry catarrh in its first stage has fluid catarrh on the second stage. One who is subject to dry headache has the dry catarrh, whenever he takes cold, instead of the usual catarrhal flow with it, he at first sneezes and then feels dryness in the air passages which is followed by severe headache and ameliorated by the starting of flow.

- The dry child is very susceptible to ear ache.

- It's headache and coryza are better in a warm room aggravated in open air. (Opposite to Nux Vomica and Allium cepa).

- Every time he takes cold there is frequent micturition and every sort of abnormality present in the urine.

- Dry teasing cough returns every winter (Dulcamara, Psorinum, and Arsenic).

- Rash before the menses every cold brings on herpes labialis, herpes preputialis, mammae engorged, sore and painful.

- Drawing pain in the lumbar region extending to the lower Limbs stiff neck from every exposure to cold.

Dr. Chowdhury

- Dulcamara varies with Bryonia and Rhus Tox in the treatment of chronic rheumatism. Its affections occur after exposure that demands Dulcamara. Sometimes this rheumatism is the effect of suppression of cutaneous eruptions and it frequently alternate with diarrhoea (Abrotanum).

- The pains are sticking tearing and drawing in character and the affected parts feel as if they have gone to sleep. The pain becomes very severe when he remains in one position and it subsides a bit when they move about. We should also think of Dulcamara in the intolerable pain in the shin bone at night time that compels the patient to get up and walk about. It is not the syphilitic pain like Aurum met and Asafoetida. It has been recommended in Lumbago when the back feels lame and cold and the patient complaints of a drawing pain from the small of the back down the thigh.

- The urine is generally scanty foetid and turbid. Sometimes it contains a tough Jelly like white mucus giving a milky appearance to the urine.

- Dr Clark recommends it in cystitis and other ailments of bladder particularly when mucopurulent urine is associated with one sided sensitiveness of the abdomen.

Dr. Tyler

- A curious regional effect of Dulcamara is around the umbilicus. Here the pinching and shooting pains occur again and again. It proved marvellously useful in pain or in skin affections of umbilicus. The pain is in the whole as a child expresses it.

Alphabet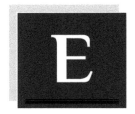

Elaps Corallinus
Dr. Chowdhury
- Chronic ottorhoea when accompanied with deafness the patient complaints of constant buzzing in the ear as if a fly were imprisoned in the auditory meatus. He is also subject to epistaxis and eruption about the nose and the face.
- This is a grand remedy for ozena, the nose feels stopped up and emits a foul smell. This is accompanied with chronic pharyngitis.
- All its discharges are black in nature.
- It is a good medicine in Cancer.
- Clerk curing a case of long standing irritating Rash in axilla which frequently used to give rise to suppuration of the axiliary gland.

Elaterium
- It is meant for Cholera and choleric diarrhoea and its stool is dark olive green froth and expelled with great force.
- At the onset of fever great chilliness is noticed with constant gapping and yawning. Sometimes the yawning is so serious that it resembles the neighing of a horse. This is followed by intense sweat with violent thirst.
- It is very useful for Jaundice of newborn baby.

Epigea Repens

- It is useful in many urinary complaints where this dysuria and strangury attending renal calculus. Hale used it in a case of strangury where the urine was full of blood and a large quantity of mucopurulent sediments in 10 drops doses of mother tincture. The patient complains of copious deposits of fine brown sand.

- Uva ursi: is another capital remedies for dysuria due to stone in the bladder. In cases were operation is deemed necessary it release the inflammatory thickness of the wall and relief suffering of the patient.

- Ipomea Nil: Cutting pain in the renal region extending down the ureter to the bladder. Nausea and vomiting that accompany the pain.

Epiphegus Virginiana

- Its headaches are neurasthenic type brought on by turner's exertion such as going on a visit during a day shopping etc. The patient suffers from a constant desire to spit a ropy viscid salivation. Vision gets a bit blurredd aggravation rising from a supine position and in open air. Amelioration after sound sleep.

- It has usually nervous headache brought on by physical and mental exhaustion and they are preceded by hunger.

Erigeron Canadensis

Dr. Chowdhury

- The hemorrhage of this remedy it is immaterial from that orifice. It may take place, is characterized by the bright redness of the discharge. Sometimes good result is obtained from local application of its mother tincture.

- Hemorrhage from the uterus associated with dysuria and irritation of the rectum.

- **Mitchella Repens:** it has also bright red hemorrhage with dysuria like Erigeron but its flow is continuous in character.

- **Phosphorus:** hemorrhage with dysuria but the menses is preceded by leucorrhoea and melancholy mood. The patient is troubled with frequent desire to urinate.

- **Sarsaparilla:** it has frequent desire to urinate with ceases as soon as the flow is established. Maturation is followed by almost unbearable Pain and the menses are ushered in by a few itching eruption on the forehead.

- **Sencio:** Menses with dysuria. Burning pain in the neck of the bladder before menses, giving rise to much tenesmus.

- Nervous women who suffer from sleeplessness due to prolapse or flexation of the uterus. She is susceptible to cold and has haemoptysis in place of menses.

- **Erigeron:** Haematuria without pain. If there is a history it is almost specific.

- Sometimes during dentition children suffer from great difficulty in passing urine. They want to urinate very frequently and they cry as often the pass urine.

Eucalyptus Globulus

Dr. Chowdhury

- Apthous condition of the mouth with excessive secretion of saliva.

- Enlarged ulcerated tonsils and inflamed throat also improve under its influence. As catarrhal remedy it comes after Aconite and Belladonna had partially relieved the virulence of the acute state but failed to arrest the progress of the disease.

- All gone sensation with pulsating of the epigastric artery ameliorated after taking food aggravated 2 to 3 hours after taking food.

Eugenia Jambos
- Great change of mental atmosphere after micturition.
- The patient becomes gay and joyful after maturation and it is short relief aggravated on exposure to sun and by closing the eyes. The eyes fill with water and tears run down on exposure.
- Nausea better by smoking.

Eupatorium Perfoliatum
Dr. Kent
- It is chilly and thirsty remedy and its prominent symptoms are vomiting of bile the aching of bones as if they would break. During fever there is severe burning of the whole body and by sweat nausea from sight and smell of food.
- Headache associated with painful joints or the headache may alternate with pain in the joints. Gout alternates with headache. Headache having a third and 7th day aggravation. The headaches are so violent that they make him sick at the stomach.
- Painful soreness of the eyeball (Bryonia, Gelsemium).
- The biggest attack often maybe ending in diarrhoea.
- It has dry hacking teasing cough that seems to rock the whole frame it is extremely sensitive to cold air like Nux vomica both are chilly and want to be covered. Nux Vomica has also aching of the bones but Nux Vomica patient is irritable in nature and eupatorium is sadness.
- After Malaria attack and gouty affections etc there is bloating of the lower Limbs oedematous swelling. It is not an uncommon thing for a malarial fever that has linked a long time to be affected with swelling of the lower Limbs. It very strongly competes with Natrum Mur, China and Arsenic. After administration of this drug it may bring back the chill and cure the case.

Eupatorium Purpurum
Dr. Chowdhury
- It is indicated in Albuminuria and diabetes is leading indication being an excessive irritation of bladder.
- The smarting and burning in the bladder is so excessive that the patient does not know what to do and finds ease nowhere. The desire to pass urine is almost constant but he passes only a few drops at a time and is obliged to renew his efforts every few minutes with each passes of urine the smarting increases.
- It is usually used after failure of Cantharis and vice versa.
- It causes importance in males and sterility and females with uterine agony.

Euphorbium
Dr. Chowdhury
- It renders excellent service particularly in gangrene of internal parts consequent on inflammation of stomach and bowels.
- The great indication of this remedy is burning pains in the bones and this symptom alone will help us in differentiating it from Acid Thuja, Silicea.
- It is a good medicine for the caries of the hip joint with burning pains at night time.
- According to Dr. Kent it is palliation in the excruciating burning pain of cancer.
- It has been used with success in cataract. Lenses become milky white and the patient sees better in the dim light.

Euphrasia Officinalis

- Chilly patient.
- Opacity of the cornea after injury of the eye.
- Wonderful remedy in measles.
- The fever occurs mostly during the day with red face and cold hands.

Alphabet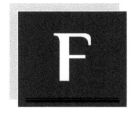

Ferrum Arsenicum

- Enlargement of the spleen with continued high fever,
- Disinclination for work, constipation.
- Sometimes colliquative diarrhoea,
- Emaciation, debility and want of thirst in any stage of the fever.

Ferrum Iodatum

- Enlarged spleen and liver without fever.
- Prolapsus uteri with amenorrhoea associated with great itching of vulva and vagina. Constant bearing down sensation as if everything is coming away. It is a good medicine for antiversion and retroversion of the uterus. The great indication of this remedy is Peculiar starchy leucorrhoea.
- It has been used in success in Albuminuria and diabetes. Oedematous swelling of the lower extremities in albuminuria. The urine is sweet smelling.
- We should think of it in haemoptysis in a phthisical patient, Great debility with emaciation. Evening chilliness followed by heat and sweat all night. Greenish discharge.

Ferrum Metallicum

When the patient talks his pale face would be bright flush, every time he talks the flash comes again. Post operative vomiting induced by only occurring after eating.

Dr. Kent

- Pains and sufferings come on during rest. Sometimes palpitation, dyspnoea and weakness come during rest. Ameliorated by gentle motion. Any rapid motion aggravates the complaints.

- Women suffering from much hemorrhage from the uterus during and after climacteric period.

- Green sickness that comes on with the girls at the time of puberty and in the years that follow it there will be almost no menstrual flow but a cough will develop with great pallor.

- Sometimes the early menstrual period is attended with a copious flow and then great weakness occurs and this goes on for years before anything like menstrual regularity is established.

- It is a very cold remedy and all its troubles ameliorate by warmth accept the pains about the neck, face and teeth which are ameliorated by cold.

- The headaches are ameliorated by pressure. Quick motion and coughing aggravate the headaches. Pain in the head and occiput from coughing.

- Chilly with thirst is a striking feature of this remedy.

- Vomiting of food without nausea sometimes there is eructation of food by mouthful (Phosphorus). Aversion to milk, meat, eggs, sour fruit, accustomed to tobacco and beer but sweet wine agrees.

- It is occasionally indicated in pregnancy, after few weeks after becoming pregnant the woman commences to throw up her food by the mouthful.

- Involuntary urination from sudden Motion, from walking, from coughing. In little children the urine dribbles all day. As long as the child plays the urine dribbles and keeps the clothing wet but this is better while keeping perfectly quiet.

- Insensibility of vagina during coition.

- Rheumatic pain in the deltoid region ameliorated by heat, aggravated by motion and by the weight of the bed clothes.
- Evening fever with chillness and thirst. Chill ameliorated by eating.
- Chaudhary: the headaches are aggravated after midnight and ameliorated by gentle motion.

Tyler
- After eating heat in stomach and regurgitation of food (phosphorus). Spasmodic pressure in stomach after the least food and drink. After fat food better eructations, after eggs vomiting. Worst from meat, sour fruits, drinking Tea, Milk, after tobacco, beer. Bad effects from drinking tea. Vomiting of everything eaten without being digested.

Ferrum Phosphoricum

Dr. Kent
- It is useful in higher potencies in chronic diseases and is deep acting anti psoric.
- It takes the symptoms among Ferrum phos and Acid phos.
- Its time of aggravation is sum in the morning, some in the afternoon, others come in the evening, night and after midnight.
- The patient is sensitive to open air and many symptoms are aggravated in open air.
- Cold drinks and Sour Food bring on many complaints.
- Complaints from lifting and straining muscles and from Sprains.
- Numbness of parts and suffering parts.
- Aversion to company and Feels better when alone.
- Confusion of Mind when trying to think in the morning, in the evening, after eating, ameliorated by washing the face with cold water.

- Fear of going to crowd, or death, that some evil will come to him of misfortune, of people. It is an excellent remedy for hysterical girls when other symptoms agree.

- Salts eat of their young.

- Pain in the face from inflammation of teeth, membrane, ameliorated by Cold application, aggravated by motion.

- Sudden attack of nausea coming at any moment so sometimes waking her out of sleep.

- Dysmenorrhoea with fever and red face.

- This is a valuable temporary remedy in the acute colds during the course of phthisis.

- Cold feet during headache.

- The rheumatism goes from joint to joint aggravated by slightest motion.

- Fever. Chilly 1 p.m. daily.

Ferrum Picricum

- Bilious patient with dark hair and eyes.

- A kind of dirty discoloration due to probably to bile pigments about the joints is another leading indication of this remedy.

- Sensation as if warts were growing on the thumb.

- Whenever any organ or any function of any organ gives out under strain or excessive use and fatigue we should always think of Ferrum pic.

- Failure of voice in public speakers, deafness arising from living in very noisy quarters and rheumatic attacks after every strenuous labour.

- It is a very good medicine for warts especially appear on the hands and they are multiple and pedunculous. The coexistence of words with deafness is a sure indication for our remedy.

- It is meant for senile hypertrophy of the prostate with frequent desire for micturition at night and a feeling of fullness and pressure in the rectum.

Ferrum Tauri

- A great tendency to sleep after eating.
- Violent peristaltic movements causing great deal of gurgling and rumbling motion in the abdomen.
- Odourless and tasteless eructation.
- Tension in the nape of neck.

Fluoric Acid

Dr. Kent
Hot patient

- It is a very deep acting and psoric, psychotic and syphilitic medicine. It is suitable in very slowest and lowest forms of disease.
- All cases of nightly fever coming on week after week and year after year.
- In the evening and night great heat sometimes to evolve the body without increase of temperature.
- All of its symptoms aggravate from warm in any form and ameliorate from bathing the face and head with cold water and motion.
- The feet burn and are put out of bad in the night. He hangs around in bed for a cool place for the feet and hand.
- A great offensive sweat of the palms and souls and makes it sore.
- It is a strong feature of this remedy to aggravate from coffee, warm drinks bring on diarrhoea or flatulence or disturbance of the stomach and cause indigestion to manifest itself in various ways.

- There is Peculiar outward sign in the nails, in the hair, in the skin, they are all imperfectly developed. It forms little encrustation here and there upon the skin that seems to have no tendency to heal. The hair loses is cluster, it falls out and if examined closely under the microscope It is seen to be necrosed. Little ragged ulcers will be found along the course of the hair. The ends of the hair are dry, the hair Mats and splits, and breaks becomes ragged in masses and lustreless.

- The nails are crippled and corrugated. They grow too fast and grow too thick, in some places and two thin in others, break easily, and brittle.

- In the evening the extremities burn and there is feverish because that is that time of fever stroke, but in the morning and day time there is coldness of the extremities.

- The patient is palled and sickly and that time becomes waxy and dropsical. Oedema of the extremities particularly of the lower extremities.

- When a debited subject suffering from bone or cartilaginous troubles contracts Gonorrhoea with it he will have a normal swelling of the prepuce or nothing seems to act upon it. Acid fluor will recover and Cannabis sativa has the same symptoms but it is seen in robust person.

- It cures fig warts. It produces hardened dry warts and dry crust upon the skin. It is useful in syphilitic sepia.

- Carries and necrosis of the long bones. It also cures the necrosis of the bones of the ears and nose. It creates an offensive acrid discharge from the ear and nose.

- It is a good medicine for antidote as well as complementary to Silicea.

- It follows trio cycle: Pulsatilla, Silicea, Acid flour. Other trio are: Sulphur, Calc, Lycopodium, Sulphur, Sarsaparilla, Sepia, Colocynth, Causticum, Sepia.

- A very serious case having Silicea symptoms should be at first started with Pulsatilla.

- The patient is over sensitive is made verse if the vowels do not move regularly. Is distressed if the menstrual flow is slightly delayed. Suffers if the call to urinate cannot be immediately attended, headache ameliorated by maturation.

- In persons who have over worked who have been working day and night to establish a business or when there has been constant use of brain it is useful.

- Persons who have destroyed the nervous system by vicious practices or by secret vice. Persons who have continuously change their mistresses. A man is never satisfied with one woman. At last they stand upon the street corners in their lust, Crave the innocent woman that go along the street. But there are some other persons who take on aversion to his children to his dearest friend and his wife that is he has lost that true and noble and orderly affections and friendship and companionship which ought to exist and he fights against it.

- Feeling of indifference towards those who love best. The above condition to found in Sepia but Sepia is relaxed to the women with uterine disturbances. Along with these symptoms there is an overwhelming sexual erethism. He is kept awake nights by erections.

- Reticence of silence sitting and saying nothing. The reticence is like Pulsatilla. A patient sits in the corner and says nothing and does nothing, eats went food is offered, it lead to her rooms when time comes resist nobody, answers nothing, such a state is found in Pulsatilla and closely allied to this remedy.

- It is suitable after Asia in the final affections that are attended with paralysis trembling and numbness in the soles of the feet.

- Numbness prevails allows the body due to feeble circulation. sensation as if the back of the head were made up of wood.

- Caries of the temporal bone, discharges offensive pus periodically, whole left side of the head retarded in growth. left eye seems smaller.
- The teeth decay or break off or ulcerate at the roots. Fistulous opening from the roof of the tooth.
- Crave cold water and is continuously hungry. Often that all gone sensation in the stomach is always eating and his relate from eating but like iodine it does not last long for soon he becomes hungry again.
- In potentized form Silicea and Merc sol are inimical, yet the high potencies of Silicea will antidote Mercury.
- Craving for pungent spicy highly season food.
- Morning diarrhoea with itching of the anus sometimes intense is present.
- Dropsy of drunkards usually cirrhosis of liver.

Dr. Chowdhury

- In inflammation of osseous tissues and in exostoses in threatened gangrene especially of the scrotum or penis and in bed sores where there is syphilitic tendency, we cannot do better than to administer a few doses of fluoric acid.
- Whitlow and panaritium which are sign of run down state of health disappear permanently under the influence of this remedy.

Alphabet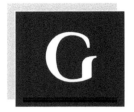

Gallicum Acidum
Dr. Chowdhury
- Dr. Nerey of New York records a wonderful cure of a case of Phthisis in a young lady with the cavity in her left lung. It was a very Grave case plural and expectoration night sweats evening fever Rapid pulse and a rapid loss of flesh he used 1X potency.
- Its principal symptoms are great weakness with a irritability excessive dryness of mouth and throat and a sensation of constriction of anus. Photophobia, epistaxis and increased secretion of phlegm in the throat.

Gambogia
Dr. Chowdhury
- The stool comes out all at once with a single and somewhat prolonged effort.
- Suddenness of the urging.
- Great relief is obtained after passing stool. (feels as if some irritating substance were removed).
- There is great burning in the anus.
- The stool a profuse watery sometimes yellow sometimes greenish and lienteric.
- There is violent itching of the canthi and eyelids.

- The pain in this remedy whenever it may be is of burning in character.

Gels: very sensitive and irritable, upset from slightest trouble which causes trembling diarrhoea and insomnia. He cannot bear opposition and contradiction, that's why he avoids society and tends to be alone.

Gelsemium
Dr. Kent
- In Gelsemium, cold develops its symptoms several days after the exposure while Aconite cold comes after a few hours.
- It is a remedy for warm climate. it has been used mostly in acute troubles in lingering acute troubles and those resembling the chronic it is very useful but in miasm it is not the remedy.
- Its complaints are congestive in nature so there is dusky and congested face. The symptoms are manifested largely through the brain and spinal cord. Hence it is a good medicine in cerebrospinal meningitis and the symptoms are: we have the neck drawn back and rigidity of the muscles of the back of the neck. There are violent pains of the back and coldness of the spine. Hot head neck and face with cold extremities (but it's use is confined to the first stage Chaudhary).
- When intermittent or remittent fever turn into continued type.
- In every type of fever or other diseases the head is hot and the extremities become cold. It has afternoon fever continuous throughout the night less in the morning.
- The heart is feeble and the pulse is feeble soft and irregular, palpitation during the febrile state. There is a sense of weakness and goneness in the region of the heart and the weakness and goneness often extend into the stomach involving the whole lower part of the left side of the chest and across the stomach creating a sense of Hunger like Ignatia and sepia.
- Involuntary loss of stool and urine during febrile stage.

- Cramping in the muscles of the back and aching under the left shoulder blade.

- As a rule the patient is thoughtless and it is the exception that there is much thirst it has profuse exhaustive sweat from motion or rather motion seems to be impossible.

- Paralytic condition of the throat and as the troubles progresses the food and drink come back through the nose.

- Sciatica with steering pains associated with great weakness of limbs.

- Numbness maybe present everywhere in the skin.

- Many times when erysipelas has spread over the face and scalp and in the most dangerous manner with the dusky red colour that belongs to gels the other symptoms of gels should be present. Sleeplessness from acute drunk.

Dr. Chowdhury

- Dr. Eriskine White was reported a case of a baby born in convulsion that he cured with gels. The symptoms to guide him were a history of pride in mother a few weeks before the baby was born and the incessant quivering of the child's skin.

- Children frequently get the sense of falling during sleep so the grass at everybody or everything around them.

- Aphonia due to paretic condition of laryngeal muscles.

- Involuntary emission of semen without an erection, spermatorrhoea from relaxation and debility, placidity and coldness of genitals and complete exhaustion of the parts.

- In female there is reflex headache due to ovarian irritation the head feels enormously and last it is excellent in congestive dysmenorrhoea.

- We think of it in threatened abortion from sudden depressing emotions as if caused by Fright anger hatred and jealousy.

Dr. Tyler
- In post diphtheric paralysis there is pricking of the finger tips and in soles in of the feet, as if shoes full of sharp little stones.
- When something swallowed went not down but up into the nose.
- Never well since "flu" Some weeks ago, tired longer, heavy cannot get well. The temperature is found to be 99 degrees Fahrenheit and there are chills.

Ginseng
Dr. Chowdhury
- In sciatica there is a bruised pain in the small of the back and thighs on rising from the bed and great languor. The pain extents as far as big toe. The patient complaints of nightly digging pain in the lower Limb from the hip to the big toe. The pain is lancinating and tearing in its character with this is noticed a frequent desire to urinate. It is a right sided remedy.

Glonoine
Dr. Kent
- The most common feature of this remedy is the surging of blood to the head and to the heart. Sense of boiling in the region of the head or in the left side of the chest. There are also wave like sensation in the head as if the skull were being lifted up and lowered as if it were expanded on and contracted.
- The pulsation is tremendous and when they are greatest in the head they are felt also in the extremities. If this continues a while the soreness in the skull is likely to come on and with the painful throbbing every throb is a pain, aggravated by jar motion and warmth and ameliorated from vomiting, cold air, and cold application. With this the extremities are cold and the head and face are flushed.
- There is no great thirst but mouth is very dry.

- When the about troubles persist for years or become chronic he will never go out in warmth of the sun without an umbrella.

- In headache he wants the head high, aggravated from stooping, from bending head backwards, after lying down, when ascending steps, the weight of the hat, (Calc phos, Nitric acid) Ameliorated from long sleep, Cold application, pressing the head from all side, holding the head firmly.

- Aggravated from wine, from stimulus, and from mental application.

- The child comes down with cerebrospinal meningitis the neck is drawn by the faces intensely hot red and Shiny. The eyes are congested and glossy, the head and upper part of the body are very warm, the feet and hands of lower portion of the body are cold and covered with cold sweat. Cold feels good to the head and heat feels good to the extremities. convulsion through out the limbs.

- Hyperaemia of the brain, a rush blood to the head. It comes in spells while walking on the street, he feels an urging to the Brain like a flush of air, and flush on the face, his hands tremble and the hands and feet become cold. He breaks out in sweat; he looks around him and does not know which way to go home. He does not know where his dwelling is. He looks in the faces of friends and they seem strange. He is a confusion which soon passes away and he feels better again.

- In threatened apoplexy and apoplexy has taken place, if the violent pressure keeps on think of this remedy and opium. A paralytic condition in one arm or leg may go on for a while and at the end of many weeks or months. In this case opium is a very good medicine but it must not be administered in large doses. The highest potencies are best and one single dose is sufficient.

- Frantic attempts to jump from the window the headache is so violent and so intense the patient wants to jump out of the window.

- Some months after being silent and jarred by body thrown from a carriage, a sensitiveness of the upper part of back and neck come on. There are two strong characteristics of glonoine in that case that is aggravated from wine and aggravated from lying down.
- These patients are sitting perfectly quiet for hours together without moving because motion aggravates the complaints.
- The whole Crown of the head feels as if was covered by hot iron as if an oven were closed by hot especially in the back of the neck and hot between the shoulders.
- When the sunstroke first comes on the face is bright red, intensely hot and shiny but as the heat increases the face glows dusky even to purple.
- When a copious flow of hemorrhage from any part stops suddenly the patient comes down with great violence and the blood rushes to the head.
- Children get sick in the night after sitting especially at open fire of falling asleep there.

Dr. Chowdhury
- Headache that app to begin in the warm weather and end at the ending of summer.
- Belladonna patient likes the head covered where as Glonoine patient is better from uncovering.

Dr. Tyler
- Numbness of lower lip (Calc carb) and right hand.
- Throbbing pain in the teeth.
- Headache ameliorated by drinking coffee and tea.
- Supra orbital Neuralgia from 6:00 a.m. to 11 or 12.
- Chin feels elongated to knee, obliged to put hand on Chin repeatedly to be sure that it is not the case.

- The difference between Amyl nitrate and Glonoine is Amyl dilates the arteries, flushing without throbbing, Glonoine - flushing with throbbing and affects the nervous centres of the circulation. Amyl usually unaltered pulse. Glonoine with altered pulse. Belladonna the circulation within the cranium is excited because the brain is irritated, with glonoine the brain is irritated because the circulation is excited. Belladonna pains come suddenly and ceases suddenly not in glonoine. Belladonna wants the head covered, Glonoine is aggravated by covering.

Gnaphalium

Dr. Chowdhury

- It has pain along the course of the Seitic nerves and its largest ramifications is intense. Numbness is generally associated with the pain. In this connection, it is similar to cold. We can compare Gnaphalium with the following medicines:

- **Graphitis:** The pain commences from the hip and rushes downward posteriorly to the feet. The left foot cramps and has to be drawn up < In damp or cold weather, usually right side.

- **Colocynth:** The pains extend from the hip down the posterior portion of the thigh into the popliteal space. The pains are sharp and shooting in character, and the patient must keep perfectly quiet as every motion < > By pressure, usually left side.

- **Ammon-Mur:** The pain is severe and long continued. It is most often left-sided, and the tendons of that side fail as if they were too short, making him lean sideways while walking > By rubbing and lying down.

- **Calc-Carb:** Sciatica caused by working underwater The pain is < When the limb is kept hanging down and hence it has to alleviate his knees constantly.

- **Euphorbium:** The tearing and tingling pain of this remedy is > By motion in respect. It is somewhat similar to Rhus tox.

- **Ferr-Met:** The pain in the hip joint is violent< From evening till midnight, the patient, though he can hardly put his leg on the ground, walks slowly to get >.

- **Kali-iod:** Sciatica with Syphilitic or mercurial history. The pain is < in the night and > by motion.

- **Kali-phos:** When the patient feels most of the pain in the souls of the foot, he is restless.

- **Ledum:** Pain from below upwards, the affected limb is cooler than the other. The left side is more affected.

- **Menyanthes:** The pain throws the affected thigh and leg spasmodically upward in a jerking fashion at every attempt to assume a seating posture.

- **Nat-Mur:** Has tensive pain in right hip and knee of remittent character, as in Ammonium Muir, the feeling of contraction of the hamstrings, emaciation of the affected limbs, and > heat are marked features.

- **Plumbum:** Chronic sciatica with muscular atrophy.

- **Ruta:** The pain is very deep-seated and feels as if it is in the marrow of the bone. There is generally a history of injury or contusion, its stomach symptoms are like Colocynth.

Gnaphalium Polycephalum

- Sciatica pain aggravated walking, lying, cold and damp.
- Ameliorated drawing limbs up, flexing thigh on abdomen.
- Alternate pain and numbness.

Gossypium-Herbaceum

Dr. Chowdhury

- This remedy is rich in sympathetic symptoms of the stomach, heart, bowel, and nervous system arising from disturbance of uterine function.

- It is generally indicated in tall women who are comparatively anemic and who are extremely nervous.

- It relieves a tardy flow of menses, especially when accompanied by a sensation as though the flow is about to start, but yet does not.

- It cures morning sickness during pregnancy. Great Nausea from the least motion in the morning soon after waking as soon as she raises her head from the pillow. The retching starts, at first very little comes, and then a little saliva and lastly some bilious matter but rarely any ingesta.

- It is a very good medicine for after pains, excruciating pain so frequently met with after labor in nervous females has been cured by me with this remedy.

- The placenta is also adherent to the uterine wall soon after the delivery of the fetus the internal OS contracts and the placenta remains inside the uterine cavity.

Graphites

- According to doctor lady doctor Dr. Tyler Graphites has Great Value in gastric or duodenal ulcers and no other drug. So far as we know has fever that little Complex of symptoms stomach pain ameliorated by food and drinks, ameliorated by hot drinks or food, lying down. In a cute pain it should be given 30C to cm to or three times for 2 or 3 days. Psorinum 1M or 10M should be given as an intercurrent remedy when Graphites we should think of Carbo veg 1m to 10m.

- It is a very good medicine in chronic intermittent fever.

- Asthma ameliorated by eating Graphites, asthma ameliorated from stools-pothos.

- Left sided medicine.

Dr. Kent

- It is a very deep acting remedy like all carbons and is accompanied by induration and burning in the base of the ulcers. Cancerous development in old cicatrices is a strong feature of this remedy. Contraction of tendons especially behind the knees.

- From eruption catarrhal discharges menstrual flow ulcers breath and perspiration there is marked offensiveness (Carbo veg, Pso, Kali.phos, Kali ars).

- When erections or discharges have disappeared suddenly from any cause and Grave chronic phenomena wave followed.

- Recurrent herpes upon all parts of the body and especially about the anus and genitals.

- Burning in any parts especially old cicatrices.

- Weakness in muscles and tendons after straining them by over lifting.

- He is sensitive to cold in winter and to the heat in summer.

- Craving for air is strong in the carbons yet often child and just as easily treated.

- Numbness is more characteristic than pain.

- Formation fissures in all the commissures and in the anus with cracked and bleeding skin in many parts with much hardening.

- The mental depression is extreme and aggravated by music.

- Motion aggravates all the symptoms except numbness.

- Extreme activity of mind in the evening and first half of night.

- Violent headaches during menstruation.

- Extreme photophobia in the sunlight with copious lachrymation. No remedy has photophobia more mark than Graphites. It has cured ulceration of the cornea.

- Recurrent pustular inflammation of cornea, cystic tumours on the lids.

- She cannot tolerate flowers.
- Ravenous appetite violent thirst in the morning with dry mouth of internal fever.
- Aversion to meat, cooked food, to fish, salt and sweet.
- Pain in the stomach ameliorated by eating. Flatulence is as marked as Carbo Veg and ameliorated from belching like Carbo Veg. Gastric catarrh with internal heat drive him to eat and drink.
- Ameliorated by warm milk. Sensitive to clothing in the liver region.
- From the anus there is copious discharge of very offensive flatus day and night.
- It has cured many cases of bleeding piles of long standing where there is extreme soreness and fissures and great burning.
- Hydrocele and small boys and baby boys.
- Aversion to coition to both sexes. Leucorrhoea instead of menses (Coccus) violent itching of the vulva before menses. Hoarseness in the evening (Carbo Veg) suffocates when falling a falling asleep.

Dr. Chowdhury

- Fat Chilly and costive patient. There is distinctly a scrofulous basis as is manifested by its tendency to lymphatic oedema.
- Most of the eruption of Graphites are seen between the toes and fingers on the scalp and behind the ears.
- Sadness and despondence are there ever present complaints aggravated by music (opposite Magnum). Restlessness is well marked. They cannot sit in one place long, but must move about. It has been recommended in impendence and idiocy. When the patient laughs all the time and laughs even when reprimanded.

- Cannot bear bad clothes around the waist due to flatulence patient who had to keep bread or some other articles of diet handy to be able to eat quickly as soon as the suffocative paroxysm asthma was about to start.
- When fat anaemic woman with disordered menstruation complain of numb and heavy feeling in the head especially in the occiput we will think of Graphites.
- Sensation of cobweb over the face another Peculiar symptom is a sensation as a skin of the forehead was drawn into folds.

Dr. Tyler
When the complications arise from the bad effects of car tissues sweet things are disgusting and nauseous.

Gratiola Officinalis

Dr. Kent
- Hot patient left-sided remedy complaints are better in the open air, but he is chilly in a warm room, with constant vapor exhalation from the body.
- There is a lack of willpower and aversion to work.
- Complaints from pride and bad effects from coffee and alcohol.
- Heat and fullness of the head sensation as though the head grew smaller. The rush of blood to the head after rising from stooping.
- Pain in the occiput from sneezing.
- Itching of the skull, ear, and eye. Mist before the eyes while reading and green objects appear white.
- Swelling of the upper lip in the morning, sensation of tension, and swelling of the face.
- Pain in the throat constantly swallowing much mucus in the throat, which he cannot expectorate, thirst, and emptiness in the stomach after eating. Craves nothing but bread.

- Nausea bitter after eating. After eating and by eructation. A feeling of anxiety in the stomach, cramping in the stomach after food, and the heavy load that seems to go from side to side as he turns from side to side. Cramp and hard aching in the stomach. The pain grows rapidly. The worst seems to extend to the back and kidneys. Marked coldness in stomach.

- It is one of our best remedies for nymphomania. Sometimes the desire is so violent that it drives her to a secret vice. (Gels, Nux vom, Phos, Zincum).

- Violent palpitation after stool.

- Vertigo during and after eating on closing the eyes while reading, rising from a seat on motion.

Dr. Chowdhury
- **Diarrhoea:** The stools consist of a yellow-greenish watery substance and are very frothy, very often there is rumbling and gurgling in the abdomen with violent colic, vomiting is particularly severe and is accompanied by pain in the head. Severe cramp in the solar plexus, intense nausea, great rectal and anal irritation in the shape of burning, cold feeling in the abdomen. Diarrhoea from taking too much water.

Grindelia-Robusta

Dr. Chowdhury
- It is mostly indicated in mucus asthma. There is an abnormal accumulation of tenacious. viscid mucus in the smaller bronchi < during sleep.

- On falling asleep, his respiratory movement ceases and does not resume until awakened.

- It is also used in asthma from heart troubles. This asthma is secondary to heart affections.

- This difficulty in respiration during sleep is due to its paretic action on the pneumogastric nerve.

- It has quite a lot of symptoms on the skin eruption. vesicular, papular Herpes Zoster. Roseola rash, insects, and bee bites are helped by it.

- Gatchell Recommends the external application of a lotion. Grindelia. R. in one in ten of water is a sovereign remedy in itches and painful erythematous eruptions.

Guaiacum

Dr. Kent

- It is a deep-acting anti-psoric and anti-syphilitic remedy. Constitution that is rheumatic, gouty, and has an inherited thesis. These patients are subject to dyadia. The tendons are too short, or they have abscesses. Catarrhal troubles, bronchitis, drawing tension, and contraction of muscular fiber. The rheumatic joints are < From warmth. (Lac. caninum, Pulsatilla) and > from cool. Gouty abscesses in joints. The leg and ankle bones are especially affected. Sensitive periosteum, stitching pains, and burning like Arsenic are characteristic.

- Every cold settles on the limbs.

- All the pains are. < From warmth and motion except for pulsating pain, which is > by pressure and walking < by sitting and walking.

- It is closely related to Causticum, Sulphur. T.B.

- Rheumatic pain in one side of the head, extending into the face.

- Sensation of looseness of the brain.

- Aversion to food and drink much thirst.

- Morning diarrhoea.

- Dry hard cough with fever > By expectation .

- Pains in finger joints and then in the whole hand.

- Shooting pains in legs from feet to knees. The knee is flexed from the contraction of the hamstring.

Dr. Chowdhury

- Carries and sponges affection of bones, especially of tibia and tarsal bones. Acute inflammation with all the redness, heat, and swelling, like Belladonna, is present.

- All its excretions are intolerably offensive.

- Inflammation of the palate grew deeper till at last perforation of the palate was threatened. It is closely related to Aci Flour, Kali. Bichrome, Natrum Sulph, Nitric acid.

- **Acid Fluric:** It has extensive ulceration of the mouth and throat. Syphilitic caries and necrosis, boring bone pains, and the offensiveness of the acrid ichor are commoners in both remedies but Guaicum wants the peculiar pungent strong urine of fluric acid.

- **Kali-Bich:** Tends to have perforated ulcers in the nose, mouth, and throat, and it differs from. Guaiacum in its stringy jelly-like discharge.

- **Mer-Sol:** Has ptyalism, flabby broad tongue, and the peculiar lardaceous appearance of the base of the ulcer.

- **Nitric Acid:** Sprinter-like pains and ulcers are inclined to spread more in circumference than depth.

- **Guaiacum:** We should think of it in syphilis sore throat and the symptoms are great burning in the throat, esophagus, larynx, and the whole of the buccal cavity in this respect it is greatly similar to Phytolacca. Its pain tends to travel backward or from below upwards.

Guarea Trichilioides

- It cures chemosis (Swelling around the cornea)of an extreme type. It helps in the case of chemosis after extraction of cataracts where the pad was so extended and thick that nothing of the eye could be seen, but the pupil at the bottom.

Gymnocladus-Canadensis

- Bluish white coating tongue is the characteristic indication of this remedy.

Alphabet

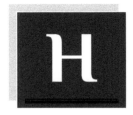

Hamamelis Virginica
Dr. Chowdhury
- In dysentery where the patient passes huge quantities of blood with the stools which are usually accompanied by crampy pain around the umbilicus. The blood discharge either maybe bright red or of tarry consistency. it is an excellent remedy in malaena when the above symptoms are present.
- It is frequently used in orchitis following Gonorrhoea. The indications are soreness and severe neurology are pain in testicles shifting to bowels and causing nausea and fainting. The enlargement of the spermatic veins, the result of violent exercise, horseback riding etc also comes under the influence of this remedy when associated with feeling of soreness.

Helleborus Niger
In brain diseases the patient beats the head or knocks the head against the floor.

Dr. Kent
- In all the complaints of this remedy stupefaction occurs in great or lesser degree. Sometimes it is complete stupor sometimes it is partial stupor but it is stupefaction and sluggishness. Its complaints are always passive and lingering.
- The patient lies on the back with the limbs drawn up.

- Sometimes the lips move without any sound the lips move as if the child wishes to say something but on further questioning the words he wish to speak are lost or forgotten.

- He is so stupor and so benumbed, he does not seem to be sensitive to heat or cold or pricking or handing or pinching.

- Sometimes there is no apparent change until that day after the medicine is administered or even the next night when there comes a sweat, diarrhoea and vomiting. These are the reactions of the medicine hence do not repeat or change the medicine.

- Sometimes after the administration of Helleborus or Zincum there is itching, tingling and formication that causes the appearance of extreme agony. This is a good sign of getting back of sensation to the paralytic or benumbed parts. In this case do not repeat or change the remedy only let it alone. They will go away.

- Wrinkled forehead, bathed in cold sweat. Paleness of the face and heat of the head. (Wrinkle of the forehead is present in Lycopodium due to lung affection but in Helleborus due to brain affection).

- There is violent thirst in these fever and unusual canine hunger.

Dr. Chowdhury

- In chewing motion of the mouth it can be compared with the following medicines:

- **Belladonna:** the symptoms are more violent indicating a higher degree of inflammation.

- **Bryonia:** certain amount of depression. Great want of secretion of the mucus surface of the body.

- **Nat. Mur:** it is only when he is covered up during chill.

- **Calc. Carb:** chewing motion is noticed during sleep and prodromal state of epilepsy.

Helonius Dioica

Dr. Chowdhury

- Consciousness of the womb: in the normal conditions due to the autonomous action of the vitality and perfect coordination of the different parts of the complex machinery. We are never conscious of the different organs of the system. When such conscious downs it means a deviated vitality and a disorder condition. The ligaments become lose and flaccid due to general exhaustion of the system, as a result of which we have uterine displacement. The uterus moves when she moves when she stands the organ dangles about. The result is a sore and tender feeling. This is reflected in the sacrum as a dragging and undefined feeling of weakness.

- Menorrhagia due to ulcerated of cervix is a common occurrence. It last long of every period and strains her already exhausted vitality to its every bottom. She loses more blood than is made in the inter menstrual period. To add to her discomfort there is the intense Pruritis of the vulva and vagina, the labia and the pudendum are hot red and swollen. They itch and burn terribly.

- Danforth: A case that Pruritis was so intense that she could tear the flesh out. The cause of this was thin albuminous leucorrhoea from a congested cervix coagulating on the surrounding parts giving rise to further irritation.

- When the affection of the kidney is secondary to uterine troubles with think of Helonius. Thus, when in albuminuria, the result of amenorrhoea, we notice weariness, languor, emaciation, debility, loss of appetite, chlorosis, constant aching and extreme tenderness in the region of kidney, especially the profuse, Char, light coloured urine. Helonius will do yloman's service.

- Sensation as though the chest was gripped in a vice. Dr Farrington reports of a case of blood spitting accompanying prolapsus uterus and a long lasting lochial discharge that is cured with Helonius.

Hepar Sulph

Chilly patient

Dr. Kent

- Extreme irritability every little thing that disturbs the patient makes him intensely angry abusive and impulsive. The impulsiveness will overwhelm him and make him wish to kill his best friends in an instant. A barber has an impulse to cut the throat of his patron while in the chair. Mothers may have an impulse to throw the child into the fire or impulse to set herself on fire and impulse to do violent and to destroy. The patient is quarrelsome, hard to get along with, nothing pleases, everybody disturbs, over sensitive to persons, to people and to place. He desires a constant change of persons and things and surroundings and each new surroundings and persons or things again displease and irritate.

- The bones even suppurate and take on necrosis and caries.

- The lymphatic glands are generally hard and enlarged. They are chronically enlarged without separation and at any cold that comes on, some particular gland may suppurate.

- The cold winds bring on sneezing and running from the nose.

- The discharge from all parts of the body have a decomposed cheesy smell. It has too sour smell discharge. Sometimes it may be noticed by the members of the family that one of the family always smells sour was a sour perspiration.

- Every cold settles on the throat causes hoarseness and loss of voice.

- He coughs and sweats. Sweats all night without relief, belongs to a great many complaints of Hepar.

- Catarrh of the bladder with purulent discharges in the urine and copious mucopurulent deposits. Ulcer of the bladder. The walls of the bladder become hardened so that it has no power to expel its contents and the urine passes in a slow stream or in drops or in the mail the Drop falls down perpendicularly. There is burning in the bladder and frequent almost constant urging to urinate. Chilly patient with gleety discharge.

- In the more acute affections of Mercury there is an aggravation from warmth of the bed But the old subjects who have been years ago poisoned with it get almost bloodless and they become chilly.

- Silicea follows well after Hepar and Hepar follows well after Mercury and thus Hepar becomes an intercurrent in this series.

- In old cases when the syphilitic miasm attacks the bones of the nose and they sink in or great ulceration takes place, those cases you sometimes see walking around the street with a big patch over the nose or over the opening that leads down into the nasal cavity. When there is severe pain in the region of the nasal bones the bridge of the nose is so sensitive that it cannot be touch and in the route of the neck there is a sensation as if splinter were sticking in.

- Ulceration of the soft palate with offensive mouth (Acid nit, Merc sol, Merc cor).

- It's a valuable purpose in its ability to establish separation around the foreign bodies and helps to make it come out (Silicea).

- Don't give Hepar, Silicea or Sulphur too often or too high in patients that have encysted tubercle in the lungs.

Dr. Chowdhury

- In hypersensitive to touch it can be compared with the following medicine.

- China off: patient with organising pain holding of his hands in apparel to anyone approaching him.

- Ruta: Starts from sleep with a scream when touched over so lightly so also is kali carb.

- Spigelia: afraid of pointed things while in Asafoetida and Sanguinaria we have pain that vanishes on touch to appear elsewhere.

- Dr Hughes experience with it "grocers itch" and Psoriasis pulmaris is worth noticing.

- In croup, the patient sits up and bends the head backwards to get relief.

- Desires for acid, wines, sour and strong-tasting things. A short of heaviness and pressure in the stomach after eating do after eating the patient says strong and comfortable. Constant sensation is felt as of water rising in the oesophagus, as though the patient had eaten something sour. A few hours after meal he feels a sort of distension on the region of the stomach and he has to loosen his clothing. The stools are soft but passed with great difficulty (Alum, Anacardium, Plat, Silicea).

- Paralytic condition of the bladder. The urine is passed so tardily that it seems that there is scarcely any expulsive power in the bladder. The patient is unable to finish it seems to him as if some urine always remains in the bladder (Alum, Silicea, Sepia), also with the above symptoms there is occasionally wetting of the bed at night.

- Fever: the time of its paroxysm is 6 or 7:00 p.m. (6:00 p.m. paroxysm is more marked under Ferrum and Veratrum) fever with great chilliness his teeth charters and he seeks to go near the warm stove. There is appearance of short of nettle rash during the chill.

Dr. Tyler

- Weeps with or before the cough.

- A case of gastric ulcer with haematemesis which cured with Hepar. The indications were craving for vinegar and pickles.

- Urging to stool but the large intestine are wanting in peristaltic action and cannot expel the faeces which are not hard. Only a portion of which can be forced out by help of abdominal muscles.

- The pains are aggravated at night.

Hippomanes
Dr. Chowdhury
- Sensation of coldness in the stomach.
- Sensation of sprain in the wrist. The arms feel as if paralyzed.
- A great pain in the wrist accompanied with great weakness of hands and fingers was frequently led to its application in chorea in young people growing too fast with remarkable results.

Homarus
Dr. Chowdhury
- It is particularly useful in patients who are awkward at night time when urgent desire to pass stools which however is ameliorated by passing a large amount of wind.
- A peculiar languid feeling in the morning (Nux Vomica). This tired feeling however passes off shortly after he starts on his usual daily avocations.

Hydrastis Canadensis
Dr. Kent
- It is a deep acting remedy where there is emaciation and ulceration, even malignant ulceration. Defective assimilation when it is noticed that stomach is the centre of the most symptoms. Complex great weakness prevails at all time.
- Catarrhal symptoms with thick, viscid, ropy, yellow mucus, sometimes white from any mucus membrane with or without ulceration.
- This medicine is very useful in the treatment of malignant ulcer. in such ulcer it is often create comfort to the patient even when it

does not cure as it remove the offensiveness, modifies the pain and restrains the destructiveness. The burning so commonly found in such ulcers is strong symptoms of Hydrastis.

- When the weakness and emaciation have progressed together for months and years in chronic stomach diseases. In chronic cases when the tissues have suffered but not cured.

- Small wound bleed and suppurate.

- Headache with stomach disorder and prolong nasal catarrh.

- The tongue is yellow, large, and flabby and strong feels as if burnt.

- No appetite no third loading of food nearly all food disorders the stomach, spitting of the food by mouthful (Phos, Ferrum, Aesculus). Vomits all food. Retains only water or milk. Eructations sour, putrid, of food eaten. Empty faint feeling in stomach with loathing of food and obstinate constipation with no desire for stool. Pulsation in the stomach.

- It has cured obstinate piles, ulceration and fissures of anus, painful piles bleeding or not.

- In prolonged constipation when enemas no longer get, when the faces remain high up or do not come down into rectum so excite desire this remedy has been great service. In constipation or diarrhoea with goneness in stomach, trembling in the abdomen and palpitation.

- The yellow viscid leucorrhoea, sometimes white, sometimes offensive, excoriation of vagina, soreness in vagina during coition, bleeding after coition.

- **By Ruddock and Dixon:** in all forms of stomatitis of children it is valuable. in simple ulceration of stomatitis matters we have found it useful in obstinate cases in which other remedies have failed. Use several times a day. In children abdominal colic with constipation child draws legs upwards, apply Hydrastis on the abdomen with a piece of wet cloth.

- Constipation
- All gone sensation.
- Stringy discharge.
- Tiredness in the morning with much yawning and straining.
- Has a dull lumbar pain such that he is inclined to use his arms in raising from his seat.

Hydrocyanic Acid

Dr. Chowdhury

- It acts powerfully on the medulla oblongata of the upper portion of the spinal cord and causes extreme dyspnoea, giddiness, dilated pupil and tetanic and epileptiform spasm.
- Suddenness of the attack and great frustration are two important features of this remedy.
- Whenever there is sudden loss of consciousness, sudden rigidity of limbs, sudden attack of convulsions and sudden stoppage of heart's action, Hydrocyanic acid is thought of before any other course is restored to.
- In epilepsy when the seizures come every three months, also and last for two or three weeks leaving the patient extremely prostrated. It is useful in those attacks where the attack last for several days at a stretch, the patient vomiting green fluid and passing green motion all the time.
- In traumatic tetanus it is reported to have done and immense amount of good especially when the paroxysms come on without any provocation and leave the patient in an extremely prostrated and exhausted condition. The patient is afraid to fall asleep or even close his eyes for fear of attacks coming on. The appearance becomes cyanotic and cold.
- Like Picric acid it is a great remedy for neurasthenia and nervous dyspepsia due to overwork and anxiety. The most important symptoms here is a great sinking sensation at the epigastrium. It

is described more as an angina felt at the pit of the stomach. Two or three hours after eating the patient complaints of burning pain in the region of navel extending to oesophagus and throat.

- Vomiting of food and a slimy bilious matter, emaciation intense Gastro-dynia and entrodynia, and above all the peculiar noise while drinking.

- It is a great help to us in the collapse stage of Asiatic cholera especially when the collapse follows the sudden cessation of all discharges. The stool ceases and vomiting decreases but the patient instead of reviving becomes remarkable cold, pulse less, cyanotic and fall of anguish. It is also thought of in threatening paralysis of lungs. The respiration being laboured coexisting with a feeling of suffocation.

- When he drinks the water rolls down audibly through the throat as though it were being poured into through an empty barrel.

Hyoscyamus Niger

Dr. Kent

- Hyoscyamus is full of convulsion, contractions, trembling, quivering and jerking of the muscles. Convulsions in women of the menstrual period. In low forms of disease it takes on the later, jerking and twitching of muscles. In low typhoid States sliding down in bed and twitching of the muscles.

- Convulsive jerks of the limbs so that all sorts of angular motions are made.

- Infants go into convulsions. Falls suddenly to the ground with cries and convulsion. Convulsion of children especially from fright. Convulsion after eating. The child becomes sick after eating. Vomits and goes into convulsion. Mother goes into convulsion soon after the child is born. Convulsion during sleep, suffocating spells of convulsion during labour. Toes become spasmodically cramped.

- Sometimes he talks to dead folks, recalls past events with those that have departed. Calls of dead sisters or wife or husband and enters into conversation just as if the person were present.

- In early state of typhoid he can be roused and he can answer questions correctly and he seems to know what you have said to him but the instant he finishes the last answers he appears to be fallen asleep. Then you shake him and ask anything he doesn't know.

- Fear of water, fear of running water (Bell, Cantharis, Stramonium).

- Stramonium has fear of water and fear of anything that might look like water such as shining objects fire and looking glass.

- Hydrophobinum has cured involuntary urination and involuntary stool on hearing running water.

- Imagine that somebody has asked a question and he answers it he will see a patient with Typhoid fever answering questions that we have not ask he imagines that persons are in the room and asking him questions. We hear nothing but his answer.

- The patient has very sensitive nerves all over the bones in the skin that he cannot bear the clothing to touch the skin and he takes it off.

- He is violent and beats people, strikes and bites, sings constantly and talks hastily.

- Patients who have come out of continued convulsions or insanity, have paralytic condition of the eyes, of the muscles of the eyes, "Strabismus" is one of the most frequently indicated remedies. The strabismus that comes on from brain diseases should be cured with this remedy.

- In fever there is much brain trouble and there is left behind a tendency to muscular weakness of the eyes, disturbances of the eyes, and congestion of the retina, and disturbance of the vision, double sight, night blindness and jerking of the lids.

- The mouth is very dry "as dry as burnt leather". The tongue tastes like soli leather because of dryness. Dryness of the mouth, nose, throat and whenever there is mucus membrane, dry, cracked, red, will bleed in low forms of fever. Twitching of the muscles of the face on attempting to put out the tongue. Catches that tongue on teeth while protruding, trembles (Lachesis). The whole mouth is dry and offensive, sometimes during fever the jaw becomes fixed as if it were lowered. Closes the teeth tightly together. Unquenchable thirst with aversion to water because there is mental fear of water.

- Like mouth there is dryness in the stomach. Burning and smarting in the stomach and when there is no inflammation, there is vomiting of blood. Stitching and quality pain with distension of abdomen wonderfully distended almost to bursting. Great petechiae upon the abdomen such as found in typhoid.

- Diarrhoea during pregnancy, typhoid passes of involuntary urine and stool. Paralysis of the bladder after labour so that the urine remains in the bladder with no desire to urinate. The routine remedy for retention of urine after labour is Causticum.

- Labour like pains from taking cold. Every cold settles on the uterus and bringing on painful menstruation. It has various cramping cramps in fingers and toes, and of muscles your and there, temporary paralysis etc.

- Hysterical Aphonia Hyoscyamus and Veratrum are two medicines that cure and make nervous hysterical women a great deal more sensible.

- Cough from cold air and from eating and drinking. cough after meals, violent spasmodic cough, sometimes spinal irritation. Spinal cough in those that have curvature of spine. A cough will sometimes last until the patient is covered with sweat and is exhausted and leans forward to get relief.

- Frequent twitching of the muscles of the feet and hands.

- Many complaints come on during sleep. The sleep is great tribulation to this nervous patient. There is sleeplessness or profound sleep.

- Jerks in sleep and cries out. Grates the teeth during sleep.

Dr. Chowdhury

- It has Loquacity and its loquacity is due to excessive animation (joy). It jumps from subject to subject. It can be compared with the following medicine:

- **Agaricus:** the patient goes on talking unmindful of all interruptions. He will hardly answer any question asked while he is in his talkative fit.

- **Lachesis:** talkativeness is most marked in the evening.

- **Lachnanthes:** talkativeness most marked between usual hours of 1 to 2:00 a.m.

- **Podophyllum and Zincum met:** most marked during the stage of chill.

- **Selenium:** talkativeness in the stage of perspiration.

- **Sordes:** appearing on the tongue and teeth. Associated with this we have rattling during breathing. The mouth remains open the lower jaw hangs down and the patient lies in a state of stupor.

- The muscles all over the body twitch intermittently this is a clear picture of typhoid state wants to escape from the room sometimes he would lie on his back his eyes quite open staring and immovable. The urine is involuntary at leaves streaks of red sand in the sheet. He constantly spits on his bed clothes.

- Convulsions begin with twitching of the mouth and face and especially of the muscles about eyes.

- In epilepsy the patient complaints of vertigo, sparks before the eyes and ringing noise in the ears.

Dr. Tyler

- Hahnemann indeed senses a twofold alternating action, much urging with rare evacuation and more frequent evacuation with rare urging, but the frequent urging with the scanty and rare evacuations is the principal alternating action.

- Involuntary stool from excitement.

- Erotomania: great mental excitement upon sexual subjects.

- Nymphomania: intense physical desire for sexual intercourse.

- Hyoscyamus is must for Erotomania and Cantharis for nymphomania.

- In Hyoscyamus auditory hallucination is marked factor as in Stramonium visual hallucination is marked(1.J.H.M 1971-46) pain in tooth which is loose.

- Hiccough after abdominal operation (Hyoscyamus), hiccough after emotion (Ignatia).

Hypericum Perforatum

According to Clarke, it is a good medicine for bleeding piles (both externally and internally).

Dr. Kent

- After surgical operation where there has been much cutting a great state of frustration coldness using of blood almost acid breath give Strontium carb instead of Carbo veg.

- When vomiting occurs in the surgical case due to application of chloroform, Phos is the remedy. Phosphorus is antidote to chloroform.

- For strains of muscles Arnica proves sufficient but is found suitable for the case for the fine weakness that persists even after Rhus tox, we have calcarea carb.

- Both Hypericum and Ledum pal are indicated after the penetration of splinters, nails etc but Ledum is suited when pain is localised where as Hypericum is indicated in neurologic pain radiating in different direction.

- The wound will sometimes yawn, swell up, no tendency to heal, look dry and shiny on the edges, red inflammed, burning, stinging and tearing pains, no healing process.

- A painful cicatrices with pain shooting up to the centre of the body following up the nerves.

- Arnica should never be used for wounds, because if it is used in full strength it may bring on erysipelas.

- Bruises of bones, cartilages, tendons, insertion of tendons, bruises about cartilages and joints, Ruta is better than any other remedy.

- Ledum acts as preventive for tetanus whether pain is localized after the penetration of splinter, nails, punctured wounds, right bites, cat bites, dog bites etc.

- A sensitive women steps on a rock during the day. When she feels all the day where the rock went in, lies down in bed and it aches so violently, she cannot keep it still. Ledum will prevent any other trouble but if that goes on until the morning the pains will be shooting up the legs call Hypericum.

- Bad effects of injury to the coccyx and spinal cord. Injury of the coccyx during labour and remains for a long time.

- When a person falls on his back and if the spine is injured, Hypericum is the remedy here.

- Old weakness of the back with painfulness on rising from a seat are often cured by Rhus tox followed by calcarea carb, but in Hypericum meningeal troubles are common from injuries of that class with drawing of muscles of back, a feeling of contraction or tightening, stitching, shooting pains in back in various directions. They should down the limbs. Injuries of the back are not so likely to end in tetanus as the injury of the sensory nerves but they are sometimes more troublesome because they linger so long.

- If you have a clear cut or incised wound made with a sharp instrument or if you have made such an opening with your knife while practicing surgery if you have open the abdominal cavity of the walls of abdomen take on unhealthy look and there are stitching burning pains, Staphysagria is the remedy. It acts wonderfully stretching sphincter or urethra. When the urethra of women stretched for stone in bladder.

- Where coldness, congestion of the head and rending tearing pains occurs for stretching sphincters or from tearing parts for the purpose of operation and Staphysagria is the remedy there.

Alphabet

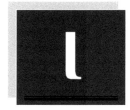

Iberis Amara

IJH April-June 1982

- Cardiac debility after influenza.
- Conscious of Hearts action.
- Palpitation with Vertigo.
- Pulse full, irregular, intermittent.
- Dropsy with enlarged heart.
- Numbness and tingling in left hand and arm.
- Whole body sore, lame and trembling, aggravated lying down, on left side, motion, exertion, warm and room.

Ignatia

Baby (Borland)

- Nervous, bright, precocious, headachy patient usually in the evening.
- Shaky writings.
- Strained expressions, Noise <, Hysterical stomach, sighing after crying.
- Worry of family matters (constant dispute between mother-in-law and daughter-in-law). Mental distress and anxiety in family matters will often produce disasters results in the organs affected. Repeat dosage of Ignatia and give greatest comfort to the patient

(Clarke). If imperturbable (calm) and not easily frightened do not use Ignatia (Dr.T.K.Morre).

- In appendicitis the patient keeps his legs moving (Ignatia), when the patient keeps his legs up gets ameliorated (R.T).

- A woman has undergone a controversy at home. She has been disturbed, is excited and goes into cramps, trembles, and quivers. Goes to bed with headache. A woman who lost her child, or husband or dear one or near ones, suffers from grief. She has headache, trembles, is excited, weeps, is sleepless, unable to control herself. In spite of her best endeavours, her grief has simply torn her into pieces.

- Useful in constitutions that have been over wrongly at school in Science art and music. Fainting in crowd.

- Children are convulsed in sleep after punishment, in the first period of dentition from fright. The child is cold and pale and has a fixed staring look like Cina. Convulsion with loss of consciousness.

- Ignatia is full of surprise and unnatural as for example, if you see an inflamed joint or inflamed part where there is heat, redness, throbbing and weakness, you will handle it with great care for fear it will be painful but you find it is not painful and sometimes ameliorated by hard pressure. Feels better lying on painful side.

- It has hysterical stomach. Cannot digest simplest food but can digest the hard and unnatural food. The patient takes raw cabbage and raw onion and feels better since that time. Cold food is craved and cold food will be digested when warm food will be disturbing and increase indigestion.

- Spasmodic condition of the larynx comes on without any provocation. Any little disturbance, a fright or distress, or a grievance, will bring a young sensitive women home and to her bed and she will go on with a spasm of the larynx.

- Ask questions not waiting for the answer. Thinks she has neglected some duty (Hell, Hyo, Aurum).

- Headache from abuse of coffee, from smoking, from inhaling smoke, from tobacco or alcohol, from close attention, from cold winds, turning the head suddenly, when pressing at stool, from jar, from hurrying from excitement, looking up, moving the eyes, from noise, from light. Ameliorated by warmth, rest, lying on painful side, better while eating but soon after it is worse.

Dr. Chowdhury

- It is suited to persons quick in perceiving (power of understanding) prompt in appreciation (expression of merit) and Rapid in execution (performance).

- Recent effects of grief (Ignatia) chronic (Ac. Ps, NM).

- It's pain is erratic in nature. Sometimes it comes gradually and abates suddenly at other times it comes on suddenly and goes away in similar way.

- Its headache is sometimes ameliorated by flow of profuse colourless urine. (Aconite, Gya, Kalmia, Sang, Silicea, Veratrum Alb)

- Dyspepsia of hysterical women with flat taste in the mouth, copious salivation, aversion to tobacco, warm food, spiritual liquor and frequent regurgitation of food.

- Sometimes the patient feels and urgent desire for stool which however is caused by mostly and accumulation of flatus and is followed by simple mere expulsion of wind with a certain amount of protrusion of the rectum.

- Constipation: desire for stool is felt more in the upper intestines. After severe straining, he passes either a hard or soft stool with certain amount of procidentia relief. Most of the straining is due to construction of anus. The prolapse becomes worse when the stools are soft.

- Toothache ameliorated while eating.

- Dr. Kent: great grief after losing of persons or objects very near, trembling of the hands disturbs her very much in writing.

Dr. Tyler

- Ignatia is the acute of Sepia and Natrum mur.
- Heat in the head. Head is heavy.
- He hangs the head forward. Lays the head forward on the table.
- Headache increased by stooping forward.
- He is apt to bite on one side of tongue possibly when speaking or chewing.
- If the right pupil is flat 12 o'clock instead of round it is due to suppressed grief (Ignatia). If the left one is Flat it is due to suppressed anger (Staphysagria).

Indigo

Dr. Chowdhury

- Epilepsy specially when associated with worms. Peculiarity of this epilepsy is that they become vehement and furious before the attack is over. These attacks apparently organised in the solar plexus and give rise to a sensation of heat over the whole head. Another sensation particularly complaint of this time is an undulating wave like sensation in the brain.
- It affects the muscles in the way similar to Rhus Tox. We find aggravation from rest and also commencement of every movement. Decided amelioration from movement and pressure is noticed. It can be differentiated from Rhus tox by the indication example aggravation after meals.
- Indigo has a characteristic cough in as much as it is almost always associated with epistaxis. It is mostly of the form of open cough where the great violence and the long duration of the attack bring about hemorrhage from the nose.

Indium Metallicum

- Severe lightning pain in the head each time he strains at his stool.

- It is somewhat like Selenium and its action over the male sexual organ where it causes a diminution in sexual desire and power. It is also used in nocturnal emission when such emission become very frequent and debilitating and as such should be compared with Acid phos. The urine smells highly offensive after it is allowed to stand for a little while.

Idoformum

Dr. Chowdhury

- It is an important remedy in the treatment of tubercular meningitis and other tubercular conditions.

- The symptoms are sharp neuralgic pains in the head, a sensation of heaviness in the head as if it would not be lifted from pillow, sleep interrupted by sighs and cries, drowsiness, distension of abdomen, swelling of the mesenteric glands, chronic diarrhoea with greenish watery and digested stools and weakness of the knees and legs.

Iodium

Dr. Chowdhury

- In pneumonia the lower lobe of the right lung is affected and the disease takes on indolent form violent chilly followed by great pressure on the chest, interruption and impediment of respiration, expectoration of tenacious yellow matter and stained with blood, and a sensation of weakness in the chest.

Dr. Kent

- This medicine is full of anxiety. The anxiety comes on when trying to keep still and the more he tries to keep still, the more the anxious state increases. While attempting to keep still he is overwhelmed with impulses, impulses to tear things, to kill himself, to commit murder, to do violence. He cannot keep still and he works night and day. This medicine carries the same feature with it into the K I., so that it makes the K I patient to walk. But there is this difference the K I patient can walk a long distance without fatigue and the walking only seems to wear off his anxiety, where in iodine there is great exhaustion, he becomes extremely exhausted from walking and sweat copiously even from slight exertion.

- Hypertrophy of all the glands except mammary which is dwindled in nature. Another peculiar thing is that when the body withers, the gland enlarges, the mesenteric glands can be felt as knots.

- Impulses to kill himself and others (Ars, H.S).

- The NV patient has an impulse to throw her child into fire. It has white diarrhoea. Bitter taste of solid food but not drinks. The patients are anxious and restless. It is a hot edition of arsenic where we see the patient with all iodum symptoms but when hungry give iodum 3x and 6x. If the patient is thin give iodum 30 (IHH-72-62). pain in the joints with no local redness.

- The patient is weak in mind as well as in body he is forgetful cannot remember the little things the pass out of mind he forgets what he was about to say or do goes of and leaves packages as he has purchased. But with all these states do not forget one thing that the patient is compared to keep doing something in order to drive away his impulses and anxiety the anxiety is wearing and distressing unless he keeps busy.

- Acute and chronic brain troubles. The head throbs, the brain throbs, there are pulsations all over. The throbbing extends to the finger ends and the toes, throbbing in the pit of the stomach, heavy pulses felt in the arms, pulsation in the back, throbbing in temporal region, there are congestive headaches with violent pain the head, pains are aggravated by motion but the patient is ameliorated by motion.

- Corneal ulcers there is oedematous swelling of the lids and oedematous swelling of the face under the eyes.

- Catarrhal condition of the nose. The sense of smell is lost. The mucus membrane is thickened. Takes cold upon slightest provocation, is always sneezing and has a copious discharge from the nose. He blocks blood from the nose. The nose is stuffed up. Every cold settles on the nose and causing stuffiness.

- There are apthous patches along the tongue and throughout the mouth. The pharynx seems to be lined with the velvety ash colored appearance. It is useful in enlarged tonsils when the tonsils are studded with exudation. Enlarged tonsils in hungry withered patient.

- Useful in chronic morning diarrhoea of emaciated scrofulous children.

- In old gouty constitutions with enlargement of the joint the history is that the patient was once in good state of flesh but they have become lean and although they are hungry the food does not seen to do them good.

Dr. Chowdhury

- Clark used iodum with remarkable success in the opposite condition of annual exam in young women who owing to nervous shock had lost all appetite and had made up her mind to start herself to death. Five drops of iodum 3 X in a wine glass of water half an hour before meal times produce such nervous appetite that she had to give up the idea of suicide from starvation.

- He trembles and is unable to move, even the exhaustion of talking brings on profuse sweating and nervous excitability. He is not fit for any violent exercise. This weakness is particularly felt when the patient makes and attempt to go upstairs. He loses his breath and has to rest several times before he gets to his destination.

- He cannot bear any hat on his head as it tends to increase his warmth.

- All its diseases are slow onset.

- The skin is rough dry and dirty with a mark tendency to papules, boils and abscess.

- Cardiac hypertrophy with great precordial anxiety necessitating constant change of position. Sensation as if the heart was squeezed together and grasped by and iron hand. Severe palpitation of the heart aggravated by least exertion. A feeling of vibration over the heart like that caused by purring of a cat is also noticeable. In this respect it may be compared with Spigelia.

- When young men and women grow fast and due to falling of off appetite, emaciates, it is time that we should be careful. A slight tickling cough, gradual but steady enlargement of glands and at least little spitting of blood showing bronchial and pulmonary congestion unless taken in hand at once may develop into TB of lungs. Iodine will form and admirable remedy and check the onward progress of the fatal malady if it is prescribed on such well marked symptoms as emaciation, weakness, profuse night sweats, tickling cough, expectoration of transparent mucus streaked with blood, diarrhoea and even strong hemorrhage from the lungs.

Ipecacuanha

Cold in the chest after suppressed eruption.

Complaints from suppressed ear discharges.

Dr. Kent

- The cutting pain in colic goes from left to right. The patient is unable to study or breathe until that pain passes off. It holds him transfixed in one position, coming like a stabbing of knife in the region of the stomach or about the navel, going from left to right and is offended with prostration and nausea.

- In cough he coughs until his face grows red and there is choking and gagging.

- Though there is sometimes thirst, it is usually absent. When it does its best work there is thirstlessness.

- In fever there is likely to be pain in the back of the head, a bruised pain through the head and back of the neck and sometimes down the back and drawing in the muscles of the back of the neck.

- Ipecac is sometimes of restless as arsenic but the Ipecac prostration comes by spells whereas the arsenic prostration is continuous. The ipecac patient tossing over the bed as much as they do when they need, patient turns and tossing and moving his hands and feet with restlessness when the spine is somewhat developed. It has opisthotonous and it has been a useful remedy in cerebrospinal meningitis with vomiting of bile with pain in the back of the head and neck and drawing of the muscles of the back refracting the head.

- It is useful remedy in epidemic dysentery, when the patient is compelled to sit almost constantly upon the stool and passes a little slime or a little bright red blood, inflammation of the lower portion of the bowel, the rectum and colon. The tenesmus is awful, burning continues urging with the passage of only a little mucus and blood with this there is constant nausea while straining of stool the pain is so great that nausea comes on and he vomits bile.

- In infants it is indicated when cholera like diarrhoea has been present and it ends in dysenteric state with continued tenesmus and the expulsion of little bloody mucus. The child vomiting everything it takes into stomach, nausea, vomiting, prostration and great pallor.

- The chest complaints of Ipecac are interesting. It is especially the infant's friend and is commonly indicated in the bronchitis of infants. It is very seldom that an infant gets a true pneumonia. It is generally bronchitis with coarse rattling, the child coughs gags and suffocates and there is course rattling which can be heard throughout the room and the trouble has come on pretty rapidly. The child is pale, looks dreadfully ill, and sometimes looks very anxious. The nose is drawn in dangerously sick.

- In whooping cough there is red face, thirstlessness, violent whooping with convulsion, with gagging and vomiting of all that he eats are the symptoms of it.

- When the uterus is continuously using but a little while the flow increases to a gush and with every little gush of bright red blood, the woman thinks she is going to faint or there is gasping and the gravity of flow is not sufficient too short for such prostration, nausea, syncope, pallor, Ipecac is the remedy.

- Severe pain in the back of the region of the kidney shooting pains frequent urge to urinate and the urine contains blood and little lots of blood with nausea and vomiting.

- The Ipecac colds often begin in the nose and spread very rapidly into the chest. With these colds of nose, there is copious bleeding of bright red blood. Every cold settles on the nose and causes copious bleeding.

- There are old in curable cases of asthma that are palliated by Ipecac. It is useful in cases of humid asthma in case of arithmetic Bronchitis when they suffer from damn weather and from sudden weather changes. Every little cold rouses up his bronchial attack and he suffocates and gags when he coughs or spits of a little blood.

- In suppressed eruptions when the eruption does not come on or an eruption has given back by cold, sometimes oozes much. Cessation of stomach and bowels follows and cold settles in the chest from suppressed eruptions. It also cures erysipelas when there is vomiting. The chill, the pain in the back, the thirstlessness and the overwhelming nausea.

Dr. Chowdhury

- General sore feeling all through the body and the bones feel as if they were broken into pieces.

- The Grand keynote of this hemorrhage consists in a steady flow of bright red foamy blood associated with nausea.

- He is full of Desire but he does not know what he wants.

- In gastric symptoms at first he brings up quantities of ingest to be followed by huge masses of bile and then mucus of grass green colour. The presence of blood like bright red pitch like colour is not infrequent.

Dr. Tyler

- Ipecac 200 is a mighty prescription.

- Chess trouble with agonies of dyspnoea and suffocation. There may be little or no nausea or again there maybe nausea with violent efforts to vomit and cough at the same time producing indescribable terrors of suffocations.

- Hale White tells us that the drug affects not only the stomach but the vomiting centre in the medulla which may account for the clean tongue.

- Gureacy says threatened abortion often with sharp pinching pain about umbilicus which runs down to uterus with constant nausea and discharge of bright red blood where there is steady flow of bright red blood give Ipecac.

- Asthma that has to stand for hours by the open windows.

- Aversion to all food no appetite, earthy taste, stomach feels relaxed, nausea.

- In uterine hemorrhage the following symptoms are very good indication. The flow was of bright red the lower limbs are built in cold perspiration, hands cold and damp, abdomen felt hot yet damp with perspiration.

- In bronchial asthma its action is one of the ramificating vagus or pneumogastric nerve. It produces spasmodic irritation in chest and stomach and is frequently indicated in asthma with violent degree of dyspnoea with wheezing and great precordial weight and anxiety.

- Dyspnoea with constant constriction of chest and from least motion. Has to sit up at night to breathe, gasps for air at the open window. Cough is suffocative. Stiffens out, turns red or blue gags or vomits. There is much coughing. We can hear the rattling of mucus in the chest yet none is expectorated. His condition is aggravated in warm moist weather ameliorated in open air. Wants fresh air with this anxious breathing his hands and feet drip cold sweat.

- Aconite and Ipecac may be given 3 X potency alternatively every 10 minutes till relief is obtained.

Iris Versicolor

- This is one of the sour remedies. Hyper acidity is the most marked feature of Iris, it is noticed everywhere that it becomes an important remedy in this dyspepsia, gastric ulcerations, gastric catarrh, duodenitis and diarrhoea when this symptom is present.

- Dr. Kidchen relieved a case of gastrodynia with Iris when this important symptom of vomiting of sour food after meals was present. This vomiting is the red strand of this remedy. There is first of all vomiting of indigested or sour fluid and cast of all yellow and green bile. The substance vomited out is thick and ropy mucus hanging from the mouth to the receptacle.

- Great burning, distress, violent pains are felt in the epigastrium. It was been used very effectively in colic which begins coming in successive shocks in the umbilical region. Nausea with straining and belching and wind, great commotion and rumbling in the vowels in the affected area much mental depression and great and wish of the mind of constant expulsion of enormous discharge of wind are symptoms indicating Iris.

- It is used with benefit in diarrhoea of cholera morbus when such trouble starts between two and three a.m. with violent vomiting of extremely sour bile and mucus and purging of profuse corrosive watery stool.

- It is a good medicine for right sided headache and this headache is due to gastric origin. It is aggravated by rest and least motion. The headache is associated with loss of spirit. Mucus and acid vomiting. It is periodical in nature. The pain is intense and throbbing as if assures in a blood state of vision or temporary blindness with vomiting at the height of attack.

- Paper Read by Surabhi Kapadia Bombay in all India Homeopathic convention in 1975.

- Drawing pain in head while coughing.

- Ropy saliva in mouth.

- Salivation while talking.

- Elongated uvula like on cone to a sharp point.

- Eosinophilia

- Expectoration at forenoon 10 a.m.

- Headache periodical in connection with rest period from our heart physical works. Sunday migraine. Many eye symptoms before or at the beginning of attack, abnormal polyuria followed the attack.

- Aggravated hot weather, spring and fall and rest.

- Ameliorated vomiting, sufficient night sleep.

Alphabet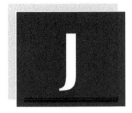

Jaborandi

Dr. Chowdhury
- Hypersecretion of all the glands of the human system. Hence, we have profuse sweating, starting on the forehead and face, and then spreading all over the body. Profuse salivation, free flow of tears from eyes and nose. Copious watery diarrhoea. All characteristics of Jaborandi. It is used with great benefit in uremia, and nephritis. Renal dropsy, otitis, pleurisy, bronchitis, coryza, glycosuria, and diabetes, when the above symptoms are present.

Jalapa

Dr. Chowdhury
- Infants who laugh and play all day, but scream and kick all night. All their troubles are < at night. It is usually a direct baby. The stool is watery, sour-smelling, and associated with colic.

- The author has cured a baby with Jalapa, with the following symptoms. Enterocolitis of a baby at > summers. The baby came to him from allopathic treatment after three months of prolonged diarrhoea. The baby was so emaciated and feeble that it was a pity object to look at. The patient was constantly undergoing contortion of the body (twitching) most probably due to a colic which it was a constant subject.

Jatropha Curcas

Dr. Chowdhury

- It is one of our chief remedies for choleric diarrhea and cholera and the characteristic symptoms are marked by a peculiar gurgling sound in the abdomen. The noise is very loud as if caused by the emptying of a full bottle inside the abdomen We may also link it to the sound caused by the sudden immersion of the empty vessel into water.

- There is a sudden expulsion of abundant alvine evacuation, sometimes containing a large number of lumbricid and Ascari. They came out like gushing torrent.

- Its third important point is vomiting. The vomiting matter is a thick albuminous glairy sort of fluid. The thirst is unquenchable. Anxiety and anguish indifference, prostration and cramps. ,make it a splendid remedy in the first stage of cholera. It needs repitation.

Juglans Regia

Dr. Chowdhury

- In Juglans Regia- The hemorrhage is from the uterus. Whereas in the Juglans Cineria. It is mostly from the lungs. In Juglans Regia, the skin symptoms are predominant, especially in scrofulous subjects we have eruptions on the sculpt behind the ear on the arms and axilla. The itching is so intense at night that he is hardly able to sleep. Many of the skin eruptions of this remedy closely resemble syphilis. The symptoms are generally aggravated by motion after fat food at night and from undressing.

Juglans Cinerea

Dr. Chowdhury

- It is a good medicine for hemorrhage in both. Gasoline scenario. And Gaglons Regia. The blood is fluid, dark, and peach-like in color.

- The headache of Jugulans Cineria is very common. The pain is sharp and shooting in character, and it is mostly an occipital headache, a headache associated with frequent micturition and it comes in the morning. Some as in Nux vom, Bryonia.

- Another feature of Jugulans is a sinking sensation felt in the epigastric region in this respect it compares well with sulphur, acid phos, Phos, with this sinking sensation is felt a sharp stitching pain in the region of the liver, extends to the right scapula as in Chelidonia and Bryonia. It is an important liver remedy like Nux vom We have also morning. < as in Nux vom, but in juglans, it is an occipital headache more than anything else, that disturbs the patient and frequently wakes him, especially at about 3 a.m., preventing him from falling asleep again, to be followed in the morning by bilious yellowish greenish jaundiced stool.

Alphabet

Kali Bichromicum

Dr. Kent

- Rheumatic affections of the joints with swelling, heat and redness wondering from join to joint.

- Ulceration is a striking feature of this remedy its ulcers are Deep and red (punched out).

- It has the sharp stitching pain like Kali Carb.

- Burning is a very marked symptom of this remedy.

- The patient is sensitive to cold; there is lack of vital heat. He wants to be wrapped up and covered warmly which ameliorates.

- His cough is aggravated in winter and emulated in warm weather but it's rheumatic troubles come in warm weather.

- All the Kalis are generally sensitive to dry cold weather.

- Many of symptoms aggravate at two or three a.m. like Kali carb.

- Generally its pains are aggravated from motion except sciatica and some of the pains in the lower limbs which are ameliorated from motion.

- It has violent headache and its headaches mostly associated with catarrhal conditions. A Kali bichrom patient always suffers more or less from catarrh of the nose and if he is exposed to cold weather the catarrhal condition will turn to dryness.

- Headache during coryza when the discharge of the coryza slacks a little. Headache often begins with dim vision headache come on with Vertigo.

- It has cured Eczema of the scalp with thick heavy crust from which oozes a yellow thick gluey substance.

- Daylight brings on photophobia.

- Yellow viscid discharge from the ears with stitching pains and pulsating in the ears. In suppuration of the middle ear with perforated tympanum eczematous eruptions on the ears itching of the whole external ear.

- Foetid odour from the nose troubled much with a sensation of dryness in the nose, loss of smell and the nose is obstructed at night with thick yellow mucus, too viscid to be blown out. Extreme soreness inside the nose.

- The bones of the face are often very sour which shooting pain in the mandible bones, pain in the molar bones on coughing. With the catarrhal condition, there is much suffering from the molar bones.

- The tongue is smooth, shiny, sometimes cracked in forms of fever like typhoid. The tongue is often thick and yellow at the base. Sensation of hair on the base of the tongue.

- The uvula becomes oedematous. (Apis, Kali.iod, Acid mur, Nit. acid, Phos, Symphytum, Tub).

- There is aversion to meat and strange to say he craves beer which makes him sick. Nausea and vomiting of drinkers.

- There is pain in the liver hard contracting pain extending to the shoulder resembling Crot.hor. Pain in the liver from motion. It is a good medicine in liver condition associated with gallstones. It corrects the action of liver so that healthy bile is formed and gall stones are dissolved.

- It has also morning diarrhoea like sulphur but with tenesmus.

- Diarrhoea and dysentery in hot weather alternate with cough and catarrhal troubles in winter.

- It has constipation with hard knotty stools followed by severe burning in the parts. Burning in anus after stool. Prolapsus of rectum. After dry hard stool there is burning in rectum. Patient suffers from a sensation of large plug in the rectum and there is great soreness in the anus. He suffers much from haemorrhoids which protrudes after stool.

- Pain from sternum to back associated with catarrhal condition and cough.

- There is cold sensation in the chest which is generally felt in the region of the heart.

- Pain in the Limbs are aggravated from cold and motion ameliorated from heat and rest but the pain in sacrum ameliorated from motion during the day and aggravated at night in bed.

Dr. Chowdhury

- Periodically attack of semi lateral headache ameliorated by pressure, open air and by eating.

- The tonsil looks large but there is hardly any inflammation and fever. There is a marked tendency to formation of ulcer in tonsil and rectum. The ulcers are seen with an ash colour slough and the patient hawks up large quantities of tenacious mucus.

- The stools are brown watery and frothy and the gush out in the morning like Sulphur, Natrum Sulph.

Dr. Tyler

- Urine is alkaline and ropy.

- Its yellowness: yellow vision (Cina), yellow sebrotics (Cheli), yellow discharges, yellow vomiting, yellow sputum, yellow discharges from ear, nose, eyes. When the tongue may be glazed, red cracked or coated with yellow. Clarke makes great point of its usefulness where large quantities of yellow watery fluid are vomited.

- Dyspepsia with Supra orbital headaches or with a peculiar headache. The patient is affected with blindness objects becoming obscured and less distinct and then headaches begin. Blindness disappears as the headache is on (Nat mur, Iris, Psorinum). With the headache Farrington says: the face is apt to get blocked and covered with pimples and acne.

- It is also shallow and yellow complexion as if the patient were bilious. The stomach seems to swell up after a full meal.

Kali Bromatum

Dr. Chowdhury

- The patient is very fretful, crying at trifles and constantly brooding. These fits of crying sometimes become uncontrollable.

- It is a splendid remedy for night terror of children. They wake up at night with some horrible dream and scream, mourn and cry. To sooth them into silence is a hard job.

- The night terrors in children due to over excitement of the brain. It is also useful in grown up men as well who have worked hard and work long and have practically exhausted themselves.

- It relieves giddiness and benumbed feeling in the brain due to merciless application over hard, difficult and intricate problem.

Dr. Tyler

- Night terrors of children not from indigestion.

- Unconsciousness of what is occurring around them. Cannot recognise or comforted by their friends. Sometimes followed by squinting.

- Frightful imagines in late pregnancy, have committed or are about to commit some great crime or cruelty such as murdering her child or husband.

Chandrashekhar Kali on his Cholera break

- It is one of the best medicines in infantile Cholera during dentition. It is most probably application in the state of reaction. Great stupid violent drowsiness and comatose sleep are the main indications of this remedy. Stupor is so violent it is difficult to rouse the child from sleep.

- Grinding of teeth, rattling breathing pale face, sunken and fixed eyes.

- Moving of the eye balls in different direction, crying suddenly to see the fearful dreams and try to wake up to open his eyes and again followed by comatose sleep. Involuntary stool and urine (In such a condition Veratrum Vir is a good medicine and it has power to remove the drowsiness and stupor) when Veratrum Vir fail he should think of Kali Brom use Kali Brom 6.

- It is also a good medicine in summer diarrhoea of children especially during the stage of reaction of the symptoms present as follows :

- Frequent rice watery stool.

- Pale face with sunken red eyes.

- Dilated pupils. Moving of the eyeballs. Convulsion spasm of the extremities.

- Dry mouth with unquenchable thirst. Apthous.

- Pain in the abdomen.

- Hardness of the abdomen due to cramping.

- Scanty urine.

- Every time there is a little urine during the evacuation of stool.

- Burning of the chest. The pulse is weak or disappearing. Blueness of the extremities. Feeling of chilliness in a warm room.

- Twitching and jerking. Great stupor. Cold body with hot head. Boring of the head.

Kali Carb

Chilli patient susceptible to cold.

Dr. Kent

- The patient is whimsical, irascible, irritable to the very high degree.

- Quarrels with his family and with his bread and butter. He never wants to be alone, is full of fear of imagination when alone, fear of the future, fear of death and fear of ghost. If compelled to remain alone in the house, he is wakeful, sleepless or his sleep is full of dreams.

- He is over sensitive to everything, sensitive to every atmospheric change. His nerves feel the cold; they are all painful when it is cold. The neuralgias shoot here and there. When it is cold and if the part affected be kept is warm the pain goes to some other place. All his pains change place and go into the cold parts if he covers one part the pain goes to the part uncovered.

- This remedy is full of sticking burning tearing pains and they fly around from place to place. Pains like hot needles sticking stinging and burning. Burning in the anus and rectum describe as if hot poker were first into that passage burning as with fire. The haemorrhoids burn like coals of fire. It's burning is like Arsenic.

- He wakes up at 3 o'clock in the morning with fear, fear of death fear of the future worries about everything is kept awake for 2 to 3 hours and then goes to sleep and sleeps soundly.

- His body is cold and requires much clothing to keep it warm but in spite of the fact that he is cold he sweats copiously. Copious cold sweat upon the body. Sweat upon the slightest exertion sweats were the pain is sweat over the forehead with headache. When puberty is late think of Nux mosch, Tuberculinum and Kali carb.

- When see the old and fatty person think of Kali carb.

- It has catarrhal congestive headache. Whenever he goes out in the cold air, the nose opens up and then mucus membrane become dry and burn when he returns into a warm room. The nose commences to discharge and the nose stuffs up. The headache is ameliorated in a warm room and aggravated in cold air. Neurologic pains in eyes and scalp and through the cheek bones from and associated of chronic catarrhal discharge. And when the discharge starts up again then pain ceases.

- With the chronic cutter of the nose there is a thin fluent yellow discharge. Dryness of the nose alternating with stuffing up. In the morning he blows out and hawks up dry heart crust that fill up the nasal passage, clear even into the pharynx and down into the throat. This Crush become dry as if they were partly formed upon the mucus membrane and when they are blown out there is bleeding. The bleeding starts from where the crusts are lifted up.

- He is subject to sore throat. Every cold settles on the throat..There is chronic tonsil and with these has enlargement and chronic hardness of the parotid glands one or both. Great nodes below the ear behind the jaw.

- He suffers mostly from dry hacking cough with morning expectoration and when coughing it seems as if the head would fly to pieces. In whooping cough there is dry hacking instant gagging cough with whooping, blowing of blood from the nose, vomiting of everything in the stomach and expectoration of blood streaked mucus. It is more suitable if that bag like swelling is present in the upper eyelid.

- The patient says I have never been quiet ever since I had pneumonia. Catarrhal stage has suffered in the chest and there is chronic tendency to take cold. These cases are throttling to go into the phthisis and be horribly be likely to recover. In such cases think of Phosphorus or Hyoscyamus.

- One of its general state is tendency to dropsies.

- Its complaints approach insidiously.

- He suffers from pain in the teeth whenever he takes cold from riding in the wind and raw weather.

- Many symptoms aggravate after eating and some symptoms ameliorate after eating. There is throbbing in the pit of stomach when the stomach is empty. After eating he feels as if stomach would burst. Great flatulence.

- Belches wind upwards and passes flatus downwards. Offensive flatus.

- Pain in the stomach after eating. Burning in the stomach after eating. Gone feeling not ameliorated by eating. The patient says Dr somehow or other I do not have a fear like other people do because I have it in my stomach. When she is frightened it always struck to her stomach. If a door Slams I feel it here (epigastric region).

- Over sensitive to slightest touch but hard pressure agreeable.

- Every time they go to the doctor's office they talk about the liver.

- It covers conditions due to psora or to the separation of eruption in childhood or to the closing up of old ulcers and fistulous opening with history of troubles ever since. It's wondering pains and chilliness are ameliorated by eruptions, by the outbreak of discharges, by haemorrhages or by ulcer flow freely.

- It is a good medicine and abdominal colic when Colocynth does not cure.

- It has most persistent and enormous haemorrhoidal tendency, that burn, that are extremely sensitive to touch, that bleed copiously, that are extremely painful making it impossible for him to sleep. He is compelled to lie upon the back and hold the legs apart because the pressure is very painful to external piles. The piles cannot be put back. There is great distension and swelling inside. Haemorrhoids that come but after stool and bleed copiously and are very painful. They must be pushed back and long after going to bed, the burn like fire and great aggravation from stool which is hard and knotty and requires great straining to expel. Fistula in anus. Burning temporarily relieved sitting in cold water.

- Diarrhoea painless with rumbling in the abdomen and burning at stool, only by day chronic diarrhoea with puffiness in eyes.

- Burning in urethra during and after micturition. Urine flows slowly with soreness and burning. Kali carb runs very close to NM in many of its old long standing bowel troubles.

- In long standing of grief and old cases of urinary troubles that follow gonorrhoea. These two remedies are useful both suitable in the white great discharge that remains. In both the urination is painful. In NM the burning is after urination but in KC the burning is during and after urination.

- All the symptoms are aggravated after coition. He has weak vision, weakness of the senses, tremulousness and is generally nervous. He is Sleepless and weak and he she was and trembles for a day or two after coition. Young man who have abuse themselves who have indulged in excessive sexual pleasure, incapacitated and then there comes a disgust as if it is not strange that there are so many divorces in the world.

- It is useful in cases of uterine hemorrhage that have been incessant and in pale, waxy hemorrhagic women. Incessant hemorrhage following an abortion. She has been curetted and has all sorts of treatment but still that oozing keeps right on. At the menstrual period the flow is very copious and clotted and then after prolonged menstruation of 10 days or so she settles back into a state of oozing and flowing until next month and then it trousers up into another 10 days of copious menstruation. Kali carb has cured a large number of fibroid tumours long before it was time for the critical period to cure.

- During labour the pain in the uterus is very weak and not sufficiently expulsive to make progress in labour pain in the back as if it would break and the woman says "my back, my back".

- Weakness of the heart cardiac dyspnoea the breath is short and the patient cannot walk or must move very slowly. Cannot lie on the left side.
- Ameliorated by leaning forward with his elbows resting upon the chair.
- In cough think of Kali carb after measles. (Carb veg)
- It has wandering stitching pains through the chest with the coldness of the chest.
- In old gouty cases, in old cases of Bright's disease, in advanced cases of phthisis where there are many troubles beware of Kali carb given too high.

Dr. Chowdhury

- A great tendency towards obesity is noticed in these patients.
- In spite of its anaemia and weakness the patient flush easily and the peculiarity of this flushing is that it is mostly one sided and partial. We find one cheek to be red and hot, the other cheek cold and pale.
- The patient yawns continuously and complaints of great sleepiness throughout the day and even in the early hours of evening when everybody around him is happy cheerful and enjoying themselves. This sleepiness however grows very intense specially after eating when they can hardly keep awake. It has been said that they fall asleep while they are having their food. During sleep they start, twitch, grind their teeth, talk and cry. The sleep is further disturbed by dreams of thieves, various diseases that people and sentimental instances.
- The patient constantly speaks of his back as if firing out. This is so bad while walking that he feels like lying on the street to obtain relief. It is pressing in and ameliorated by rubbing. One strange indication of aggravation of the backache from eating.
- The cough is dry and paroxysmal one peculiarity about the cough is that the viscid mucus or pus whatever happens to bring up is

swallowed. The expectoration usually consists of hard white mucus which practically flies out of the throat while coughing or less the patients follows them without being able to throw it away. The cough is usually aggravated after eating and drinking and the patient complaints of a feeling of weakness and faintness in the chest especially when walking.

- In chest troubles usually the right side of the lung is affected.
- Sensation as if the heart where suspended by a thread.

Dr. Tyler
The time of aggravation of Kali carb is as follows:
- At 2:00 a.m. vacant with stomach pains or dry cough.
- At 3:00 a.m. asthma terrible attack or dry cough, whooping cough, must get up and walk.
- 3 to 4 a.m. Diarrhoea.
- 5:00 a.m. suffocating and choking cough (NS).
- 9:00 a.m. headache worst.
- 10:00 a.m. gets hungry and faintness.
- Noon chilliness and stubborn sensation.
- In asthma must lean forward with head on knees.
- Violent colic pain before menses constipation during.

Kali Chloratum

Dr. Chowdhury
- It produces destructive degeneration in the kidneys. Hence, it is a useful remedy in nephritis and hemoglobinuria with albumin and blood in the urine. It is usually indicated when the secretion of urine decreases in quantity and becomes highly aluminous, with a great percentage of hematin and casts. The urine either looks black or greenish-black and has to be frequently drawn off by the

caterer is great. Its greatest application, however, is to be found in ulcerative and Follicular stomatitis.

- The whole mucus lining of the mouth becomes a red turbide. Even The tongue becomes full of ulcerations. These ulcers have a shot of grey's base. Salivation becomes profuse and acid submaxillary glands become swollen. Red and oedematous. The smell from the mouth is very offensive. The secretions are excessively tough and stringy. Epistaxis difficulty following incessant cough and difficult respiration are a few indications of Kali. Chlor.

Kali Cyanatum
Dr. Chowdhury

- Ugly-looking ulceration of the tongue. Chronicity of complaints, offensive salivation. Hemorrhage from the affected parts with neurologic pain at the greatest indication of this remedy. The neuralgic pain is particularly felt in the temporal region, sometimes between the temporal region and ciliary arch. It may be also felt in the orbital and submaxillary regions. It is almost unbearable < after a full meal > by motion in the open air.

- The breathing is very slow that at times we feel that they are hardly breathing.

Kali Iod
Dr. Kent
Hot patient

- It is an antipsoric and antisyphilitic remedy.

- Mental: There is a very strong degree of irritability, coarseness, and harshness of temper. He is harsh with his family and with his children, abusive. It will take all the sense of refinement of his mind, and then he will become sad and tearful, extremely nervous, and must walk and be on the go if he remains in. the room he becomes weak and tired and feels as if he could not stir < In the warmth of the house > In the open air and movement.

Nervous and mental exhaustion comes from resting. Walks long distances without fatigue.(Iod), but in Rhus tox, movement brings on relief, but walking long distances brings on fatigue.

- Head: bipartal bone pains < By warmth of. House and > By walking in the open air, the scalp breaks out with nodular eruptions, tuberculosis, and Syphilitic eruptions. Great disposition of hair to change color and fallout. Coldness of the painful parts. Iritis of the most severe type.(Staphysgharia, Nitric acid, Merc Sol). There is copious thick green expectoration greenish discharge. Mucus from the nose, from the eyes, from the ear. Thick greenish dish. From the ulcer. The thick green or yellowish-green discharges are very fetid.

- It is constantly taking cold sneezing and continuously copies water discharge from the nose. Excruciating the passage and causing burning In the nose, this coryza is <In the open air. But all the rest of the patient is > In the open air. Incorriza he gets> in a warm room. Repeated attacks of violent acrid coryza from the least cold.

- Its external symptoms are > By cold and open air, whereas its internal symptoms are < By cold things such as cold milk ice cream, ice water, cold drinks, and cold food. Cold things in the stomach < all the symptoms.

- It has flatulence and belching like Carbo Veg and Lycopodium.

- It is a good medicine for the liver, the patient is covered from head to feet with an eruption that forms great nodules, fairly burning. She cannot tolerate covering, the intense heat of the body without the rise of temperature. Rough nodular manifestation all over the body it disappears in a few hours but returns in a few days like weeks or months. A single dose of very high potency of Kali iod will turn things in order.

Dr. Chowdhury

- Loss of appetite completely even sometimes death may occur by the suppression of psoriasis or other similar skin diseases by the application of crude drugs. Extreme sensitivity of the parts affected. It is not localized sensitive. Sensitiveness, as is seen in boils and ulcerations. The whole surface is tender. The slightest touch and pressure cause pain. Which is more or less diffused over the whole area.

- Dr. Kent has reported a case of supraorbital neuralgia. He was cured with Rhus tox simply on the indications of diffused soreness over the whole head that was accompanied by paroxysm neuralgia pain.

- Like other Kali, it has < after coitus.

- It is generally suited to pale delicate subjects with a tendency to flatulence, distension, depression of spirits, and pronounced emaciation with progressive weakness.

- We also think of it in children with big heads emaciated limbs and big teeth. The youngster generally cannot bear any jerk or jolting because of any definite lesion in any of the limbs but on account of a general sense of tenderness.

- It is a good medicine for hydrocephalus, where there is a history of syphilis. In acute hydrocephalus, it should. be prescribed where there are strabismus, elaborate respiration, convulsion, paralysis, and dilation of the pupils with automatic movement of the limbs.

- In Iritis, the pupils despite repeated administration of atropine contract to a pinpoint Chemogis edema of the lids with lachrymation, [urulent secretion and injection of conjunctiva.

- After most pneumonic symptoms have disappeared. We sometimes have a peculiar harassing cough to deal with a cough that is sometimes dry often accompanied by profuse expectoration of profuse greenish sputum. This mucus purulent matter whenever it may be is frothy and has the appearance of soap suds. There is sharp stitching pain from the sternum to the back, Kali carb, Stanum, and Sanguinaria are the two other remedies that may be needed in a similar condition of cough. In all these three remedies, the expectorations are copious. With Stanum and Kali, it is greenish. In Sanguinaria, it is frothy, sanguineous, and fluid and the taste of sputum is fetid, but in Stanum its taste is sweetish.

- Ait is a good medicine for tinnitus overium with a patient mercurae syphilitic constitution and a lot of bone pains to which he is a constant subject.

- Noises in the ear from chewing (Kali sul, Nitric acid).

- Noises before menses (Kreosotum).

- Noises after menses (Ferrum, Petroleum).

Kali Nitricum

Dr. Chowdhury

- The pains of this remedy are stitching in character. Such pains may be felt everywhere. And whereever found. They generally tend to impede respiration on this indication, it may be used in pleurisy as well as pneumonia.

- Its indication in the above complaints are severe cough with shortness of breath, expectoration of blood, red or turbid urine. And great and constant thirst. A very great symptoms here as well as its asthma, is a peculiar dyspnoea that prevents the patient from drinking as drinking brings on suffocations.

- It's menstrual flow is ink blue. All its symptoms are < from eating veal, wine and beer.

Kali Phos

Dr. Kent

Chilly patient

- The symptoms of this remedy are < Morning, evening, and night. over sensitive, nervous persons (delicate) worn out from long-sufferings, much sorrow and vexation, and prolonged mental work, such as broken down from sexual excess and vices.

- It is a long-acting antipsoric.

- More symptoms are < During rest and > Gentle motion and slowly walking about. Generally, the patient is sensitive to cold. And its complaints < From the cold, aversion to cold air < after coition

- The weakness emaciation anemia and tubercular tendency are strong features of this wonderful antisoric remedy.

- Emaciation wasting diseases with putrid discharge and putrid stoles.

- Pulsation feels all over the body and in the limbs.

- Symptoms are one-sided.

- The high and highest potentials have served best, and it should be used in a single dose.

- She takes an apathy towards her husband She is cruel to her baby and husband. Perverted affections.

- Fear in the evening fear of a crowd or death, of disease, of evil, of people of solitude. Weak memory. Forgetful.

- It is a great remedy for imbecility. She is impatient and impetuous, indifferent to surroundings, to joy and her family, to his business matters, and then comes in. indolence and lassitude, quarrels with her family, the irritability is very marked.

- Easily startled from a fight. During sleep from touch and noise, he is. Indisposed to talk or to be talked to, racking in sleep, vexation brings on many complaints. Weary of life.

- Vertigo afternoon and evening < After eating on looking upwards> In open air, vertigo with a tendency to fall forward. Objects turn in a circle on rising when standing when stooping, or turning the head when walking in the open air.

- Congestion and fullness of head-on coughing.

- This has been a useful remedy in high and may bring affection when associated with putrid diarrhea.

- The headaches from mental work in students, and brain fog from overwork are cured by this remedy.

- Neuralgia of left mastoid process < by motion and open air.

- Burning in the forehead during stool.

- Perspiration on mental exertion of the forehead, cold sweat.

- Anaemia of the optic nerve.

- Discharge from the ear, bloody, offensive, putrid, and purulent.

- Epistaxis in the morning on blowing the nose.

- Brown patch from the edge of the brows to the eyebrows three inches wide, lasting three months. Chlorotic. Face dark circle under eyes.

- The tongue is dark coated and bleeding.

- The appetite is increased and sometimes ravenous, But goes off on the site of food. Hungry soon after eating, from nervous weakness, hunger during menses, and aversion to food. To bread, to meat.

- The sensation of coldness in the stomach, desires cold drinks, sour things, sweat,

- Constipation with very difficult stool hard large knotty.

- Diarrhoea copious stool, dark frequent, large light-colored. stools. Often smells putrid and purulent like rice water, yellow or yellowish-green mucus.

- In tired nervous women who are subject to abortion. Abortion to coition, desire increased intense for four or five days after menses, itching from Leucorrhoea. It cured a chronic abscess discharge periodically through the vagina and rectum. A copious orange-colored fluid.

- Leucorrhea, burning copious greenish yellow offensive putrid after menses in young girls pain in ovaries on going to sleep. Pain in the uterus and ovaries at night. During pregnancy.

- It has been a great service in hip-joint disease.
- Burning feet, souls, and toes.
- When skin is drawn tight over the wound after the removal of cancer, (Dr.Ghosh).
- Neural pain occurs in any organ with depression, failure of strength, and sensitivity to noise. And light > In gentle motion, but < When white and alone.

Kali Sulph

Dr. Kent
Hot patient

- It has cured most obstinate cases of chronic intermittent fever.
- More symptoms are.< In the evening > By fresh and open air.
- Predisposition to pthysis, is frequently indicated after T.B. and when well-selected remedies fall Short in action.
- Pulsation all over the body touch < Complain. Many symptoms. < On walking.
- When pulsatilla has acted well for a time, and because of opposite modalities, Silicea does good work for a while and then the patient swings back to the original state, symptoms, and modalities, then it is, then that Kali sulph is of great usefulness.
- Quite unlike Pulsatilla, this patient is easily angered obstinate, and very irritable.
- Vertigo < In the morning in a warm room and looking upwards.
- Much dandruff eruption on the scalp, crusts, and eczema, most sticky pimples. Scaling fullness in head and hair. Falls out.
- It has cured polyps.
- Great desire and distress in the stomach appetite. Appetite increased, ravenous or wanting. Aversion to bread to eggs to food to meet. To hot drinks. And warm food. Coldness of

stomach and Catarrah of the stomach desire. Desires are things sweet, cold drinks, and cold food sensation of emptiness in the lower abdomen after stool. > By displacing flatters.

- Impotency induration testes orchitis after suppressed gonorrhea, itching of genitalia and scrotum, sexual desire diminished or entirely lost.
- It builds a woman who has been subject to abortion abortion to caution.
- Asthma or other respiratory trouble < In warm room > in the open. Air. Catarrh of the chest-rattling of the chest from every cold change in the weather. After bronchitis. In children when every cold causes rattling in the chest and there is no expectoration.
- It has cured, swollen, sensitive mammae coming every month before Menses.

Kalmia Latifolia

Antipsoric, sycosis, syphilis.

Dr. Kent

- The symptoms that indicate this remedy show themselves especially in the muscles, in the tendons, in the joints, along the course of the nerves, in rheumatic complaints.
- All its complaints are aggravated from motion, sunrise to sunset, first half of the night, sometimes during whole night.
- Palpitation aggravated from lying on left side and bending forward, ameliorated lying on back and sitting erect.
- It is suitable in old troublesome recurrent headaches associated with cardiac disturbances. A headache will come on easily if the sun comes out but it will not come on if the day is clouded. Aggravated from the light of the sun and increasing brightness of the sun's rays.

- Kidney disease associated with heart disease, in albuminuria with heart disease, difficulty breathing, difficulty heart action. It is often indicated in Bright's disease (albuminuria) with disturbance of vision during pregnancy.
- Neuralgic pain appears after the sudden disappearance of hepatic eruptions.
- In herpes, ringworm, cold sore or isolated vesicular eruptions.

Dr. Chowdhury
- Hypertrophy of the heart and valvular insufficiency. The heart action is tumultuous, rapid and feeble. Dyspnoea and anguish are extreme. The patient is propped up in bed. He complaints of very sharp pain in the heart and pain that pretty nearly takes his breath away and shoots down into the abdomen and stomach. There is also a remarkable slowness of the pulse sometimes coming as low as 40 beats per minute.
- We think of it and rheumatic fever. Almost all the muscles of the body are affected. The fever is high. Every attempt to move is attended by excruciating pain, presence of albumin in the urine.

Kreosotum

Diabetes with carious teeth or history of caries of teeth, cancer of the uterus with terrible offensive bloody foetid oozing. It has at least palliated and made the neighbourhood of the patient bearable (Dr. Tyler).

Dr. Kent
- It has three characteristic symptoms:
    - Excoriating discharge
    - Pulsation all over the body
    - Profuse bleeding from small wounds.
- A prick of a pin will cause the oozing of bright red blood. Any pressure upon the mucus membrane will cause oozing, hence in case of sore throat while examining the mouth with a tongue

depressor it bleeds easily from the mucus membrane of the mouth.

- The lachrymation is excoriating. It excoriates the margins of the lids and cheeks and they become raw and red and smart.

- The corners of the lips and mouth a red and raw and the saliva burns and smarts.

- The leucorrhoea causes smarting and burning about the vulva so that the mucus surface of the labia are red and raw, sometimes inflamed but always burning. The vagina burning during coition and there is bleeding after coition.

- Granulations of the vagina and os uteri so that the pressure of the act of coition brings on burning and bleeding, smarting and excoriation. The male organ will smart and burn after coition in contact with the secretion of the vagina during coition. The urine burns and smarts.

- Every emotion and exciting circumstance is attended with throbbing all over the body. Pulsations to the end of the fingers. Every emotion is attended with tearfulness. Pathetic music will bring out tears that are acrid and palpitations and pulsations that are felt to the extremities.

Alphabet

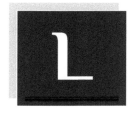

Lachesis

Dr. Kent

- Lot of symptoms in the spring season or goes from a cold into a summer climate. The warm south winds excite the symptoms. The patient cannot bear warmth in any form, faintness, and palpitation of pulsation from a warm bath, The patient may be cold or chilly, yet a warm room increases or brings out the symptoms. Cold extremities with hot heads.

- Upon the face, there is an appearance of anxiety. The face is purple-spotted. The eyes look suspicious. If there is an ulceration, it bleeds black blood, which soon coagulates and looks like charred straw, and all-round the ulceration, there is a purple-matted appearance.

- Varicose veins that come after gestation.

- From the slightest exertion of minds or slightest exertion. The extremities become cold. The heat becomes very feeble and the skin is covered with sweat and the head becomes hot.

- Complaints that affect the left, upper, and right lower.

- Mind: all sorts of impulsive insanity jealousy without reason. Unwarranted jealousy and suspicion. Many times, this medicine has cured the suspicion of girls when they are simply suspicious of their friends. She never sees a whispered conversation going on, but they are talking about her, suspects that are continuing to injure her and she will resort to any scheme to see if they were not talking of her to her determinant. A woman imagines that her. Her friends, husbands, and children are trying to injure her and her friends are going to put her in an insane asylum apprehensive of the future, thinks she's going to have heart disease and is going. Insane imagines. Her relatives are trying to poison her, and she refuses to eat. She thinks sometimes that it is only a dream and she can hardly say whether she dreamed it or whether she thinks it. She thinks she is dead or dreams that she is dead and, in the dream, preparations are being made to lay her out of that. She is about to die and thinks she is somewhat else and in the hands of a stronger power. Thinks that she is under some human control. She is compelled to do things by spirit. She hears a command partly. In her dream, she must come out. Sometimes it takes the form of voices in which she is commanded to steer to murder or to confess things she never did, and she has no peace of mind until she confesses something she has never done. Imagine she is pursued imagines that she has stolen something, or that somebody thinks she has stolen something, and fears that. It is the last. It is full of religion, and insanity. In many cases, a close connection between mental symptoms and heart symptoms will be there, especially in young women and girls who have met with disappointment and have been lying awake in the night because of disturbance of the affections or from disappointment, shattered hopes, or grief. All gone sensation in the heart with difficulty breathing.

- Surging of blood to the head. With cold extremities > after moving.

- The cardiac symptoms are frequently connected. The heart symptoms, it is seldom that the headache. Without cardiac difficulty.

- The touch of clothing is very painful, while the pressure from a hard bandage is agreeable.

- Four sensitiveness to noise motion in. motion in the room 2. Conversation to others. To others walking over the floor.

- Violent pain in the eyes from touching the throat.

- Fistula, Lachrymatis, which is accompanied by long-standing eruptions about the face.
- Anything introduced in the canal of the year will cause a violent spasmodic cough.
- Syphilis, where it has affected the nasal mucus membrane. Producing crust and finally affecting the bones.
- It is a good medicine for the old. Drunkards who have Red nose.
- It has spring saliva, which can be pulled out from the mouth.
- It has cured the suppuration of the ovaries.
- The menstrual sufferings are before and after the flow > during the flow.

Dr. Chowdhury

- He suspects everyone around him serves. Wife, children. With no exception. Even the poor doctor attending to him is looked upon with dread.
- Like Natrum Mur at times believing in robbers being in the home, whom he would try to avoid by jumping out of his window.
- A case of perpetual insanity of a lady whose entire menses phenomena revolved at around one idea of her husband being faithless to her.
- Cutaneous hyperesthesia is very prominent despite the great depression of the vital force The least touch makes the patient unconscious.
- Malaria fever: The chill starting from the small and the back seems so violent as to make the teeth chatter. Another prominent proximity Of these patients during chill is that they want to feel tightly pressed. A lady wanted her daughter to. Lie with her full night across her during chill. The sweat is profuse and makes him garlic. Trembling and mapped tongue intolerant. To pressure on the throat and chest, burning in palms and soles. The internal

sensation of heart with cold feet, restlessness, ice coldness of years, lips and nose shriveling, and lividity of the skin. Morning and incessant signing are some of the other symptoms to be found in this patient.

- It is indicated when the urine becomes dark. This is due to the presence of decomposed particles of blood in the urine.

- Sensation of a ball rolling loose in the bladder, especially while turnover, the sensation of the ball may occur elsewhere as. throat abdomen and other organs or cavities of the body.

- Diarrhoea of drunkards and during climaxes, the stools are watery, chocolate colored, and cadaverous smelling. The tongue is smooth, red, and shiny. They suffer from a tormenting urging but cannot pass anything as the anus feels closed.

- Throat: The indications are elongated uvula, swelling, and purple color of the faces. sensation of a lump in the throat, which descends on swallowing, but returns soon. Difficulty with swelling, swallowing liquids, especially saliva, sensation as if something lodged in the throat, and sometimes > the pain in the throat extends even to the ear and is < On degeneration.

- It is a very good medicine for ulcers, carbuncles, abscesses, malignant cushions, etc. They are usually very sensitive to touch. The affected parts look bluish, discharges are Icarus and offensive in carbuncles. The most important symptom is intense burning. They must rise at night and bathe it with warm water to relieve the burning The surrounding parts are always covered with numerous small boils.

Lac Caninum

Dr. Kent

- It is a deep and long-acting medicine.
- It makes ulcers very red, and it has cured such cases.
- A general hyperesthesia of the skin and all parts is marked.

Dr. Chowdhury

- In forgetfulness, it can be compared with the following:

1) Forgetfulness after sexual excess. Acid Phos, Natrum Phos, Calcarea at times.

2) Forgetfulness after mental exertion and < in the morning.

3) Forgetfulness after waking from sleep: Thuja, Kali-Bich.

- He has a strange delusion about snakes, he imagines he is surrounded by snakes. He falls asleep thinking of snakes during sleep, dreams of snakes, and wakes up from sleep in fright, as if about to be beaten by snakes.

- He thinks he's wearing someone else nose.

- Pains too repeatedly shift from side to side and shoot to the ear in each attempt of swallowing profuse salivation and internal sensitiveness to the throat are guiding symptoms.

- Great sinning feeling in the epigastric and faintness in the stomach.

- Intense unbearable backache felt more in the suprosacral region, like. Rhus tox. This backache is < from rest and on first moving. The whole spine becomes a painful coccyx to the back of the brain and is very sensitive to touch and pressure.

Lac Dedloratum

Chilly patient

Dr. Kent

- The chronic milk subject is very cold and bloodless and cannot get warm, even in warm rooms and in warm clothing. She is so chilly and so sensitive to cold that she feels air blowing on her in the rooms as if she is fanned even when there is no possible draft and others feel the room warm.

- The complains are < by motion > from rest.

- All who have diarrhea, nausea, vomiting, sick headaches, eruptions, or food eructation from the stomach after drinking milk and in time the general idea of milk sickens will be known.

- She becomes faint and dizzy when raising her hands high to thread her needle. vertigo on turning in bed or moving the head from the pillow. On opening the eyes when lying. Vertigo when stretching up with the hands. Standing to fall to the right when standing and walking.

- It has cured many violent periodical sick headaches that have been present since childhood. And said to be inherited. During a violent headache, there is sometimes a sensation as though the head is expanding. Headaches come before and after menses.

- Grinding teeth during sleep with pain in the stomach and head with vomiting.

- Entire cases of appetite. Great thirst in stomach and head with vomiting irritations, empty. or sour, distention from gas, nausea after drinking cold water in the evening, vomiting of undigested food immensely acid taste of bitter water, and lastly a brownish stool which in water separated and looks like coffee grounds.

- Involuntary urination when walking in cold air when riding a horse and when running to catch a train.

- Soreness of the chest with oppression, rheumatic pain in the chest in cold damp weather. Tubercular deposits in orifices of both lungs.

- Ends of finger ice cold, rest of hand warm.

Lac- Felinium

Dr. Chowdhury

- The headache is terrible and it penetrates the left eyeball to the center of the brain. A sensation of constriction along the bridge of the nose. It is prominent. One of the Proverbs felt her head down so that her chin pressed heavily on the chest. And in her agony, which was great, she rushed from room to room, holding her head firmly in her hands.

- In headache its indications are sharp lancinating pains in the center of the left eyeball, extending externally to the temple and frontal region over the eye, with intense photo. Redness of the conjunctiva and lacrimation.

- Dr. Berridge used it with great success in a case of. Keratitis, where the pain was so excessive for three nights and days that the patient did not have wind or sleep. pain felt like a knife running from the affected left eye to the occiput.

Lachnanthes

Dr. Chowdhury

Chilly patient

- It has headaches of great intensity. The pain is splitting bursting pain< on the movement of the head which is associated with a disposition over a carpet, terribly disturbs the patient.

- The patient has a sensation of a piece of ice laying on their back between his shoulders, which causes him to shiver and gives him goosebumps hot flat iron is the only thing that > the chilliness.

- It is a great remedy for torticollis. The neck becomes stiff and the head gets drawn to one side. The pain in the nape of the neck is so great that gives him a sensation of dislocation when this occurs. With sore throat. It is a very good indication.

- Circumscribed redness of the face with an abnormal brilliance of the eyes in loquacity, it resembles Lachesis to some extent.

Lactic Acid

Dr. Chowdhury
- It is corrosive that eats into every tissue of the bones, except the enamel of the teeth.

- It is generally suited to this pale anemic woman who loses much blood at each menstrual period.

- It is a great remedy for diabetes mellitus, morning sickness during pregnancy, and chronic arthritis.

- Its nausea is just like Ipecac but in lactic acid, a constant water brash, continued discharge, or profuse saliva. The saliva brought up feels hot and exceedingly sour and corrosive. So must so it leaves an acute burning all along the passage from stomach to mouth in its progress upward.

- In diabetes: large quantities of foamy strong-smelling dark urine voracious appetite, great thirst, dry past, sticky tongue, chilliness of extremities, a feeling of emptiness and sinking in stomach, and distress and pain in renal region.

- According to Nash, in diabetes with rheumatic pain, the other symptoms are acid and profuse, sweat, and rheumatic inflammation of the elbow. Knees and small joints of upper and lower extremities., nocturnal <.

Lactuca Virasa

Dr. Chowdhury

- Its most characteristic symptoms are sensations of constriction and tightness, affecting the whole body, but more especially the chest.

- Crampy, stitching pain in the left chest, extending to the left scapula. An indispensable tightness of the whole chest at night. obliging to sit up with anxious suddenness and feeling of terrible suffocation., lend to its indication in angina. A similar sensation, caused him to wake up suddenly with pain and cough, leading to the indication of asthma.

- The cough is most incessant and spasmodic. Threatening almost to burst his chest. It feels as if his chest would fly to pieces. The cough is caused by. A peculiar sensation of tickling in. tongue.

- Another symptom is the sensation of lightness. The whole body feels light as if swimming in the air. Dreams of swimming in the wind and walking above the ground.

Lauroccrasus

Dr. Chowdhury

- It is particularly useful in long faint. The patient suddenly loses consciousness which he does not recover for a long time. His lower jaw drops. Arms to side. Respiration becomes suspended, and the pulse weak and scarcely palpable. The eyes remain wide open and stoned. There is hardly any forming from the mouth. The patient takes a deep breath. After long intervals.

- It has a dry harassing cough, it is particularly useful in the spasmodic cough to be seen in the later stages of whooping cough, when the patient becomes frustrated, it is useful in cough with vascular diseases of the heart

- It has green diarrhoea. Drinks roll through audibly through the esophagus and intestine. Coldness of both pulses, cloudiness of the brain, faintness suppression, and retention of urine. The sensation of constriction of the throat when swallowing. Complete paralysis of the sphincter muscle. It is almost specific in certain conditions of cholera with choleric diarrhoea.

Ledum Pal

Dr. Kent

- Air is an irritant to raw parts and will keep up an unnecessary discharge of pus, even from a perfectly healthy sore.

- The patient is constitutionally cold, cold to touch, coldness in the body. Coldness in the extremities with a hot head. And again, we see the other extreme where the whole body is overheated and the head is also in great heat.

- Pain < From motion at night and from the warmth of bed > From cold application with copious pale urine.

- It is suitable in old prolonged cases of inflammation of the knee joints of pneumatic knee joints. Such a patient sitting. With the joint exposed to the cold, fanning the joints or putting evaporating lotion upon the joint.

- It counteracts the effects of whiskey and takes away the appetite for whiskey.

- Phagmonous erysipelas of any part of the body, but particularly of the face or injured part.

- Urination frequent. quantity diminished or increased. Stromas often stop during the flow, burning in the urethra after urinating, itching, redness, and discharge of pus, it has red. Sand in the urine. As marked in lycopodium according to Lippi Copious color. Urine light specific gravity.

Lilium Tigri

Dr. Kent
Hot patient

- From every motion the heart flutters and is irregular and excitable.

- The mental symptoms, the heart symptoms and uterine symptoms often rotate or alternate.

- She can hardly speak a decent word to anybody. She will snap an event spoken kindly. She is so irritable that her friends cannot specify her. She. Lies awake at. Nights and is tormented either by fanatical religious ideas or a. religion. Is melancholy and seems inclined to dwell. To dwell upon insane ideas. Concerning religion and mode of life has wrong. Ideas concerning everything receives wrong impression and everything is inverted She sits alone and roots over imaginary troubles when spoken to is crabbed.

- A slight tingling comes up at the back of the head and goes to the top and is associated with Vertigo. The pains in the forehead are very marked, and they are associated with disturbance of vision, a loss of vision, the room looms darker, the eyes are unable to focus very often with the complaints of the head, the eyes are turned in a convergent strabismus, or there is a threatened syncope with pain in the forehead.

- The patient suffocates in a crowded room in the theater. Like (Apis iodine, lycopodium Pulsatilla).

- Its diarrhea is just like sulfur because it has great heat on the head emptiness in the stomach and great burning of the palms and souls. It has also a dysentery-like mark core, but it has great tennis mills, mucus, and blood burning in the passage of the rectum during stool. Recurrent dysenteric attack with. Every cold in those who suffer from pelvic and abdominal relaxation, mental irritability, palpitation, and fluttering of the heart with nervous constitution.

- Hemorrhoids after delivery (Kali Carb) with relaxed uterus and vagina.

Dr. Tyler

- Constant hurried feeling as if imperative duties and utter insanity to perform them during sexual excitement.

- A sensation in the pelvis, as though everything was coming into the world through the vagina, the dragging downwards towards the pelvis is felt as high as the stomach, even shoulders worst standing not> by laying. Wants to place their hands on the hypogastrium and press upwards to relieve the dragging sensation, and wants to draw long breaths inward to raise the abdominal contents.

- Craving appetite for dinner, increased desire for meat, abortion to bread, coffee to. The usual cigar. It is a good medicine for the relaxed condition of the pelvic organ.

- Bearing down sensation. < by standing (Sepia).

- Bearing down sensation > by standing (Belladonna).
- Bearing down sensation by sleeping (Pulsatilla).

Lithium Carb

Dr. Chowdhury

- It is an invaluable remedy in chronic rheumatism, especially when accompanied with valuable troubles.
- Any little excitement causes fluttering of the heart, and pain in the heart, very frequent and is felt when the patient bends forward > When he passes water.
- Another peculiarity of rheumatism consists of the appearance of an eruption on the affected parts. The small joints are especially involved. Great tenderness, swelling, and tenderness of the cast joint of fingers. The skin of these patients is dry harsh and rough.
- It has soreness like Arnica, bones joints, and muscles feel bruised as from falls or blows. Even the eyeball feels sore.
- Pneumatic soreness of the cardiac region are trembling and fluttering sensation of the heart after mental agitation and induration of aortic valves.
- The urine is strong, scanty, frequent, and full of uric acid deposits. Deposits while passing urine flashes of heat. Felt in the region of the bladder extending into spermatic cord.
- Headache of females brought on by sudden cessation of menses. It is felt in the vortex head of the eyes. The eyes feel very sore, and they find it difficult to keep the eyelids open. The headache is. > By taking something but it returns and remains still food is taken again.
- Loss of vision cannot see the right half of an object. It is due to excessive use of the right eye, insufficient light, and direct exposure to the blinding effects of strong sunlight. Also, we find chronic hardening of the membrane gland.

- The nose is swollen red. A bit puffy, but it is dry. When inside the house and moist when he goes into open air.

Lycopodium
Dr. Kent

- It is anti- psoric, Sycotic, and Syphilitic remedy with chili patients.

- All the symptoms are < By cold except head and spine, which are > by cold < Buy exertion. He cannot climb and cannot walk fast. The rheumatic pains are.> by motion, he is extremely restless and must keep moving. If there is inflammation with the aches and pains, the patient is > From the warmth of the bed and motion. And he will keep tossing all night. He turns and gets into a new place and thinks he can sleep. But the restlessness continues. All night, the headache is worse from lying down and from the warmth of the broom, and better from cold air and motion.

- After a mere mouthful, he becomes flatulent and distended. That he cannot eat anymore. While the abdomen is distended, he is so nervous that he cannot endure any noise. The noise of the cracking of a paper ringing the bells or slamming of doors goes through him and causes fainting. (Antim crud, Borax, Natrum Mur).

- There are painful ulcers, ulcers beneath the skin, abscesses beneath the skin, and cellular troubles, the chronic ulcerations are indolent with false granulations. Painful burning stinging and smarting, after > applying cold things < with a warm poultice hives come out in the warm room and a warm bed. It comes out either in nodules or in long and irregular stripes, stitched violently. The sites of old boils and pustules become indurated and form nodules that remain for a long time. Ulcers bleed and form great quantities of thick yellow offensive green pus.

- Poor tone and poor circulation numbness in spots emaciation of single members.

- It has religious insanity which. has a mild and simple beginning. This religious insanity grows greater and greater until he sits and brutes. It has a dread of solid solitude and people and when. He is fully carried out in the lycopodium patient. You see that she deals with the presence of a new person or the coming of Friends and visitors, she wants to be lonely with this that is constantly surrounding her. Sadness with weeping comes over the patient on receiving a gift at the slightest joy. She weeps. Is very nervous. Emotional, Sensitive patient. She picks at imaginary things in the air and seizes flies and all sorts of little things flying in the air.

- Wakes up in the morning with sadness. There is sadness and gloom. The world may come to an end or the whole family may die. The house may burn up. There seems to be nothing cheering, the future looks black after moving about a while, and this passes off.

- Extensively merry and laughs at simplest things.

- This trustful suspicious and funniest finding.

- If he goes beyond his dinner hour, a sick headache will come on. He must eat with regularity, or he will have a headache, which he is subject to. This is somewhat like Lachesis headache. Cactus has a congestive headache, which becomes extremely violent, with a flushed face, if he does not eat at a regular time, the Lycopodium headache is > by eating but in Cactus < by eating.

- Lean emaciated boys are subject to prolonged pain in the head every time. The Little Fellow takes cold. He has a prolonged, throbbing headache. And from day to day and month, he becomes more emaciated, especially about the face and neck. This remedy is especially suitable in these withered lads with a dry cough, and a prolonged headache in children who wither after pneumonia or bronchitis. Emaciate about the face and neck takes cold on the slightest of provocation. Suffer with a headache from being heated, have mighty headaches, and a state of congestion that affects the mind more or less which they rouse out of sleep-in confusion. The little one screams out in sleep, weakens frightened looks wild, and does not know the father and mother, or maybe, or family until after a few moments, when he seems to be able to collect his senses and then realize where he is lies down to sleep again. This thing is repeated again and again.

- Upon the scalp, we find eruption in patches, smooth patches with the hair off, patches on the face, and eczematous eruptions behind the ears, bleeding and oozing a watery fluid. Sometimes yellowish watery, the eczema spreads from behind the ears up over the ears and to the skull.

- Eczema in a lean hungry withering child with more or less head troubles. Moist oozing behind the ears like red sand in the mine. Dry tossing cough in a child that kicks the lower of a child whose left foot is cold and the other hot with copious appetite eating much with unusual hunger at times and great thirst and yet losing steadily. It will throw out a great amount of eruption first and then subside later.

- It often suffers from a thick yellow discharge from the nose. The nose is filled with yellow, and green crushed blown out of the nose in the morning, and hawked out of the throat. Now, when the patient takes a cold, the thick discharge to a great extent seizes and he commences to sneeze and has a watery discharge. Then comes Lycopodium headache, great suffering, and hunger pain. Finally, the coryza passes away, and the thick yellow discharge returns and the headache subsides.

- The nose troubles often begin in infancy. The little infant will be at first with a peculiar rattling breathing through the nose and finally, it will only bleed through the mouth as the nose is obstructed. This goes on for days and months. The child breathes only through the mouth. And when it cries, it has a shrill tone, such as is found when the nose is plugged up.

- In old chronic categories of adults, they must keep continually blowing their noses. The mucus discharge is almost as thick and tenacious as in Kali- bich.

- In deep-seated chest troubles, bronchitis, or pneumonia. But the chest is filled up with mucus. It will be seen that the face and forehead are wrinkled from pain and the. wings of the nose are flapped with the effort of breathing in the brain troubles of Stromonium. The forehead is wrinkled.

- The face is often covered with copper-colored eruptions, as found in syphilis.

- After eating he's distended with flatus and gets momentary > from belching yet he remains distended. Pains immediately after eating, vomiting of bile, coffee-ground vomit. Black inky vomit. Lycopodium patients are always belching. They have. Irritations that are occurred like strong acid, burning the pharynx. The stomach symptoms are < brought on by cold drinks, beer, coffee, fruit, and diarrhoea flows. Everything later turns into the wind.

- Infectious urging to stool, stool hard difficult, small, and incomplete. The first part of the stool is hard and difficult to start, but the last part is softer, thin, and gushing, followed by faintness and weakness.

- It has wetting of the bed in little ones, involuntary micturition in typhoid, and low fever is guiding symptoms of this remedy.

- Absence or suppression of menses for many months, the patient being withered, declining pale and shallow, becoming feeble. It seems that she does not have the vitality to menstruate. It is also suitable for girls in Puberty when the time for the first menstrual flow appears. She goes on 15 to 18 years without development. The breast does not enlarge, the ovaries do not perform their functions. Worry about lessons (Lycopodium, Silicea).

- The extremities are cold, while the head and face are hot, with much coughing and trouble in the chest.

- There is a restlessness of the lower limbs which comes on when it thinks of going to sleep. And this prevents sleep until midnight.

- Sulphur, Grapities, and calcarean carb are no longer acting and deeper acting than Lycopodium.

Dr. Chowdhury

- Lycopodium is a sour remedy, whereas Nux vom is a bitter remedy.

- The tongue is quoted white, the patient complains of blood and, a putrid taste in the mouth that sometimes changes to sour.

- It has cured many cases of dyspepsia with heartburn that commences at 3:00 PM and ends with vomiting of intensely sour food and bile at about 7:00 PM.

- Lycopodium patients are generally costive. They suffer from frequent ineffectual desire for stool. This is not due to irregular peristaltic as in Nux vom, but to the presence of construction in the rectum Each evacuation causes a terrible amount of pain and urging that leaves the patient in a very prostrated condition. In some bad cases, we may see, after the stool, the most striking symptom is the persistent pain after evacuation. It is so severe as to arrest breathing. The pain is cutting, tearing, stretching, and cramping in nature.

- It is also serviceable for the constipation of young men who, are tormented by night pollution or addressed to masturbation.

- It is a very good medicine for diabetes insipidus where thirst is very great. The patient took an enormous quantity of water and passed an equally last quantity of pale watery urine.

- The female sexual system discharges blood from the genitals during every passage of heart and soft stool.

- During labor, the patient dances up and down in the pain. She must keep constantly in motion, labor pains run upwards, and are temporary > By placing her feet against a support.

- In fever, the paracetamol may come on between 8 and 9:00 AM or in the evening between 6 and 7:00 PM. It is ushered in with shaking chill and incessant yearning and nausea between chill and heat. He vomits an extremely sour fluid in typhoid. The tongue is swollen, so that it cannot protrude when you. ask the patient to do so. It only rolls from side to side like a pendulum. In his attempt to talk, which at most is indistinct, stammering, and heavy.

Dr. Tyler

- Whole abdomen distended after a stool.

- The first part of the stool is lumpy, and the second. is soft.

- Gray salty tasting expectorations

- Stitches of the left chest during expectorations.

- Burning as if glowing comes between the scapula. (Phosphorous, Kali-bich)

- Hungry when waking at night.

- Desire for hot things and sweet.

Lycopus- Virginicus

Dr. Chowdhury

- These patients generally show signs of exophytes. Their thyroid glands become enlarged. They suffer from pain. Tachycardia and tremors. Their eyeballs protrude. This protrusion is at times so excessive as to amount to a practical discoloration of the eyeballs from their sockets.

- It is a great remedy for erratic pains. Generally, the pain begins on the left side and jumps from place to place. And at last, return to its original site. It is > from warmth < from cold air and movement. For erratic pain, it can be compared with the following medicines:

- Kali-Bich: The pain shifts like Lycopus, but it is a pain that is generally in small spots and can be covered with the tip of the fingers.

- Lac caninum: The changeability of sides and location of pain is the red strand of this remedy.

- Ledum: It has also erratic pain, but it shifts in an upward fashion.

- Pulsatilla: Pain which is erratic in nature is accompanied by chill and shivering. The intensity of which is determined by the intensity of the pain.

- Another peculiarity about Lycopus pain is that the patient is more sensitive to it when he concentrates his thoughts upon it.

- Sometimes the pain is located in the precordial region and at the apex. But the peculiarity about it is that the paint shifts to the left, wrist, and inner side of the right calf, and then comes back to its original location. Many of the important symptoms of this remedy are similarly characterized. Thus, for example, the pain in the testicle shifts to the supraorbital region, sometimes from one testis to another.

- It has been recommended very highly in diabetes mellitus. The patient passes a huge quantity of urine daily. Thirst is exceedingly great. The patient drinks large quantities of water. It is a thirst that nothing but the coldest water would satisfy. The specific gravity is much diminished, and the urine shows deposits of mucus epithelial cells abundance, spermatozoa, and oxalate of lime crystals. Sometimes the urine is very scanty. It is accompanied by the edema of the feet.

- Patient is very allergic to dust.

- One peculiar symptom is that so long as the bladder is full, it does not trouble the patient at all. But as soon as he passes urine and the bladder becomes empty, he feels a great distended sensation for that reason.

- The menses are very scanty and last from half an hour to six or seven hours, and generally intermittent for 10 or 12 days. (Euphrasia).

- It is useful in the tickling cough of phthisis when accompanied by hemoptysis and tumorous action of the heart. Dr. Hale recommends it is the greatest palliative in advanced Phthisis.

Borland: In gradual cardiac failure with dilation of the heart:

- The patient is pale and restlessness.
- Horrible tumultuous sensation of the heart which radiates up to neck and head.
- Complains < laying on the right side.
- Aversion to all foods, especially the smell of them.
- It is a good medicine for high B.P with enlarged thyroid.
- It is good medicine for diabetes mellitus with enlarged thyroid.

Alphabet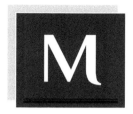

Magnesium Carbonate
Dr. Kent
- It is deep-acting and long-acting and permeates the economy as thoroughly as sulphur > From motion, desire for open air yet very sensitive to cold air wants to be covered during all stages of fever. Daily evening fever symptoms occur every 21 days.

- Sensation of heat even sweat from eating and drinking warm things. Evening thirst.

- It is especially related to the left side of the face, neuralgia in the night, driving him out of bed, and keeping him in constant motion.

- It has varied eruptions upon the skin, dry scaly, dandruff-like eruptions upon the skin very unhealthy hair and nails, particularly it affects the teeth and roots of the teeth in every change of weather, the roots of the teeth become violently painful burn, shoot and a continuous toothache before and during menstruation during pregnancy She suffers all the time with toothache, tearing pain in the left side of the face, although the roots of the teeth are perfectly sound. The hollow teeth are usually sensitive and painful. Magnesia carb and China when no other symptoms are present, are prominent remedies among the affections of the teeth during pregnancy.

- In tuberculosis patients, parents, and the child tend to into marasmus. The child's muscles are flabby. The child will not thrive, despite feeding. Finally, it emaciates and the back of the head begins to sink in as if from the entropy of the cerebellum. The appetite increases for milk and meat and animal broths And yet they are not digested. And when the milk is taken, it continually passes the bowel in the form of white potter clay or putty. It is a complete picture of a magnesium carb stool composed of putty-like undigested stool.

- The magnesium carb baby smells like the Hepar baby. The. perspiration is sour and the whole baby smells sore. It is not especially the stool. The stool smells strong and pungent and very often the whole child has a pungent order like an unclean baby, though it would be well washed.

- It produces inactivity of the rectum and anus, apheresis, the stool is large and hard, requiring great straining to expel. It is dry, hard, and crumbling. The stool will remain partly expelled and then crumble, breaking out into many pieces. Its diarrhoea is greenish, and the green parts float upon the watery portion of the stool.

- The face of the chronic adult case is pale, waxy, sickly, and shallow. And this patient will not write up and will not thrive. She becomes so tired; that she sweats upon little exertion. She is disturbed by every change of weather and is worse at the beginning of the menstruation. She seems to take cold whenever menstruation is coming on. It has coryza every month before the menstrual period.

- Violent craving for meat and aversion to vegetables.

- Tendency to dryness of the mucous membrane and dryness of the skin. Dryness is a marked feature of this remedy.

- The magnesium carb patient always complains of a sour stomach, and sour eructation. Food comes up, sour. There is nausea and vomiting up in the throat, there is pain in the stomach after eating an ordinary amount of food, bloated after eating, and much flatulence after eating, the stomach digests the food slowly and it becomes sour.

- Patients suffering from dry cough before the evening chill like Rhus tox. Some persons have simply this tendency, go along year after year in this withered state with the little locking cough spasmodic in the night from tickling in the larynx.
- Sleepiness during the day and. Sleeplessness in the. night.

Dr. Chowdhury

- The patients are extremely sensitive, both bodily and mentally.
- The slightest touch causes startling. The slightest noise irritates the slightest pressure <Almost all symptoms and the slightest exposure to droughts of cold air bring in untold miseries.
- Extreme acidity. This sourness runs throughout the length and breadth of magnesium carb. The stools, the vomited materials, and the sweat have an acid taint. The absence of the symptoms is a great contradiction of magnesium carb < Of all the symptoms, especially pains from rest and > from walking about.
- Tumors and bone growth have also yielded to magnesium carb. Dr. Dr. Kent was cured with a tumor of the right malar bone by an aged sea carpenter, on whom he tried various other remedies, but without much avail.
- Cutting pain about the naval distinction of the abdomen and. Rumbling and gurgling, followed by loose diarrheic stools are present. The stools are green watery frothy.
- It is full of dreams of dead persons of fire and thieves.

Magnesium Muriaticum

Dr. Kent

- It is a deep-acting anti-psoric suited to nervous patients with stomach and liver troubles. It has enlarged glands and irritation of the nerve centers and brain.
- Many of the complaints are > by open and fresh air except head which is > from warm applications and covering.

- He is extremely restless only with great difficulty can he keep still as if forced to keep still, he becomes anxious, restless, fidgetiness throughout the body, coupled with anxiety. It may come at any time, but < at night at bed and Steelworks on closing the eyes to go to sleep.

- While reading she feels as if someone were reading after her and she must read faster and faster.

- Vertigo.> Walking in the open air.

- Hunger, but knows not for what. Ravenous hunger, followed by nausea< from salty things, from eating salt food, from salt baths, from sea bathing and at sea shore from inhaling seashore, chest complaints, liver complaints, and constipation of constipation and the patient has urticaria at sea shore, Arsenic will cure the case.

- The right lobe of the liver painful sore while laying on it. When it turns towards the left, he is uncomfortable. He feels as if lever dragged over the left (Natrum Sulph, Ptelea).

- Attacks of gastralgia in the evening.

- No power to expel the contents of the bladder, so he presses with the abdominal muscles on the full bladder and passes a little. Lack of sensation of the bladder, so that sometimes he cannot tell in the dark, whether he is passing urine or not.

- Numbness in the extremities, tearing pains in the upper limbs, and marked restlessness in the lower limbs.

Dr. Chowdhury

- It is particularly a woman's remedy. Women who suffer from hysterical paroxysms are complicated with uterine distress.

- A coated large flabby yellow tongue, accumulation of water in the mouth, continual rising of frothy, sour, severe hiccup after dinner, causing vomiting. Regurgitation of food while walking. Rotten, rancid irritation, water brash, oppression in the pit of the stomach intolerance of milk are the guiding symptoms of the remedy < from mental exercise, res, meal and coition.

- Constipation is mostly common in children during dentition. The stools are sometimes covered with mucus and blood. They are so hard and dry that they seem as if they were burnt. Such constipation is very common in poor, puny, rachitic children with enlarged abdomens Quite a lot of urging is necessary before defecation.

- The menstrual pain is generally > by having back pressure.

- There is a frequent desire to pass urine and it can only be passed by bearing down with. Abdominal muscles show an atonic condition of the bladder.

- They sleep a lot during the day with a great deal of sleepiness at night.

Magnesium Phosphoricum

Dr. Kent

- There are times when a nerve in which there is considerable pain becomes sensitive to pressure and becomes sore.

- Convulsion in adults or children followed by extreme sensitiveness to touch to the wind to noise to excitement to everything, such convulsion, children have during dentition.

- Cramps from prolonged exertion. Stiffness numbness awkwardness and deadness of the nerves from prolonged aversion. There it applies to the long use of hands and fingers in writing and gives a fair sample of the writer's cramp. It is especially useful in cramps that come in the fingers from writing, playing instruments, and piano practice. Pianists suddenly break down with stiffness of the fingers after several hours of labor for years. A laborer's hand will sometimes cramp and become almost useless. The Carpenter after prolonged use of the tool has a cramp. This is a strong feature of this remedy in all sorts of over-exertion.

- Violent cramps in dysentery and cholera morbus that may make him scream out.

- Violent attacks of headache with a red face when > from pressure, heat, and dark Magnesium Phos is a good medicine instead of Belladonna.

- It has cured more face-aches than other pains.

- It is a wonderful medicine in spasmodic hiccupping. It should be prescribed if no other symptoms are present.

- Spasm of the stomach with clean tongue.

Dr. Chowdhury

- Is pain a neuralgic in nature and rapidly changes its place, its pain has also been described as crampy pain. It comes on spasmodically and bends our patient double with colic, it is mostly a nocturnal pain. It comes on almost every night and leaves him with the light of the dawn< by motion and drought of air.

- Cedron: Neuralgic pain, supraorbital neuralgia, periodicity is well marked < after caution during menses laying on the left side.

- Chin-ars: Violent neuralgic pain in the left mammary region.

- Plumbum: Neuralgia at rectum.

- Rhodotron and Hamamelis: Neuralgia of scrotum.

- Magnesium Phos: This is a splendid remedy for headaches of schoolchildren suffering from optical defects. It is neuralgic in character and > by hot application. It is a good medicine for the headaches of young mothers after childbirth. Sudden flushes of pain in the back part of the. mouth and head, then spreading all over the head and involving the eyes are a frequent occurrence necessitating rest darkness, and tight bandaging.

- It is a good medicine for flatulent colic in children < At 3 to 4:00 PM. The flatus passes neither upward nor downward.

- It has been used with great success in spasmodic hiccups and persistent vomiting. The patient spits up what he had eaten, even while at the table with little or no nausea.

Dr. Tyler
- Magnesium Phos and Colocynth: Should present many points of resemblance, since Colosseum, which belongs to the. the vegetable kingdom contains 3% of magnesium phos. It acts best when given in single dose of C.M. per day.
- Spasms or cramps in the stomach with a clean tongue, as if a. band was tightly laced or drawn around the body.
- Flatulent colic of children and the newborn with drawing up of legs, remittent colic cramps, crampy pains with acidity.

Magnesium Sulphurica

Dr. Chowdhury
- Diarrhoea: Copious tool in cholera vomiting of food copious yellowish slimy sticking stools and the presence of large quantity of watery serous fluid.
- The toothache comes on as the patient enters a warm womb after being in fresh cold air for some time. It is < By the least contact of food either. hot or cold.
- Dr. H.T. Webster finds it a good medicine for warts.

Malandrinum

Dr. Chowdhury
- Allen advises not to use this remedy often then once in a fortnight, as it is deep acting one. It should be used both in preventive and during the attack,
- According to Burnett: The lower half of the body is affected. Greasy skin and greasy eruptions slow prostration never-ending healing one, another appears. Excluding Burnett, the following symptoms should be noted:

- Diarrhoea Acrid: Yellow offensive discharge followed by burning in the rectum and anus.

- Dark brown foul-smelling stools almost involuntarily pain in the abdomen may supervene.

- Black foul-smelling diarrhea with malaise and weariness.

- Child constantly handles the penis.

- Pain along the back as he was beaten.

- Soles of feet bathed in sweat, scald, and burn when covered or warm. Deep cracks, sore and bleeding, or soles of feet> by cold weather and after bathing. Restless sleep, dreams of troubles and quarrels.

Magnum Opus

Dr. Kent
Chilly patient

- It is preeminently a drug that causes a species of chlorosis, and it is suitable for chlorotic girls in the broken down constitution, waxy, anemic, pallid, sickly, and threatening, phthisis with necrosis and caries of bones and organic affection. There is a history of long periods of scanty menstruation or the menses have been delayed until the patient was 18 or 20 years of age.

- A strong feature is the greatest soreness of the periosteum, especially of the skin bones. The a tendency for ulceration and eruptions around these. There is thickening and infiltrations, chronic eruptions. Invertebrate like psoriasis.

- Repeated attacks of laryngitis, each leaving the patient in a worse state than before. T. B. that begins in the larynx.

- Aversion to food, no appetite, nothing will tempt him.

- The bones are sore from walking and Arnica relieves a day or two. But in this remedy, it is deep-seated and prolonged, and we would not think of Arnica, which would give relief only a day or so.

- Vesicular eruption infiltrating deep-seated with a tendency to crack and bleed, roughness of the skin, and psoriasis.

- Complaints < In cold damp weather and before storm.

- Anxiety and fear, great apprehensiveness, something awful is going to happen. Restless and anxious. The more he walks, the more he becomes anxious, and anxiety in the daytime while moving about > by lying down, sad. Weeping and silent nothing can console him to lay down and get peace. It is a good medicine for bedridden women who love to keep steel and it is said of them that they love to lie in bed.

- Agglutination of the eyelid eyelids. It is a suppurative and catarrhal remedy. The eyelids are swollen. Aching of the eyes on looking at near objects, especially a near light. Pain in the eyes from sewing, reading the fine print, and doing anything that would concentrate vision. Ruta is nervous gout constitutions, when there is pain in the eyes and complaints from sewing, and reading fine prints for a long time. It is especially for artists who work with reading glasses.

- Ears: Offensive discharge from the ears. Dullness of hearing > by blowing the nose. Stopped sensation > By blowing the nose, catarrh of the eustachian tube, the external ear is painful to touch, which seems to many patients that all their trouble settles in the ears. All the pains and aches in the upper part of the body settle in the ears. The pain in the throat shoots to the ears. Pain in the eyes, that centers in the ears. Catarrhal condition with increased deafness < During cold and damp weather he is deaf when the cold rains come in the fall, then there is soreness, rawness, and burning in the auditory canal with much itching.

- Silicea and Kali carb: These are the two principal remedies for the paroxysmal cough that comes on from scratching the auditory canal. But in. Maganum, itching in the ears from talking, swallowing, coughing, and doing anything that brings the throat into operation. It is sometimes present in laryngeal phthisis, in chronic ulceration of the larynx that shoot to the ears.

- It is just like Dulcamara, as their complaints < about damp cold air and weather.

- Small wound suppurate and every bruise remains sore for a long time. There is not much bleeding. There is not much blood.

- Colic pain in the abdomen. < In the damn cold weather. > by dabbling up. Cold things create much distress in the region of the liver, in the stomach and bowels.

- Cramps in the anus while sitting> laying down.

- Very scanty menstrual flow. It lasts for a day or two, and it comes too soon.

- It is a wonderful remedy for speakers and singers like Argent Met. Constant accumulation of mucus, more forms as soon as he clears it. Humming all the time and annoying everybody (Argent Met, Phosphorous, Siicea, Sulphur).

- The cough is > by lying down < during the day, from walking, laughing, talking, deep inspiration, and cold damp weather.

- The limbs are full of distress even to gout, sore bones, and burning in soles. Arthritic, enlargements, painful peritoneum, sore joints. It has rapid Inflammatory rheumatism like pulsatilla and Belladonna. But the tenderness of the joints with not much swelling and < From damp weather.

- This remedy does not usually come up in fevers. But in the case of low typhoid, after the fever is somewhat abetted, the bones are sensitive and sore all over.

Dr. Chowdhury

- All its symptoms are < at night time from cold In cold rainy weather and by change of weather.> From lying down in the open air. By eating and by swallowing.

- It has a particular affinity for the ankles and ankle joints. Many of the complaints of this remedy begin in the lower limbs and generally run upwards.

- Catarrhal deafness over the ears, it is also used in catarrh of the Eustachian tube with stitching pain and wheezing noise in the ears. The dullness of hearing is always > By blowing the nose and is < By cold damp rainy weather.

- Cough with an irritation is felt about the middle of the sternum > by lying down.

- Cough > by lying down. It can be compared with the following medicine.

- Ammon Mur: Coffee is caused by the tingling in the throat, whereas in many the tickling is felt deep down. Thick yellow matter is present. Stitches in the chest. Though its cough is. > By laying on back but < Or turning on the sides and always marked with a strange coldness between scapular.

- Euphrasia: The < Is more marked in the morning hours when the patient gets out of bed sometimes it is so harassing, that he has to lie down again for relief. Always > after eating. The cough comes only during the day, nor at night.

- Sepia: Its cough is found mostly in women suffering from uterine derangement < by walking fast.

- Zincum Met: Cough spasmodic in nature and is caused by a sensation of tickling in the larynx <after eating and drinking milk. We think of it particularly in that spasmodic variety of cough in children. When. During a fit of coughing, the infant automatically puts his hand on his genitals.

- Unhealthiness of the skin around the. joints very often we notice suppuration of the skin around the joints.

Mancinella
Dr. Chowdhury
- Its chief action is centered on the skin and throat. Intense redness of the skin with numerous small vesicles containing yellow serum, which desquamate on the following day. Large vesicles appear all over the body, and especially on the soles.
- Affection of the throat after scarlatina and past diphtheria ailments.
- Tongue coated white as in opthal.
- After drinking water, colic pain in the abdomen.
- When waking hands go to sleep and feel as if too thick.
- Icy coldness of hands and feet.

Medorrhium
Dr. Kent
- The infants soon emaciate and become marasmic, or a child becomes asthmatic or suffers from the vicious catarrh of nose or eyelids or has ringworm on the scalp or face, are dwarfed, and after some waste of time, it comes to mind that the father was treated with gonorrhea that was obstinate and perhaps had condylomata on the genitalia.
- The woman married several years ago desires to become a mother. She was healthy when she married, but now she has ovarian pains and menstrual troubles. She has lost all sexual response is going pale and waxy and becoming violently sensitive and nervous constant state of worry.
- The mental symptoms are < during night.
- The rheumatic inflammation is < from motion. But where swelling is not present, these patients act like the Rhus tox patients.

- Most psychotic patients suffer from colds, and some are sensitive to heat.

- Trembling and quivering, growing weaker, intense formication starts from the slightest noise, feels faint, and wants to be fanned. Extremely sensitive to cold damp weather subject to neuralgia, stitching, and tearing pains > by heat, the patient is extremely sensitive.

- Wandering neuralgia of the head < In cold damp weather, sharp pains come and go suddenly. No part of the head is free from pain. Intense itching of the scalp. Herpetic eruption on scalp, ringworm. Copious dandruff, hair dry and crispy.

- The mouth is full of canker sores and ulcers in the mouth and on the tongue. The breath is foul, string is mucous in the mouth and throat. The catarrh of the throat and thick white mucus are constantly drawn or drawn from posterior nets.

- Children of psychotic fathers are especially subject to attacks of vomiting diarrhoea and emaciates. They resist well-selected chronic remedies, but after giving Medorrhinum they improve.

- Sensation of coldness in the chest and mammae, stitching pain in the chest, the chest is sore to touch, and < by the motion of breathing. Burning in heart, extending to the left arm.

- Lame back is the common complaint of these patients, with pain across the back from left to right shoulder. Great heat in the upper part of the spine, stiffness in the back on rising or beginning to move< in cold damp weather tender spine. Burning palms and soles, trembling hands and arms, and burning palms, want them to be fanned. Right-hand cold, then the left.

- Legs cold up to knees. Contraction of muscles of the posterior part of the thigh down to the knee. Cramps in soles and calves, and burning feet want them to be uncovered and fanned. Legs swollen to knees and pit upon pressure. More bruised legs. Ankles and soles. sore and bruised. Look blue. He cannot walk on the soles, swelling, and itching of the souls. It cures the tenderness in the souls. So common in chronic gonorrhea, rheumatism, and tenderness of soles, that he had to walk on his knees, cold, sweaty feet.

- Sleep: Can sleep only on the back with hands over her head, and sleeps on her knees with her face forced into the pillow. Terrible dreams of ghosts and dead people sleepy, but cannot sleep. Sleep loss for part of the night.

Dr. Chowdhury

- Great pallor yellowness of the face, particularly around the eyes, as if occurring from a bruise. A yellow band across the forehead close to the hair, the greenish shining appearance of the skin, peculiar, serrated talk, offensive odor about the body, scaly, surfy, margins of the eyelids, and falling eyelashes are all characteristics of Medorrhinum.

- In Medorrhinum: The patient feels much better in sea sore, but Syphilis> takes place from high altitude.

- In dysmenorrhea, there is intense colic causing drawing up of the knees.

Dr. Tyler

- Coldness of the breast when the rest of the body is warm.

- Agonizing pain in the solar plexus, he applied his right hand to his stomach and left hand to the lumber region.

- Its cardinal symptoms are:

1) Better at seaside.

2) > laying on abdomen

3) > in wet weather

4) < daylight to sunset

5) Continuous watering from the ice sensation of sand under leads.

6) Can only pass tool by leaning far back. Very painful as if a lump on the posterior surface.

Melilotus

Dr. Chowdhury

- For congestive headache It can be compared with the following medicines:

- Ailanthus: Passive congestion of the head and > Buy nosebleed.

- Amyl Nitrosum: Marked congestive Headache and hemicrania But in this remedy, the affected side looks paler than the other.

- Belladonna: Has marked congestion of blood to the head. > The headache is not > by lying down but by sitting propped up.

- Ferrum Met: Congestion of the hand of people who are debilitated and anemic and is associated with sudden vertigo. The headache is momentarily > by pressure and entirely by open air.

- Gelsimium: Passive congestion of the brain and is associated with dizziness and blurring of vision before headache.

- Glonoine: Crushing weight across the forehead. This is mainly a sun headache, increasing and decreasing with the sun.

- Sanguinaria: Congestion is associated with dizziness in the head and is > By quiet rest in a darkened room from pushing the head deep into the pillow.

- Veratrum Viride: It is an excellent remedy when the congestion is most intense.

Mentha Piperita

Dr. Chowdhury

- It has marked action upon the respiratory organ.

- Hence it is remarkably helpful in cough caused by irritation of the respiratory passage.

- The voice is Husky, and the tip of the nose is sore to touch. The inhalation of smallest quantity of smoke at once induced the most distressing persistent cough. The least breadth of air and the slightest attempt at singing or speaking < the trouble.

Menyanthes Trifoliata
Dr. Chowdhury

- Its most prominent symptoms are general chilliness. This is felt in the head, ears, abdomen, feet, legs, and fingers. There is a sensation of chilliness felt even in the area of the esophagus. I have seen it as prescribed in various ailments on the simple indication of the extreme coldness of the nose.

- The next important indication is a sensation of tension. This tension is felt in the roof of the nose, arms, hands, fingers, and head, and, in fact, over the whole body. The skin fills tight. Everywhere it is a feeling as if he has been cramped and crowded into the tight fitting of his skin.

- Fidgetiness: Spasmodic jerking and physical twitching are found everywhere. These are always worse during rest as soon as the patient lies. His legs jerk and twitch so that he has to sit up. This spasmodic jerking is usually seen in gouty persons with deposits of Calcareous tissues in many of their joints. It has been used with great success in sciatica, where stitching and contractive pains are felt in the region of the hip joint, causing spasmodic jerking of the thighs and legs when in a sitting posture.

- It is generally adopted where there has been great abuse of quinine.

- The Chilliness is felt most severely on the back and. Back, and generally > By the warmth of the stove. As soon as he rises from his bed in the morning, he feels coldness creeping over his abdomen back, and sides of his hands and his feet are ice cold as if they have been kept immersed in ice water. There is shivering with the awning.

- These patients are ravenously hungry and show a marked desire for meat. Fingers and toes are cold, although the rest of the body retains its normal heat.

Mephities

Dr. Chowdhury

- The patients seem to have the power to withstand extreme cold. They thrive in cold weather, washing in ice water, very agreeable to them, and relieves all their suffering.

- The author met an elderly lady suffering from asthma, who gets relief from bathing, which. she would do it 5 or 6 times a day.

- They frequently wake up at night time suffering from a peculiar congestion of the legs, which gives them a sensation of heat in those parts. This brings on an easy feeling in the legs and makes them fidgety (Zinc).

- The patient is very talkative in nature (Lachesis, Strombomonas). They are led from subject to subject by the vividness of their fancy.

- The cough is brought on by reading aloud, talking, and drinking. (Rumex, Stricta, Phosphorous, Kali-bich, Ambra gresia).

- In Huffington, when the cathedral symptoms are more or less absent and spasmodic, symptoms are most prominent. The cough is < At night and after laying down and is attended with a suffocative feeling. Food has been taken hours before vomiting. It thus resembles. Drosera, Corallium rubrum.

Mercurius

Dr. Kent

- The breath especially is very fitted, and it can be detected upon entering the room. The perspiration is offensive. It has a strong, sweet penetrating odor. The perspiration is offensiveness and runs all through, offensive urine, and sweat. The odors from the nose and mouth are offensive.

- The glands are inflamed and swollen induration is also with general inflamed parts. If the skin is inflamed, it is hard. Inflammatory glands are hard. Induration with ulceration, ulcers, sting, and burn and have a lardaceous base. An ashy white appearance looking as if spread over with a coating of lard chancres that on that form. A whitish cheesy deposit on the base.

- With inflammation that is burning and stinging and the rapid formation of pus. < By both heat and cold. Abscess burn and sting.

- Steady emaciation with trembling < at night and warm up the bed. Great restlessness cannot find peace in any position. The sufferers may be psoric, syphilitic or psychotic.

- At times there is a gangrenous condition. This may be seen everywhere, especially on the lips, cheeks, and gums.

- A marked feature running all through is hastiness and hurried, restless, anxious, impulsive position, coming in spells in cold, cloudy weather, or damp weather. The mind will not work. It is slow sluggish and forgetful. He cannot answer questions right off looks and things. And finally, grasps it. Imbecility and softening of the brain are strong features. Desires to kill persons contradicting her, impulses to kill or commit suicide, anger with impulse to do violence.

- Head troubles that have come on from suppression. Discharges such as suppressed otorrhea after scarlet fever, or when there are head troubles in scarlet fever. If you are called to a child with sweating of the head, dilated pupils rolling of the head. < at night, for those who have had scarlet fever and suppressed ear discharges, it may cure lingering typhoid cases, but the history of suppressed ear discharge should be there.

- There is tension about the scalp as if it were bandaged. Nervous girls have headaches over the nose and around the eyes as if filled with a tap, or as if a tight were pressing the head, the catarrhal headaches are very troublesome. Headache in those suffering from chronic catarrh with thick discharge, the thick discharge becomes watery, and the pain in the forehead face, and ears, very distressing, chronic, rheumatic headache from the suppression of discharges from any part or foot sweat, suppressed alteration of foot, sweat, and headache. (Silicea)

- It is a wonderful remedy to ward off acute hydrocephalus after missiles and scarlatina. The child rolls the head and moons, and the head sweats. It is closely related to Apis.

- The whole external head is painful to touch. The scalp is tense and sore and filled with sweat on the head. Children have moist eczema and excoriating offensive eruption.

- Every cold settle in the eye in gouty and rheumatic patients. Cataracts of eyes < from looking into the fire, or rather sitting close to the fire. The radiating heat causes smartening. The rule nowadays is to use a mydriatic in iritis to prevent adhesion. I have. I have treated many cases, and I have no desire to dilate the pupil. Sometimes you will see a little fine growth on the iris. Growing across the pupil and attached by a pedicle. It is a syphilitic Condyloma.

- It is not deep enough to cure the whole constitution in certain cases that are constantly taking cold. It kicks off the cold at once, Kali iod Is the best for the same cold. Do not give many doses of Merc to psoriatic patients. Look for a deeper one.

- Aversion to meat, wine, brandy, coffee, greasy food, butter, milk disagrees and comes up sour, sweet disagrees.

- Merc, Ipecac, and Aconite are frequently indicated in epidemic dysentery in hot weather. Ipecac, Dulcamara, and Merc are frequently indicated in epidemics of cold weather.

Merc-Sol (Mercurius Solubilis)

Dr. Kent

- Itching of the genitals from the contact of the urine. It must be washed off in general. The genitals burn after urinating, and they are always carrying their hands to the genitals. Little girls have acrid leucorrhea, causing burning and itching and much trouble.

- Boils and abscesses at the menstrual period.

- A woman while pregnant has been eliminated. Stroking of the genitals, diffused inflammations, soreness, and fullness of the genitals and pelvis, cause difficulty in walking.
- She must take to bed with pelvic cellulitis in the early months of pregnancy.
- Merc is an important remedy. Repeated miscarriages from sheer weakness, prolonged lochia, milk's scanty and spoiled. It is one of the palliative for cancer of the breast.
- Jerking and quivering of the paralyzed parts.
- Rawness between the thigh and between the scrotum and thigh.

Dr. Chowdhury
- In toothache, he feels better by rubbing his cheek.
- It is a great hemorrhagic remedy, we think of it when the blood coagulates easily.
- Its most pronounced and prominent symptoms are tremors, trembling of the whole body, and even tremors of the tongue, is present. Thus it is a suitable medicine for paralysis patients.
- It is a good medicine for Syphilitic sores. the prepuce of glands, pains with a great deal of phthisis and pora- phimosis The chancres are indurated with a lardaceous cheesy base and inverted edges red. It spreads both in circumference and depth and secreting a yellow excoriating discharge.

Dr. Tyler
- It is notable, especially for its foulness and offensiveness of breath, of his profuse, saliva, of his drenching sweat, but curiously enough, stooled urine menses, Licoria are not especially offensive, excepting the stool in Markcore.
- Sweetest taste in the mouth.
- Green slimy accrete stool that. Excoriate the anus.
- Frequent sneezing without Coryza.

- A weight hanging from the nose.

- Mania throws off clothes at night, fears and scolds Leaps up high, talks and scolds much to herself. Does not know her nearest relationship. Frequently spits, spreads the saliva out of her feet, and licks some of it again, often like cow dung and mud of ponds. Takes little stones in her mouth without swallowing them, yet complains they're cutting her bowels. Does not. harm anyone but resist when touched. Does things she is told to do and while taking a walk she feels a strong inclination to catch passing strangers by the nose.

Mercurius Corrosivus

Dr. Kent

- It has more excoriating and burning.

- More activity and excitement. It is violent and active in its movement. In Merc Sol, we have slow spreading ulcer. But in Merc cor, there is great eating. It will spread over an area of large as a hand in in a night.

- In dysentery, there is more violence, copious blenching, and great anxiety, can scarcely leave the stool for a second.

- It is one of the most frequently indicated medicines for albuminuria in pregnancy, and a very useful remedy when gout is present.

- From the slight irritation of the foreskin of the male organ, the mucous membrane and the skin contract, and phimosis takes place.

Dr. Chowdhury

- It is good medicine for cyclitis, choroiditis, iridocyclitis, episcleritis retinitis, iritis, and peritonitis. Most of these troubles are syphilitic in origin.

- Its characteristic symptoms are faintness, weakness, and shuddering.

Mezereum

Dr. Kent

- The outer surface of the body is in constant irritation. Nervous feeling, biting, tingling, etching, changing place from scratching, even when there is nothing to be seen. There is violent etching at the patient rubs and scratches until the parts become raw and thin burns. The parts become cold after scratching, itching < in the warmth of the bed. It compels the patient to move and change position.

- Vesicular eruptions upon the skin running a certain course, itching, burning like fire. Dries into a crust and disappears, a new crops up near the same place.

- Eruptions with much itching, dark red rash with violent itching, biting, tingling, crawling, changing place by pressure, rubbing, or scratching. Cases with a history of suppressed eczema, or syphilis, are useful when eruptions have been suppressed by zinc ointment, mercurial, etc. Eruptions on the face, eyes, ears, and scalp in children or adults that have disappeared under the use of some ointment and in vertebrate catarrhal conditions have resulted, or in which eye symptoms have developed. Ear troubles from suppressed eruptions, thickening of the mucus membranes of the ears, degeneration of the drum of the ear, deafness, and diarrhoea. Any trouble in the nose and throat. Any trouble in the nose especially when there is a history of suppressed eruptions.

- If skin symptoms are.< by warm but its neuralgic parts or < by cold. The eruptions < by washing. When the eruptions are not out. The skin is hot and he wants something to cool He is better from cool water. There is simply a redness at this time.

- Sensation of goneness, fear, apprehend, faintness in the stomach as if something would happen, every shock, pain, and hearing bad news. It comes on when the doorbell rings. If the patient is expecting the postman in waiting for a friend or departure of the cars on being introduced to someone, he experiences a thrill, beginning in the stomach, is frightened in the stomach (calcarean, Kali carb, pulsatilla). These solar plexes individuals often have a deep cracked tongue and are hard to cure.

Dr. Chowdhury

- He takes no pleasure in anything everything seems to him dead, vanishing of ideas He looks through the windows for hours without being conscious of objects around. He forgets what he is about to say.

- A general unhealthiness is seen all over the body. The skin gets wrinkled and folds. Intense itching all over the body, as though. thousands of insects were creeping, scurfs like fish scales to be seen all over the back chest, thighs, and scalp. It is a first-rate remedy for itch-like eruptions, which appear after vaccinations for eczema. There is intolerable itching and copiousness severe exudations. The ulcers are extremely sensitive. A thick, yellowish scab and a band of vesicles appear around the ulcers.

- Its pains are very characteristic. Its pains are lightning. They come suddenly while talking or eating and disappear, leaving the part numb. This pain starts in the infraorbital foramen sometimes in the zygoma, travels to temple, corner of the mouth, and down the neck to the shoulder.

- It is an admirable remedy for certain types of constipation after confinement, it should be prescribed when. The stools are hard as stone and are immense in size. It feels as if they would spit the anus open. They keep coming in sections and exhaust the patient so that she trembles. The stools are preceded by chill and followed by long stitches in the rectum.

- Antim Crud: It is indicated in the constipation of old people and the stools are hard and the feces too large. Same as Mezereum, but it has suicidal despondency with quoted tongue anorexia and the dyspeptic condition is prominent.

- Apis Mel: Admirable remedy in chronic constipation, the stools are hard, large, and difficult to pass and are evacuated only once or twice a week. The feeling in the anus is as if it were stuffed full of heat and throbbing.

- Graphities: The stools, which are very large in size are passed with great difficulty and are covered with mucus. The. physician is rendered difficult by the fissured condition of the anus and the great dryness of the part.

- Lachesis: It has a large stool. The stools of legacy are simply enormous, while evacuation takes place the sprinter is nearly paralyzed. And after evacuation, they close very slowly. After evacuation, the patient feels as if 1000 hammers were beating inside the anus.

Dr. Tyler

- Its action is characterized throughout by violence. Violent itching, sudden violent pain in the face during sleeping, violent sensation of hunger, violent burning in mouth, violent pain in stomach and esophagus. Violent inclination to cough, violent acute fever, etc,

- It has annoying quieting of eyelids, twitching and jerking of muscles of the right cheek twitching of muscles in the pit of the stomach.

- Salty and pepper test, bitter and. Smartest. Especially beard taste, bitter and causes vomiting.

- It has a reputation for gastric ulcers and even induration and carcinoma. Constant desire to eat without hunger and take something into the stomach whereby he has less pain and nausea disappears after eating.

- Dr. Nash says "He once cured a very obstinate case of facial neuralgia with Mezereum worst by eating only relief was to hold face as near as he could to a hot stove". No other heat applied wet or dry relieved.

Mitchella Repens

Dr. Chowdhury

- Persistent hemorrhage from the uterus with frequent desire for urination, which was not very satisfactory (Dysuria hemorrhage).

- We also use it for false labor pains in the last month of pregnancy, when the pains are slow, feeble, and inefficient. It stimulates and completes labor.

Morphinum Muriaticum

Dr. Chowdhury

- Vertigo is very intense and it is felt from the slightest movement of the head. Everything turns dark and the patient becomes unconscious.

- It has a few important gastric symptoms, such as tympanitis and vomiting of green substance. Delusion of vision on closing his eyes he sees a man standing at the foot of the head, he also finds the room full of white and colored babies. Anxiety, restlessness, delirium, and terror make him cry out in alarm.

Moschus

Dr. Chowdhury

- A great indication for Moschus is his frequent tendency to faint, even from the least excitement.

- The nervous hyperesthesia is the most intense. Is manifested by extreme tremulousness and restlessness of the patient. She faints even when talking and eating. She's so prone to it that the slightest disturbance of her mental equilibrium or the least emotional changes brings on a state of fainting. Even the fragrance of a sweet flower has brought about this condition The most noted indication of Moschus for hysteria as well as for epilepsy and hystero- epilepsy is, however, a sensation of cold and shivering before and during such attack, the patient shudders as from a great chilliness, spasm of the larynx and spasm of the chest accompany these convulsive fits.

- Its mental symptoms are somewhat like Palladium. She cries one moment and bursts out the next in uncontrollable laughter. She is very frightened and exhibits a great dread of death.

- Quarrelsomeness, malic, and rage bring her to the same pedestal of ugliness as palladium. When angry she keeps it for a long time, an inner rage keeps on scolding her till her lips turn blue, stares, and she falls into a long spell of fainting.

- Under its action sexual desire to be greatly excited in both sexes and even in aged persons. It is a good medicine associated with diabetes. The patient emaciates daily and suffers from an. Insatiable thirst. Large quantities of urine, commencing sugar passed daily. Spasmodic crop in nervous children after punishment.

Dr. Kent

- It cures many historical girls who have come to adult age without ever learning what obedience means. They are. Self-willed obstinate and selfish.

- One cheek red and cold the other pale and hot. It indicates certainly some historical perversion mind of the patient.

- Very sensitive to cold and complaints < from cold.

- Let things fall from her hands.

- Fear of laying down least she died .

- Vertigo on moving head or eyelids > In open air with nausea vomiting and fainting.

- Craves for beer and brandy. Aversion to food, the sight of it makes her sick, fainting during meals.

- Involuntary stool during sleep. copious watery stool during the night, stitching in the anus to the bladder. Copious colorless watery urine. Urine passed during the night is offensive and full of mucus. Violent sexual excitement, emission without erection.

Millefolium

- A hemorrhagic patient should have a dose of a Millefolium or Lachesis before having teeth extracted.

- A woman predisposed to hemorrhage should have a dose of Millefolium before going into confinement.

- Oppression of chest, palpitation, surging of blood from chest to head.

Dr. Chowdhury
Another name for this plant is nose-bleed.

Murex Purpurea

Dr. Chowdhury

- It is used in ovarian cyst prolapses, Dysmenorrhea, carcinoma uteri, and in bad effects of abortion.

- It is just like Sepia, but the difference is as follows:

- Murex: Excessive sexual desire. Excited by the slightest desire.

- Sepia aversion to intercourse.

- Murex: Profuse and excessive hemorrhage, during this period of hemorrhage, she passes large clots and blood coagula. It is an important remedy for hemorrhage during climaxis.

- Sepia: The flow is always scanty.

- It has a distinct sensation in the womb as in Helonias, but the patient is constantly aware of a heavy substance dragging about the pelvic cavity. It is more a sensation of bearing down than anything else. It has a sinking and all-gone sensation in the abdomen.

- It is an admirable remedy in the prolapses of the uterus when displacement is associated with sore pain in the uterus. The pain extends upwards from the right side of the uterus and crossing the body goes to the left mammae. Sometimes the uterus feels as if it is cut by a sharp instrument, this myalgia pain in the uterus generally comes on when the patient is in bed and is > by sitting up or walking about. In this respect, it can be compared with Lilly Hgh but in Lilly Hgh the pain originates from the mammae, traversing downwards to the uterus.

- Greenish irritation discharge but it generally comes in the daytime and disappears at night.

- Constant desire to urinate. She has to rise several times in the course of the night to pass water.

Muriatic Acid

- When treating a low form of continued fever with extreme prostration, we should think of Arsenic, there has been anxious and restlessness. With phosphoric acid, there has been the mental Frustration and with the muriatic acid, the muscular weakness comes first. And there has been history of restlessness, and the mind has been stronger than could be expected. With this great muscular exhaustion, with. Jaw hanging down, and the patient. Sliding down in red and soon the involuntary story and urine.

- The Vertigo comes on moving the eyes on laying on right side. This Vertigo is sometimes associated with the liver disease > by lying on left side.

- Burning extending right to left eyes > washing. Itching in the eyes.

- The nose is top nose bleed in pooping cough in Zymotic fever in diphtheria and scarlet fever.

- Great thirst during Chile and thirstless during. Fever aversion to meet emptiness in stomach from 10:00 AM till evening. Emptiness in abdomen in the morning after the usual normal stool.

- Heaviness of arms, numbness of coldness of fingers at night. Lower limbs dusky, putrid ulcers on legs with burning margins, swelling of right Tendo Achilles feet cold and blue, burning of palms and sores, swelling and burning of tips of toes, peering in limbs > By motion. Pain in the limbs during intermittent fever.

- Perspiration during first sleep symptoms< when perspiring.

Dr. Chowdhury

- Unconsciousness with constant moaning.

- Pain in the stomach while talking.

- Like Nitric acid, Muriatic acid is powerful antidote to Murietic and it meets condition caused by Mercury also similar condition otherwise arise. Like other disinfectants, it causes as well as remedies.

- Rapid decomposition of tissues and dynamically cures low putrid condition met with in disease.

- It not only corresponds to low febrile states it also meets many of their sequel. Deafness otitis and glandular swelling about the ears often require Muric acid.

- Jerking, beating, tearing pain from the left half of the occiput to the forehead soon followed by similar pain in the right half.

- When writing a spasmodic pain like cramp, on the ball of the right thumb which went off on moving it.

Myrica Cerifera

Dr. Chowdhury

Itching of the whole body during jaundice.

- There is a constant aching pain in the liver immediately below the ribs.

- The tongue is thickly lined with yellowish white coating, bitter taste, offensive breadth, and want of appetite.

- Yellowness of the skin, dark-colored urine.

- Drowsiness, tenacious, thick, and nauseous secretion in the mouth.

- Extreme lassitude, jaundice, and pain under the scapula are clear-cut indications.

- It is good medicine for cancer of the liver (I.J.H.71-25).

- It produces abundant secretions of tough tenacious mucus.

Myrtus Communis

- Its chief indication consists in the sharp stitching pains in the upper portion of the left lung, going right through from the front of the left scapula < On taking a deep breath, yawning, and coughing.

- This Indication is used in phthisis and pneumonic affections. The cough is dry and hollow and caused by tickling in the upper interior of the lobes.

Alphabet

Naja Tripudians

Dr. Kent

- The patient is disturbed by the coldness of the collar < after sleep. There is exhaustion and trembling, trembling of the muscles His direction is somewhat like Lachesis from left to right. For example, ovarian pains, diphtheria, and joint affections go from left to right, like Lachesis < In damp weather or on inflamed surfaces, it produces grayish exudation. Naja is not as subject to hemorrhage as either Lachesis or Crotalus.

- There is trembling of muscles aromatic diathesis and a tendency of all complaints to settle about the heart. It is used in valvular troubles of the heart in young persons who grow up with cardiac valvular diseases If the valvular trouble is congenital, it can be cured in school boys and girls who have no symptoms. This is the genetic remedy for this kind of complaint. Always prescribe Naja unless guided away from it by some specific symptoms. It is more nervous but Lachesis has more septic symptoms and a tendency to hemorrhage and sepsis.

- There is much sneezing with running up of water from the nose, inability to lie down at night, and dryness of the air passages of the nose here. Knows hay fever. The patient has a suffocative attack in August.

- The whole state is in a state of congestion, emptiness of the left side of the chest. Low pulse or intermittent pulse with all the complaints of the chest that is inability to lie down on the left side. Numbness of the left arm, there is dyspnea. If you go to sleep, he wakes up with suffocating.

- There is a dry hacking cough with sweating of palms. The extremities are cold and blue, and the head hot copies sweating of the hands and feet. But the sweat is not offensive. There is a sense of fullness and puffiness of the hands and feet showing a slow circulation in the veins.

- Deep profound sleep with strenuous breathing.

- Naja has all the symptoms of lactose, except the following. Acute stitching paints that go right through the chest from the precordium to the region of the scapula are associated with very marked numbness. Where that numbness is pronounced, one would give Naja in presence in. preference to lactases. Stitching pain is more marked in NASA, but in legacies, the feeling of constriction is predominant (Borland).

- She wakes with a headache every morning. < By exhaustion.

- It has rawness in the throat and larynx, dreadful aching in the throat, extending to the larynx, which is not > By swallowing but the legacies. The state is expressed more by a lump in the throat.

Dr. Chowdhury

- The drug has a strong affinity for the medulla oblongata and cerebellum.

- The sensation of hot iron running through the chest and the sensation of heavyweight has been verified repeatedly by several pro-overs. Constrictions and pressure of the throat. A sensation of choking, spasmodic stricture of the esophagus, and dyspnea. Fluttering of the heart, and stitching pain in the region of the heart are always to be remembered.

Natrum Carbonicum

Dr. Chowdhury

- It has a very marked irritating action over the skin and mucous surface of the body, the skin of the whole body becomes dry, rough, and cracked in places, and itching with a sensation of formication is always present. Eczema, herpes, words, and ulceration are everywhere present.

- It has ulceration on the heels, but in Lycopodium, ulceration on the in steps, rather than on the heels.

- The most important feature is a strong bearing down feeling, as if everything would come out. This is partly due to the passive congestion of the uterus noticed particularly during and after coitus > Rubbing is an important characteristic of Natrum Carb. It is used in weak and efficient labor pains having been guided to it by great desire on the part of the patient to be rubbed while in pain. It expels moles or the product of false conceptions.

Dr. Kent

Chilly patient

- Persons who are in the habit of taking carbonate soda, have old dyspeptics, are always belching, and have sour stomachs and rheumatism. After 20 years, they are stoop-shouldered, pale, sensitive to cold, chilly < by list draft require much clothing, unable to register the cold or heat, require a medium climate, a state of trepidation, from the slightest noise, the slam of a door, weakness from slight exertion of mind and body. The rattling off. paper causes palpitation, irritability, and melancholy. Separate from family and friends. Aversion to mankind and society, feeling a great diversion between himself and them. Music causes a tendency to suicide. Great weakness with an increase of religious insanity. < from the slam of a door, a pistol shot, which causes headache and complaints in general < many symptoms from drinking cold water when overheated.

- Urine offensive like that of a horse from a vegetable or milk diet.

- It throws out eruptions upon the knuckles and fingertips, as well as the toes and vesicular eruptions open up and form ulcers on the joints or fingertips (Borax, Sepia. Arsenic). Vascular eruption on the body in patches and circles. The herpes family is especially related to Natrum carb, the herpes is as large as a dollar on the hips, thighs, and back. Smaller patches show vesicles containing a white serum burning. Smarting and itching> from scratching the eruption passes away with a crust, but will often ulcerate.

- Bookkeepers lose the ability to add figures in reading a page. The one previous to it soon goes out of the mind. The memory will not hold out from the beginning to the end of the sentence. Confusion of mind follows, and then he is unable to perform any mental labor.

- Leucorrhea <, by coition.

- The body troubles are < from cold and in winter. As if he had no blood in his body. Extremities are cold, and he cannot get them warm. Cold as ice to knees and elbows, the body and extremities are < In winter and head in summer.

- Anxious trembling and sweating during pains.

- Its catarrh, discharges are usually thick, yellow, and purulent. And the discharges are commonly offensive.

- Almost a constant headache over the eyes in the forehead at the root of the nose, congestive headache < from the change of weather, cold room, damp weather increases by every storm, most fetid edema, mucus membrane ulcerated and destroyed.

- There is puffiness in general, the hands, feet, face, pit on pressure. Infiltration of the cellular tissues.

- Thrush in infants, little white aphthous patches, especially in nervous withered infants who cannot stand any kind of milk > By eating when chilly, he eats and can keep warm. The pains are > by eating he has an all gone feeling and pain in the stomach, which. drives him to eat. He gets hungry at 5:00 AM and 11 PM.

5 AM is the favorite time for its <. He becomes so hungry at this time that he is forced out of bed to eat something. Headache, palpitation, and chilliness > from eating.

- Prostatorrhea after urinating and a difficult stool.
- Sterility, she's unable to conceive and is cold to knees and elbows. Cold body in winter and hot body in summer. Relaxation of the sphincter vagina, causes a seminal fluid to gush out as soon as ejected by the male. She is a dyspeptic woman, but not hysterical.
- Menses Is too soon or too late.
- Palpitation at night when ascending and while lying on the left side. Pains in the hollow of knees on motion. Ulceration of the heel from blisters.
- Nervous hunger in pregnant women who cannot sleep.

Some other symptoms
- The patient cannot bear any change in diet (H.G. Nov 73). In labor pains, the patient wants to be rubbed, which seems to relieve her.
- She's full of anxiety with tremors and perspiration during every pain. She will often say rub me, rub me.
- Headache if he delays his meal (Sulphur) but not > from eating, < from eating (Antimonium crudum).
- The greedy nibbling (eats little at a time) nervously exhausted patient.

Natrum Muriaticum

Dr. Kent
Hot patient

- It is a deep and long-acting medicine and requires much time to manifest its action.

- Unrequired affection, she is unable to control her affection and falls in love with a married man or coach, though she thinks it is foolishness.

- Aversion to bread, fat and rich things.

- Both Natrum carb and Natrum Mur have vesicular eruptions, but the former is chilly and later is hot patient.

- It's discharges from the mucous membrane is watery and thick, whitish like the white of an egg. There is gluey oozing from the edges from the ears flows a thick white discharge.

- Pain in the head < From 10:50 AM till 3:00 PM.< In the later part of the night, she sleeps late in the night and wakes on the later part of the night, having pain in the head> From sleeping and sweating. Sometimes all the pain seizes from sweating, except headache, sometimes greater the pain in the head, more the sweating, but sweat does not >.

- In spinal trouble when there is great sensitiveness to pressure and irritable spine the vertebrae are sensitive. And there is a great deal of aching along the spine < From coughing and walking> From lying. On something hard or pressing the back against something hard. They may sit with a pillow or the hand rest against the back.

- In menstrual trouble the woman lying with some hard object under the spine.

- The stomach is distended with flatus after eating. There is a lump in the stomach. It seems to take a long time for to food to digest. < from eating > from vomiting of whitish slimy mucus. There is a great thirst for cold water.

- There is a great variety of menstrual complaints too scanty, too free, too soon or too late.

- Condition of pregnancy: Wasting of the mammae gland. The uterus intensely sore, the Leucorrhea, which is at first white turns green, there is pain during sexual intercourse. Dryness of vagina,

- a feeling as though sticks are pressed into the walls of the vagina, pricking pains.

- Useful after labor, when the mother does not progress well, the lochia is prolonged, copious and white. The hair falls out from the head and genitals. The milk passes away. Useful in after pains, when there is subinvolution of uterus.

- The cut finger bleeds only water.

- Awkwardness characteristics, all their movements like Apis and Bovista they feel nervous. Drop things and break them.

Dr. Chowdhury

- The headache is sometimes violent and maniacal. During the maniacal headache the tongue becomes dry and cling to the roof of the mouth and the pulse becomes intermittent.

- Displacement of uterus is a common factor every morning after getting up the peering down becomes. So accentuated that they have to sit to prevent prolapses. This is accompanied by this backache is so troublesome that they have to lie down on their back or press a pillow against it to obtain relief. A characteristic urinary symptom that generally accompanies this prolapse is an increased desire to urinate. The suffer weakness of the bladder. In consequence of this, they suffer from involuntary. Escape of urine every time they cough. Cough, sneezing or in any other way, exert themselves. Urine flows instantly negotiating frequent, frequent change of clothes.

- In the female sexual system, there is diminished sexual appetite. This loss of desire sometimes amounts to a regular aversion to Coitus. This may be partly due to grid dryness of the vagina, which renders the act painful and coughing, smarting and burning after act.

- Aversion to bread, meat and coffee and desires bitter things. There is a distress in the stomach after eating > from tightening of the clothes.

- She is constantly weeping and does not know why she is weeping.

Dr. Tyler
- Burnett's Nat-Mur was a very chilly patient with special coldness of knees. Coldness of legs, knees to feet. This chilliness over and over again disappeared after taking Natrum Mur, muddy urine or urine very pale. He found that Natrum Mur will clear the urine.
- Lachrymation with headache, great lachrymation is a feature of this remedy.
- Great longing for bitter things beer or bitter things or farinaceous food, sour, salty, oysters or fishes.

Other Symptoms
- Wasting is the result of demineralization. Every demineralization is due to an intoxication. If there is wasting without apparent reason and without the patient being a tuberculum, think of cancerinic. Demineralization may be autogenous (Psorinum). Give Natrum Mur and weight is restored. If not restored, then immediately start treatment of cancerinic state.
- The patient wants to bathe, every time he perspired, warm patient, craving for salt, perspiring profusely with constipation.
- She sheds tears in solitude.
- It is a good medicine for long standing chronic diarrhoea. The patient is usually an elderly person. A brownish or yellowish complexion with fullness and discomfort in the gastric region. Following this, there develops a diarrhoea which comes on early in the morning as soon as the patient moves in. an attempt to arise, the desire is sudden and urgent, necessitating with utmost haste on the part of the patient.
- The stools are thin and watery without form and yellowish or brownish in color as a rule, there are three or four stools in early morning or four noon, and as many more during afternoon and

evening, but very seldom, if ever any at night, unless the patient has been very in. discrete during her evening meal, the stool is re practically painless.

- He cannot forget the evil someone has done to him. He went on thinking about revenge.
- It is a good medicine for biting finger nails.

Natrum Phosphoricum
Dr. Chowdhury

- On waking in the morning, the patient experiences an acid taste in the mouth, which practically persists throughout the day. Sour eructation and sour vomiting are also frequent. The stool and perspiration smell of acid. It is a good medicine for chronic dyspepsia.
- Golden yellow creamy coating of the roof of the mouth and back part of the tongue.
- A diarrhoea, especially in children with green sour-smelling stool caused by an excess of acidity is a frequent occurrence. Flatulent colic, vomiting of curdled masses, much straining of stool. A constant urging to stool with the passing of jelly-like masses of mucus,
- Pricking up the nose.
- Itching at the anus.
- Inability to retain urine.
- Sensation of hair at the tip of the tongue.
- Dropping of the thick yellow mucus from the posterior nerves.
- Consumption characterized by an intense acidity of the expectoration, so much to cause soreness of the lips and rawness of the tongue and mouth. A similar acidity also secrets from the uterus and causes sterility.

- Leucorrhea with watery creamy yellow acid discharge causing itching, rawness, and soreness of the part found in Natrum Phos, a speedy cure. The discharge smells sour and sickening.
- Inflammation of the eyes when there is a golden yellow creamy matter. The eyes are glued together in the morning with a creamy discharge.
- Like Cina, Natrum Phos is highly efficacious.
- Ailments from worms.

Dr. Tyler

- Pain based at heart > by pains by limbs and the great toe or vice versa.
- Eczema, which symptom of acidity.
- Ulceration of stomach pain in one spot after food face red, blotched, yet not feverish.
- Sclerosis of the liver and hepatic form of diabetes, especially where there is a succession of boils.
- Colic in children with symptoms of acidity, green sour-smelling stool, and vomiting of curdled milk.

Dr. Kent

- The tongue is quoted yellow. Yellow at the base or dirty white. The roof of the mouth is coated golden, yellow, or creamy.
- Urging to urinate at night after coition, emission of prostatic fluid during stool seminal emission after coition without dreams, without erections.
- Cold hands, legs and feet. Ice cold during menses in the daytime, burn at night in bed. Contraction of extensor in the forearm while writing.
- Sore stinging corns.

Natrum Salicylicum

Dr. Chowdhury

- Giddiness associated with intense tinnitus ovarium and deafness.
- It is a good medicine for dyspnea.
- He gasps like fish out of water This later symptom also.
- Aids to its application in those types of chronic bronchitis where life becomes an agony. Mostly due to the intensity of dyspnea that practically chokes life out of him every second. of his existence.

Natrum Sulphuricum

Dr. Kent

Hot patient

- This is one of our most frequently indicated constitutional remedies. The symptoms appear in the morning, evening, and during the night, especially before midnight complaints < In the wet weather it especially belongs to patients with neuropathic and bilious constitutions. He suffers from universal catarrh and the discharge is generally greenish.
- Strong desire for open air and feels better by it.
- A woman during gestation attempted several times to hang herself, after this remedy she was cheerful, and there was no disposition of suicidal disposition, cheerful after stool.
- Sadness in the morning, which passes off after breakfast. Extremely irritable in the morning. Violent anger, which is followed by jaundice, and fear of a crowd, of evil people, startling from light or noise and in sleep.
- The pains are < From thinking of them and > by pressure laying down an open air.

- Complaints < on the right side, heat on the right ear, evening catarrh on the right ear. Stopped sensation in the right ear. Purulent discharge from right ears.

- Pain in the liver from laying on the right side. Dragging in the right hypochondriac region. When lying down (Natrum Mur, Carduus Mariannus, Ptelea) sores and itching on the liver while walking. Sharp pains in the liver on deep inspiration. The liver is disturbed by mental exertion and anger. It causes the liver to make healthy bile, which is natural. In the event of gall stones, when given at long intervals, it has removed gall stones in many cases.

- Sensitive to clothing over the hypochondria.

- Distress and emptiness in the abdomen. > by passing flatus and by eructations, cramps, and many pains from obstructed flatus, pain, and distension in the ascending colon. Pain in the region of the. sacrum. It has cured many cases in the first stage of appendicitis. Feeling in the abdomen, as if a diarrhoea would come on > by eructation and passing flatus. Distress in the abdomen that hurries him to stool, but only flatus passes.

- It has cured sugar in the urine and polyuria. Urine loaded with bile.

- Tendency to suppuration around the nails. It has cured cases. Bad cases of psoriasis of the palms, and ulceration. Pain under the nails and in the tips of the fingers. Pain in the right hip joint or motion. Stitching on the left hip. Pain in the hip extending to the knee. Sciatica by motion.

- Drowsiness in the forenoon while reading. Chili from 6 to 9:00 AM with fever, then dry heat until 1 am.

- It has been the epidemic remedy in cerebrospinal meningitis, with pain in the back of the head and neck, and the head was drawn backward, piercing pain between the scapulae in the evening while sitting, and tenderness of the spine. Sore pain in the small back and sacrum pain in the small of the back during the night, compelling her to lie on the right side. It passes away in the morning.

Dr. Chowdhury

- Violent pain felt in the great depth of the brain, and it feels as if the bones at the base of the brain were crushed. A great deal of congestion is felt in the brain, and there is often bleeding from the nose associated with great heaviness of the head. It is a good medicine for salivation with headache. During a headache, her mouth used to get full of saliva, coughing. to spit continuously.

- Stool: The stool Starts after he gets up in the morning and begins to move. The urging is sudden, and the gushing is accompanied by flatulence. There is quite a great deal of rumbling in the bowels due to flatulence. This rumbling is mostly located on the right side of the abdomen in the ileocecal region. The stools are dark, bilious, or, greenish. The stools are involuntary while passing flatus or urine or during sleep. Before stool, we notice a contractive pain in the abdomen extending to the chest, violent colic, as if pinching and a good deal of rumbling characteristics of the stool.

- Better and cheerful after stool.

- Disagrees with bread and desires for ice cold water.

- Looseness of bowels with each asthmatic attack.

- Fever.: Any kind of fever with icy coldness of the limbs, absence of thirst in all stages bilious vomiting and < in wet weather.

- Dr. S.M.Peace cured An intermittent fever with the following indication when the patient took off his boat at night, the ball of the right great toe invariably itched.

- His dreams are mostly about fight.

Dr. Tyler

- Its chest troubles are < early in the morning from 4 to 5 am.

- Cannot digest starchy food milk and potatoes. (Aloe)

- Nosebleed before and after Menses.
- Thirst for something cold desires for ice or ice-cold water.
- Flatulence, colic, and flatus passed with difficulty causing bellyache and bruised pain, waking her at 2 am.
- Cannot bear tight clothing about the waist.
- Excruciating pain in the right hip joint. < Stooping and from some motion when stretching or walking feels nothing. Most felt when rising from a seat or moving in the bed.

Niccolum Metalicum

- It is a good cough medicine.
- When the patient coughs, he must sit up and hold the head with both hands or else the shooting pain in the head becomes agonizing. This would very naturally suggest Bryonia but minute analysis suggests that it is not holding up the head that > but the act of sitting up. That is > another peculiarity of this cough is that the patient puts arms on their thighs while coughing.

Nitric Acid

Dr. Kent
Chilly patient

- Old scars become painful in cold weather and when the weather changes.
- The discharges are thin, bloody offensive, and excoriating. Sometimes a dirty yellowish green, strong odors from the body.
- Anger from trembling starts from fright on falling asleep.

Nitric Acid

- The whole mental state is from riding in a carriage.
- Subject to Coryza every winter violent pain in the throat extends to the ear on swallowing.

- Longing for fat pungent things herring, chalk, lime, earth, aversion to bread and meat. Generally thirstless.

- The relaxed condition in weekly infants and boys that so much disposes to inguinal hernia is often overcome by Nitric- Acid and the hernia cured.

- Itching and burning anus. Constant acrid moisture about the anus. periodical bleeding in the rectum and pain in the sacrum. The piles are so painful, that she breaks out in sweat.

- Ulcers that destroy the frenum. Paraphimosis and phimosis and great swelling. The female is greatly troubled by the constant itching and burning and sexual desire.

- In T.B with night sweats and hemoptysis. The pulse is rapid and irregular and every fourth beat is missed.

- Pain in the back, nights, compelling to lie down or abdomen. Sharp pains in the back on coughing.

- Emaciation of upper eyes and thigh.

- It is a good medicine for fever. They are thirstless during all stages, with cold hands and feet. Copious night sweats are taken into account.

Dr. Chowdhury

- Extreme fetid and corrosive discharges are the characteristics of this remedy.

- In the acute primary stages. We have flat suppurating ulcerations which are irregular in shape and zigzig edges. The least touch or movement cause bleeding from it. In some of the cases, we notice sloughing of the entire integuments of the penis, which leaves the organ entirely divided.

- In the female's similar destruction of the tissues is also seen. The pubic region has sloughed away, leaving the muscular structure entirely bare. Its ulcers are spreading in circumference but not in depth.

- He must stand and press a long while before urine appears, but once the stream starts it comes uninterruptedly.
- The liver is seriously affected, as a result of which we have obstinate jaundice.
- With this there is persistent diarrhoea. The discharge from the bowels is offensive, green, and watery. They frequently contain long pieces of mucus.

Dr. Tyler

- The patient is chilly, depressed, indifferent, intolerant of sympathy.
- Sensitive to noise, pain, touch, joy.
- Irritable, suspicious, obstinate, restlessness.
- Fears death.
- Aggravation from wind, thunder, and wet.
- Desires fat and salt.
- Profuse sweat of hands and feet.
- Profuse falling of hair, especially vertex, from congestion of blood to scalp from syphilis.
- Wakes at 2'0'clock- every night and is unable to fall asleep again.

Nux Moschata

Dr. Kent
Chilly patient

- The patient appears to be dazed. There is complete loss of memory.
- She is automatic in her motion actions.

- She goes about the house, performing her duties, but if interrupted forgets what she has been doing, forgets that she was already in conversation with her son.
- She has no collection of past events.
- This is a singular state of mind, sometimes found in hysterical women.
- She lies with eyes closed and yet knows everything that is going on, but remembers nothing.
- She speaks with intelligence about the things of the moment but knows nothing of the past.
- In coma of typhoid and intermittent fever, they give an answer, that has no relation with the correct answer.
- Faintness even fainting when standing long, such as occurs in a nervous woman standing to have a dress fitted.
- The hemorrhages stand out in bold relief.
- Hemorrhages from the nose, uterus, and bowels.
- There is vomiting of blood.
- Often there is a sensation of dryness even when that is moist
- In women the breasts are flat.

Dr. Tyler

- Dryness, drowsiness, and chilliness with a tendency to faint.
- Sensation as if all vessels were pulsating, especially in the head. A throbbing, pressing pain, confined to a small spot, principally to the left supra-orbital ridge.
- Vomiting, spasmodic during pregnancy from irritation, pessaries, acid, and stomach flatulence.

Dr. Chowdhury
- The sight of blood, even standing for a long while, a strong odor of flowers or scents, and slight emotional disturbances will cause the patient to swoon away.
- The tendency to swoon or faint is more marked after stool.
- It is good medicine for chronic diarrhoea during pregnancy.

Hering reports a case of impending abortion in a female after six months of pregnancy due to a severe kick in the lower part of the abdomen from a child who was sleeping with her. Nux Moschata stopped the semi-sanguineous, foul-smelling discharges from the vagina which was accompanied by a strong bearing down pain. Abortion looking almost imminent.

Nuphar Luteum

This medicine is 1st proved by Dr. Pitet

- Weakness of the sexual sphere.
- There is an entire absence of erection of sexual desire. Volumptous ideas fill the imagination but do not cause excitement.
- The penis is retracted and the scrotum is relaxed.
- Involuntary seminal loses is frequent during sleep.
- We also notice involuntarily emission during stool or when urinating.
- It is also a great remedy for entro colitis.
- The stools are extremely yellow.
- It also has morning diarrhoea like what we find in Sulphur quite early, long before it is time for the patient to get up in the morning.
- He experiences intense urging which obliges him to go to the bathroom.

- He gets two or three passages of liquid yellow stool and no more till the next morning.

Nux Vomica

Dr. Kent
Chilly patient

- Hemorrhages occur at a certain time every day.
- The patient of Nux Vom is oversensitive to medicine.
- Suppose a person is oversensitive to a drug, maybe as a result of previous poisoning aggravating it, and every time it is administered, he suffers too much.
- A dose or two removes the sensitiveness.
- When all medicine disagrees, Nux Vom will cure the morbid sensitiveness and other troubles.
- Some symptoms are aggravated by cold like piles, asthma.
- It is the medicine when the patient thinks that something should come out by an anger outburst.
- In children's jaundice, start with Nux Vom 6 or 30 followed by Chelidonium.
- Very often Natrum Sulphuricum patient cough compels the patient to hold the abdomen.
- Patients are never contented, never satisfied, and disturbed by their surroundings and they become irritable so that they want to tear things, to scold.
- Impulsive are strongly marked at times.
- The woman has impulses to destroy her husband or to throw her child into the fire.
- The impulses are intermingled with a violent temper. Cannot be contradicted or opposed.
- If a chair is on the way, she kicks it over.

- While undressing if a part of his clothing should catch on a button he would pull it off, because he is so mad at it.

- Skin oversensitive to touch to draft.

- Full of pains and aches.

- He sweats easily on the slight provocation.

- A drawing on the back like a pulling or tension in the muscles.

- A drawing pain in the back and neck forcing the patient to let the head go back.

- Drawing pain down the spine, lumbago.

- Backache as soon as he lies down as if it would break (Bryonia, Phosphorus), must get back to walking.

- Pain in the region of the kidneys and liver.

- Pains draw so that he cannot turn over in bed. The only way he can get over is to lift himself up by his hands and then turn over and lie down.

- Drawing pain in the sacrum in connection with dysentery.

- Cannot bear reading or conversation, irritable, and wishes to be alone.

- Nux is an old dyspeptic, lean, hungry, withered, bent forward, prematurely aged. Always selects his food and digests almost none.

- Aversion to meat. It makes him sick.

- Craves bitter, pungent things and tonics.

- Sensitive to least draft.

- Sneezing caused by itching in the nose. This itching goes to the throat and trachea.

- Dry teasing cough with great soreness of the chest.

- Sharp liver and sweat or a hot sweat like opium.

- Thirst is not a marked feature.
- Sometimes it is found in the treatment, tendency to jaundice in all the febrile stages.
- The minutest touch of the throat causes urging.
- It is given as a routine medicine for the decrease in appetite (decreases after eating. Graphites, Kali bromatum, Nux Vom) IJH. 70-64.
- Heat on the head when eating.
- Diarrhoea from leaving off beer (Aloe)
- In chronic cases Sepia is more apt to be indicated and follows Nux Vom well.
- It is closely related to Sulphur and often antidotes the overaction of Sulphur.
- One menstrual flow is prolonged to the other.
- Useful to persons who say they have asthma from every disorder stomach.
- Asthma associated with cough, rattling in the chest, chest fills up with mucus.
- Cough with gasping, and retching, appears as if he had taken a fresh cold.
- Coryza every time he disorders his stomach.

I have a patient, who has coryza every time she eats sausage.

Dr. Chowdhury

- Nux patients are always in the front rank of all enterprises and in consequence, they generally occupy the topmost places in all occupations and all departments of life.
- They are the topmost scientist, best doctors, best lawyers, the commercial managers.

- These are the people who are bidding high to buy the universe with their whole life, body, and entity.
- They never pause and they never think of the enormous price they are paying for their success.
- It has violent headaches. It is generally felt in the morning on waking as if they did not sleep well at night.
- Sometimes it is described as a feeling of confusion, and stupefaction aggravated by eating, exposure to open air, mental exertion, anger, chagrin, menstruation, constipation, and debauchery aggravated from warm room, from pressure and wrapping of the head.
- The diarrhoea generally comes on in the morning, after rising from bed or immediately after eating some food.
- The stools are either papescent or watery, sometimes frothy and sour. Intense backache is felt before and during stool.

Dr. Tyler

- It seems as if he would like to strike anyone in the race who speaks a word to him. So irritable in his disposition.
- Aching pain in the occiput in the morning, immediately after rising from bed.
- Cough which brings on headache as if the skull would burst.
- Short pressive pain in the rectum after a stool and after a meal especially on exerting the mind and studying.
- The slightest touch of the hand immediately brings a spasm.

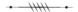

Alphabet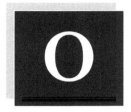

Ocimum Canum
Dr. Chowdhury

- It has calculable value in. renal colic due to calculus where the symptoms are. excruciating. crampy pain in the region of the kidney with violent vomiting every few minutes.
- The patient twists and turns in agony and wrings her hands with the intensity of colic.
- Urine is thick and purulent with an intolerable smell of musk.
- Often it is full of brick dust sediment indicating the presence of blood.
- It is a good medicine for bilious remittent fever. Dr. Biswas of Pabna who experimented with it extensively found it an admirable remedy for those types of bilious fevers that were accompanied by slight catarrh or congestion of the bronchial tubes and a certain disturbance of the gastric functions.
- Acute redness of the tongue with a slight coating at the back. Aphthous sores in the mouth.
- Moist mucus rakes in the chest.
- Slight pain while breathing, dyspnoea aggravates from lying down.
- Loose fetid stool and great irritability of the spine are some of its indications.
- It is a good medicine for Autumnal fever and asthma.

Oenanthe- Crocata

Dr. Chowdhury

- It is generally indicated in nocturnal epilepsy and epilepsy arising from sexual disorders.
- Most of the cases occur in women mostly during the menstrual time where the absence of menstruation at the allocated time leads to disturbance and subsequently to epileptic from convulsion.
- The spasm of this remedy comes in quick succession and with entire unconsciousness.
- The eyes are half closed, and alternate redness and paleness of face.
- Involuntary urination and defecation.
- Want of aura, redness, and swelling of face and neck.
- Foaming from the mouth and tight closing of jaws and hands are important symptoms.

Oleander

Choudhury.

- Great rolling. And rumbling in the abdomen. With emission. Of foul-smelling flatus
- The stools are yellow, undigested, and involuntary. The presence of undigested particles. Of food taken on the previous day is very characteristic.
- The stool is apt to occur during a meal as in Ferrum. Chloline---
- It resembles Graphities, --------------------------------, and violation about the unhealthiness of the scalp.
- It has violent headaches and the curious feature of this headache is aggravated looking sideways and crossing eyes.

Oleum Animale

Dr. Chowdhury

- It has stitching pain like Kali Carb, Carbo Animals, and Bryonia, but the stitching is associated with a burning sensation.
- The part feels as if it is being stitched with a red-hot needle.
- The pain shoots from behind upwards.
- Also, we have a pulled upward sensation connected with some of its pain aggravated after eating and aggravated from rubbing pressure in the open air.
- It is a remedy for migraine and in this respect, it is very similar to Gelsemium, Sanguinaria, Ignatia, Natrum Mur, Spigelia, and Kali Brom.
- There is polyurea of clear urine accompanying this attack.
- Toothache of irritable patients invariably aggravated by pressing the teeth together.
- The mucus membrane of the buccal cavity is very relaxed; hence these patients are constantly biting them.
- They can hardly eat without biting their cheek.
- Profuse accumulation of snow-white mucus within the mouth (Nux Moshcata).

Oleum Jecoris

- It is a useful remedy in the atrophy of infants with hot hands and heads with a great tendency to catarrhs, rickets, and bone affections.
- It has also been found to be useful in diseases of joints in pale thin cachectic (people who are tubercular, scrofulous in their temperament).
- Scrofulous abscesses, ulceration of glands, and cold abscess in similar subjects.

- Hectic fever, night sweats, and chronic persistent diarrhoea with marked emaciations.
- Cough and hemoptysis have been helped by this medicine. It is thus seen to be a T.B. remedy.
- It has caused pain in the liver.
- General soreness not only in the liver but also all over the body.
- Occurrence of palpitation with the other symptoms of the heart.
- Great burning of palms.
- Yellowness of the expectoration, leucorrhea discharges and other secretions.
- The tongue is yellow-coated.

Onosmodium

- The patients are lacking in the eye. Proper ideas of Inability to focus eyes on an object.
- They want objects held. At distance. To be able to look at.
- It is. Also. A good medicine for. Headaches. Brought on by I strain.
- Headaches due to myopia and also in catarrh of the middle year with constant roaring.
- It has impotency with the entire loss of sexual desire.
- Dryness of the throat, nose, and mouth are its guiding symptoms.
- Aggravation of headache in the dark and laying on back.

Opium
Dr. Kent
Hot Patient

- Perfectly painless Ulcers do not granulate and do not eat or spread with numbness or lack of sensibility opium will often heal this ulcer.

- Insensibility in parts that are in a high grade of inflammation.

- When drinking the esophagus seems to have no action and the fluid does not go down but passes out through the nose.

- The patient wants to be alone; she tells. You she is not sick, and yet she has a temperature of one. 105 to 106 degrees centigrade. Is covered with a scorching hot sweat and has a rapid pulse. Is delirious. You ask her how she is and she says she is perfectly well and happy.

- The stomach is in a state of undue warmth sinking all gone. Hungry, and this is aggravated by eating.

- In cerebral epoxy with stertorous breathing and jaw-dropping pupils. Dilated or contracted generally Face is mottled, purple, or hot hot sweat.

- One-sided paralysis with high blood pressure. This causes a flow of blood to the brain. And when given. Homeopathic. Lie. Homeopathically It checks this in six hours. He will become rational.

- Nervous headache. Beginning in the back of the head and spreading over the whole face. Aggravated in the morning.

- He feels as if his head wear held down on the pillow by the intense aching pain in the base of the brain. And yet, when he gets up, he is unable to lie down again.

- This is common in women. A false plethora, excitable. Excitable going through pregnancy. Or menstruation.

- The pain begins in the morning and so. Violent that the patient cannot move. Wink the eye, turn the head cannot bear the least noise on the ticking of the clock.
- It is difficult to get symptoms from her opium will. Aggravate at once.
- It is full of convulsions, Opisthotonos, cerebral meningitis, and aggravation in warm and stuffy rooms.
- Washing with hot water, with other characteristics of opium. (Apis)
- Fear and it's restful the object of the freight. Continuously looms up before her eyes. Epilepsy darting back to fright.
- Complaints from sudden joy, anger, shame, sudden freight.
- Opium eaters like whiskey, and drinkers are constitutional liars. Pulsatilla cures the diarrhea following the abuse of opium.

Dr. Chowdhury

- It checks all the secretions of the body, except those of the skin which is generally covered with a peculiar hot sweat.
- This want of secretion render. Opium such an admirable remedy for Constipation, especially for children and corpulent good-natured women.
- It is also meant for diarrhoea, a diarrhoea brought about by fear, sudden joy or other emotional disturbances.
- The stools are generally involuntary black and offensive.

Dr.Tyler

- No doubt abnormal painlessness is a grand keynote for opium. But in the pathogenesis, many acute pains will be found. And among them, this. Recorded by Hahnemann himself, horrible. Labor-like pains in the uterus compelled her to bend the abdomen during stool and urine which is infectious.

Opium in abdominal Colic (Borland)
- There is an apt to be a definite area of distension.
- The patient may say that he gets a feeling as if everything simply churned up to one point and could not get past it or as if something were trying to squeeze the intestinal contents past some obstructing band or as if something were being forced through a very narrow opening.
- Its arch of distension is likely to be in the center of the abdomen, when the pains are developing and coming up to the head, he develops an extreme hyperesthesia to noise.

Oxalic Acid

Dr. Kent
- It has got a peculiar radiation. The pain comes suddenly and goes very quickly and settles on the left shoulder through the left clavicle.
- The violent action upon the heart racks the whole system, trembling convulsion, loss of sensation, numbness, in the body and limbs, and blueness of the lower limbs, fingers, and lips. Paralysis of limbs are symptom showing how violently this remedy takes hold of the body affecting the heart spinal cord and brain.
- < From exhaustions and motions symptoms come on paroxysm, palpitation alternates with loss of voice. The patient is sensitive to cold.
- No remedy produces more violent cutting, stitching, and tearing pains in many parts. Soreness and bruises all over the body including the forehead, stomach abdomen, throat, urethra, hands, and feet. Painful spot on the scalp. Sore to touch also in other places, the body is mottled in pieces.
- Complaints come from eating sour fruits.
- The symptoms, especially the pains, come on from thinking.

- Fainting during stools.

- There is marked hyperemia of the brain. And surging of blood from body to head. Flushes of heat mount upward. He becomes dizzy and there is a vanishing of sight. The head feels empty, with headache in spots < from wine, laying, after sleep and on rising and better after stool. Sore tender spot on the scalp.

- Pain in stomach > After eating, eructation, nausea, the pain of the navel colic, rumbling in the bowels, urging to stool, sugar increases, pain in the stomach. Coffee causes diarrhoea, and heartburn < In the evening. Paroxysmal pains in the abdomen in the night. > Great pain in the region of the umbilicus. < stitching pain in the liver > by breathing.

- The tenesmus during stool causes pain in the head. Constipation with difficult stool and the straining causes headaches, and obstructed flatus in the splenic flexure of the colon, causing pain in the left hypochondriac region.

- Tearing pains in the spermatic cords < from motion. Marked tenderness in the testes < from walking. Strong sexual desire and erection, when in bed. Seminal emission and sexual weakness, shooting pain along the spermatic cord.

- Benumbing pains in the small of back > after stool, numbness in shoulders, to fingertips, pain in the point of flexed fingers. The cold sweat of face, hands, and feet.

Acute cardiac Failure- Borland

- The patient always complaining of a feeling of the most intense exhaustion, very often associated with a sensation of numbness. They frequently state that their legs and feet feel numb and paralyzed as if they had no legs at all. The skin is as cold as carbo veg, but there is a peculiar mottled eynosis in Oxalic acid. Which is not found in other drugs.

- The fingernails fingertips and toenails will be eynotic, But in addition, there is a peculiar mottled appearance of hands and feet.

- There is a somewhat similar mottled appearance on the face especially over the molar bones. These patient wants to keep still <By movement these patients complain of very definite sharpness. Precardial pains. These pains are not typical angina pain, but more of sharper pricking short of pains, which usually come through from the back and may run up the left side of the sternum towards the clavicle or down the left side of the sternum into the epigastrium. It is a good medicine for cardiac failure after influenza.

Dr. Chowdhury

- It is a left-sided remedy. It makes a natural selection of the lower lobe of the left lung. Sharp lancinating pain in the left lung is extremely characteristic.

- Terrible pain in the lumbar region, extending from the thigh and over the region of both kidneys.

- Pains return as soon as the patient thinks about it. This is not only true about pains but of the symptoms as well. When he thinks about his urine, it becomes imperative for him to urinate. Thought of stool or diarrhea brings an urgent desire to deficit. Its pains are felt in small spots.

Alphabet

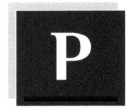

Paeonia Officinalis

Dr. Chowdhury
- It is mostly used in anal abscesses, fissures, fistules and boils.
- The leading indications are intolerable pain during and after stools and oozing of a kind of moisture from the rectum, leaving it constantly damp.
- The hemorrhoids are intensely painful. The pain goes from the anus to the testicle.
- There is usually a complication of fistula with piles.

Dr. Tyler
- Dreams of ghosts who were sitting upon his chest and oppressing his breath, so that he frequently woke up groaning.
- Burning heat in eyes, face, throat and anus.
- It can compare with Hamamelis in varicosis, Silicea in ulcers, and Sulphur in diarrhoea.
- It is curative in nonsyphilitic ulcer.

Palladium

Dr. Tyler
- Sensation of tallness, while the things around them look small and insignificant. (Platinum). Proud and haughty (Platinum). Stramonium also imagines he is large and tall and surrounding objects small.

- Both platinum and palladium have a bearing-down sensation in the uterus. While platinum acts upon the uterus and palladium upon the ovary.
- The sensation of something active bounding about inside the body. (Thuja, cocculus, Theridion).
- It has a crawling sensation as if fleas on the back, arms, abdomen, thigh, and ankles, and actual spots like flea bites appear in various places. Lips, nostrils, etc.
- It has also violent itching.
- Pain in the right ovarian region > by pressure. < From cold motion after exertion after social. Excitement > From touch. (headache) Pressure (pain in the ovary). Rest, rubbing, open air, and sleep.

Chowdhary
- Its headache is quite characteristic. It is felt across the top of the head from ear to ear. The pain is flitting and transient.
- Sensation as if the head had grown taller as if something terrible would happen, as if something was hanging in the throat, and as if the uterus would prolapse. The pain is shooting in character from periphery to center.

Pareira Brava

Dr. Chowdhury
- It acts upon the bladder and urinary organs. Constant desire for urination but cannot evacuate easily.
- He can emit small quantities of urine by going down on his knees and pressing his head firmly on the floor.

Paris Qudrifolia

Dr. Chowdhury
- Sense of expansion felt principally in the head. The head feels as if it is badly distended or the skull has become too tight.

- Its headache is of spinal origin. It arises from. the nape of the neck and produced a feeling as the head was immensely large. Pathologically. It is due to acute congestion of the head < from close thinking. The eyes too feel as if they are too large for their sockets and that the lips would not cover them. The sensation is as if the eye is being tightly drawn backward using a string to the middle of the brain.

- Loquacity, garrulous. He jumps from subject to subject (Lachesis).

- Disorder of the sense of touch everything feels rough to touch. Numbness and pricking accompany this feeling of roughness.

- Very sensitive to offensive orders. At times, this sensitiveness is so exaggerated that the patient experiences foul smells everywhere. Milk, bread, butter, and every other item. Of food discarded due to the imaginary foul smell of putrid scent everywhere.

- It has been used in the affection of cerebral spinal nerves, pain in the nape of the neck, increasing in times to great acuteness and associated with numbness, heat, and heaviness. The pain begins in the nape of the neck and shoulder. Extended over the whole side and renders even the arm powerless. Moving hands and grasping everything excite pain in the Occiput and nape of the neck.

Passiflora-In

- It is a good medicine for insomnia.

- The insomnia is not due to pain or distress but to a nervous erethism. It must be used in bigger doses.

- Its most important indication is a clean tongue.

Petroleum

Dr. Kent

- The tendency is to throw out vesicles, herpetic vesicles, which are isolated, and the vesicles tend to form a thick, yellow crust with Considerable moisture.

- There is a special tendency to produce vesicular eruptions about the back of the neck.

- All eruptions each violently.

- He cannot rest until he scratches the skin off.

- When the parts become moist, raw, and inflamed he scratches the skin until the moisture Use's 4th. Encrypts on scratching until the skin blades and the parts become cold.

- Coldness in spots, coldness in the stomach, abdomen, in the uterus, between Scapulae, coldness in the heart.

- The mucus membrane or Internal skin has little patches of ulcers and induration about the patch, and hence useful in syphilitic ulcers.

- Diarrhoea during the day and cough during the night.

- There is an all-gone-hungry feeling after stool. Which drives him to eat with the diarrhea. There is constant hunger, yet he cannot eat without pain.

- Chronic gonorrhea, itching is common to the internal skin and a striking feature in gonorrhea is the itching in the posterior half of the urethra with the discharge.

- It almost drives him wild and keeps him awake at night.

- He rubs and manipulates the perineum to relieve this itching.

- Sore bruised feeling all over the body, especially in joints.

- Rheumatic pain in joints from motion.

- Sore to touch, sensation as if bruised it is like Arnica.

- It is suitable for old stubborn occipital headaches.
- Silicea is a routine remedy in the offensive foot sweat with periodical offensive sweats all over and especially under Adilla Where it is so pungent that it can be observed on the patient entering the room.
- It is not closely related to Silicea, but it has relation with Graphites and Carbo veg.
- It suits occipital headaches from riding in a carriage or from such motions with nausea like sea sickness.
- Cracks in the leads.
- Caterial state of the Eustachian tube. The Mucus membrane is thickened and deafness results. It is. Catarrhal state.
- Heat and burning skin hot in places with the sensation of coldness in spots.
- Paretic conditions, especially left-sided weakness of muscles, and weakness of the lower extremities, especially the left side.
- The eruptions on the surface and the state and the state of Induration are like Graphites but the oozing in petroleum is thin and watery.
- Its wonderful use is complementary with. Rhustox in eczema of the genitalia of either male or female.
- Eruption on the scrotum penis Vulva.
- Rhustox produces violent inflammation of the skin of the genitalia of men and women.
- Erysipelatous inflammation, nodules, vesicles, and large blebs.
- Petroleum produces small vesicles, which itch, sting, and burn.
- Herpetic itching, redness, and moisture on the scrotum, skin cracked, rough, and bleeding extending to the perineum and thigh.

Dr. Chowdhury
- In the eye its use is confined to blepharitis marginalis (less of eyelashes), fissures of canthi, and scurfy and dry appearance of the skin around the eyes should be considered its leading indication.
- The stools are yellow, watery, gushing and contain particles of undigested food.

Dr. Tyler
- Strong aversion to fat food, meat, and open air.
- Stitches in the heels as if a splint were lodged in it.
- Vertigo comes on from stooping and rising.
- Great anxiety about his family.
- When going on a short journey the anxiety increases till he becomes inconsolable.

Petroselinum Sativum
Dr. Chowdhury
- Sometimes the physician is sent in a hurry to attend to a small child, jumping up and down with pain and screaming, inquiring into the cause of the child's suffering, he Is informed that the poor thing is unable to pass urine.
- A single dose of Petroselinum will relieve all the suffering.

Phellandrium Aquaticum
Dr. Chowdhury
- It is a right-sided remedy and has got special affinity for the female mammae, especially the right one.
- The nipple pains each time the child is put to the breast.
- The pain shoots upward and backward to the shoulder and the sacrum.

- It removes abnormal sleepiness in women after childbirth.
- It is very useful in the treatment of bronchitis and phthisis.
- Continuous cough for hours in the morning accompanied by dyspnea and prostration.
- Coarse rales are present and they compel the patient to remain in a sitting posture.
- It relieves the cough, even in the last stage of consumption.
- When a cavity has formed in the lungs and edema of extremities, copious diarrhoea, difficult respiration, and profuse sweat have started.

Phosphoric Acid

Dr. Kent

- Mental enfeeblement is the greatest indication of. Acid phosphoric patient.
- The mind seems tired.
- When questioned, he answers slowly or does not speak, but only. Look at the questioner.
- He is too tired to talk or even think he says do not talk to me. Let me alone.
- In acute diseases, especially. In typhoid fever. Is averse to speaking or answering questions. He merely looks, finally, he rises and says do not talk to me. I am so tired. He can. Not think what he wishes to say cannot frame his answer to questions.
- In every case, we find the mental symptoms are first to develop. The remedy runs from the mental to physical form to the muscle (reverse muriatic acid.)
- He says he is all right. Physically can work. Can exercise even violently but the mind is tired.

- There is mental apathy cannot read newspapers, and carry the trend of Thoughts.

- He forgets the names of those in his family. A businessman forgets the name of his clerks He is in confusion.

- It has also a great physical weakness, so tired in the back, so tired in the muscles so tired all over. A paralytic weakness.

- Later there is sexual impotence, aversion to coition, loss of sexual desire, no erection, the penis becomes relaxed amid an embrace and he cannot finish the act (Nux Vom).

- Ailments from business care, prolonged grief young man suffering from unrequired affections, or the loss of loved ones. Ailments from care, grief, sorrow, homesickness, or disappointed love, particularly with drowsiness. Night sweats towards morning emaciation. Grow weaker and weaker, withered face. Night sweat catches cold in the slightest provocation.

- During the weakness there is Vertigo. Vertigo while lying in bed. Seems like floating while lying in bed. Limbs seem to be lifted while the head does not seem to move as if the limbs were floating.

- Congestive headache in school girls from the slightest exhaustion of the mind and use of eyes. Peritoneal pains. Bones ache as if scraped. Aggravated by motion. When lying the pain shifts to the side laid on.

- Most of the complaints are > From keeping warm from absolute quiet from being alone at peace < from exertion, mental and physical from being talked to. He is sensitive to cold weather and sensitive to warm rooms.

- In low type of fevers, the complaints come on slowly Slow decline, and a slow increase of prostration Such appearances are found in advanced typhoid. It has a prostration lymphatic abdomen and, a dry brown tongue. Sort this on the. Teeth. Gradually approaching unconsciousness. Little thirst. Increasing to intense thirst wants to be left alone. Look, at the questions with glassy eyes as if slowly comprehending the questions. Pupil's contracted, dilated eyes sunken. Hippocratic countenance. Continued fever, bleeding from the nose lungs, bowels, hemorrhage from any mucus membrane discolored lips.

- Pains and aches all over the body < from motion. The pain seems deep-seated often along the nerves. The pains are extremely aggravated at night. Severe bone pains.

- Hypertension is accompanied by prosthetic enlargement. Give (A.P).

- When hypertension appears in place of menopausal symptoms. When the patient says, I have stopped Menstruating. 5 months back, but suddenly I'm getting giddiness. If it is detected, there is high BP. "Sumbal".

- Enlarged Thyroid with high BP (Lycopodium) Without enlargement of thyroid but there is a toxic condition. Thyroid, high B.P., after childbirth, especially after. Toxemia. Give Hydrocyle .(I J H 72.5)

- Its complaints are > from diarrhoea copious thin watery stool. From the quantity, it would seem that the patient would be exhausted. Diarrhea without debility. The mother wanders. Where it all comes from and yet the child seems well. If the diarrhea slacks up the patient is worse and on comes symptoms of tuberculosis weakness, prostration and brain fag. Some patients say they are never comfortable unless they have the diarrhoea.

- Diarrhoea: Abdomen much bloated. Tymphanetic. Great soreness of the bowels, as if. In typhoid state white or yellow water diarrhoea. Chronic or acute without pain or any marked ability.

- Prostatorrhoea: Immediately after every erection discharge or prosthetic fluid, even when passing a soft stool, the prosthetic fluid is discharged.

- It is a good medicine for. Troublesome leucorrhea. Yellow mostly after menses with itching profuse, yellow, thin, acid with chlorosis. It suits women who have been who have been nursing their children for a long time.

- The tendency of these patients. Ending in brain fag and weakness is run to the chest troubles. If a diarrhoea comes on, then chest trouble is everywhere. If a diarrhoea comes then the chest troubles are averted. Acute typhoid, pneumonia, low form of fever, ending in chest troubles.

- Prolonged fever, ending in a feeble heart with palpitation and mental symptoms. Palpitation during sexual excitement, the tendency to abscesses after a prolonged fever.

- Red spot appears whenever the flesh. Is thin over the bones after fever, abscess in the muscles, and state of molecular weakness. About the ankles over the tibia, where the flesh is thin. Boils, abscess, pustules of other. Moist eruptions separate eruptions. Tissues become weak.

- Creeping tingling. And crawling all over the body. Formication over whole body spot. In the spine backache.

- It is good medicine for diabetes Mellitus. And no other indication is detected. Usually, there is a history of shock and disappointment or pain in the leg after eating.

- In Typhoid Hering quotes, the following points itching of the nose from irritation Peyer's patches. Left side abdomen sensitive to touch.

Dr. Tyler

- In the navel, a periodical aching squeezing. Loud rumbling in the abdomen, especially upper part.

- Quite pale urine which immediately forms a thick whitish cloud.

Dr. Chowdhury
- The patient is originally strong. Gives away to the confinement rain upon it and has broken down. Stoop-shouldered, slender, shy almost maidenly boy.
- They tremble in all their limbs at all times.
- While walking. They make Missteps and Stumble easily.
- Due to the great thickness of urine the flow is interrupted, it stops and flows again. Stringy gel-like masses at a time. Looking like cuddled milk or a cheesy substance blocks the passage. The smell of urine is like raw meat.

Phosphorous

Dr. Kent
- Its complaints are found in such as emaciated and in those who are rapidly emaciating. In children who are going into Marasmus and in persons who have in them the foundation of consumption fairly well laid.
- In pleuritic girls who have grown too rapidly and have suddenly taken on weakness. Palllar, green thickness with menstrual difficulties.
- The prick of the needle will bring forth much bright red blood.
- Blood settles beneath the conjunctiva, or the skin, anywhere.
- Bloody saliva. Small bruises take on broad blue spots.
- Petchiac all over the body. Such as occur in Typhoid Fever.
- Fungus growth. General dropsical condition.
- The Mucus membranes are pale, such as found after bleeding in low forms of disease.
- Stiffness is a marked feature of phosphorus. Stiffness on beginning to move limbs. Stiff like a. foundered horse, especially in the morning.

- Weak relaxed condition of the joints following spasm.
- It has cured Poly of the ears and nose.
- Glands enlarge especially after contusions like. Belis. Glandular affections of weak pale sickly individuals such as suffers from diarrhea. Exhaustive conditions abscesses. Fistulas opening with hectic fever. Abscess with copious discharge of yellow puss.
- Always wants to be rubbed. He's generally better after sleep. Always wants to be rested.
- Apprehensive during thunderstorms, which brings on many complaints. Palpitation, diarrhea, and trembling. Fear in the evening, fear of death, fear of strange. Old faces. Looking at him from the corner.
- Weeping sad hysterical, will uncover the body and expose his persons. Violent. Loquacious.
- The headaches are most violent and are attended with or preceded by hunger.
- The scalp is covered with dandruff. The hair falls in patches living in bald patches here and there. Great soreness of the. Scalp. Most of the hair hangs down during headaches.
- Objects look red and often blue in the field of vision or objects. Sometimes looks green or gray as is observed in the incipient phthisis. Momentary Blindness is like a painting that seems to suddenly become blind. Paralysis of the. 3rd pair of nerves, where there is falling off the lids. Swelling of the eyelids.
- Bright red hemorrhage after the extraction of teeth.
- Violent hunger must be eaten during the chill. Must get up in the night to eat. Violent thirst in both. Acute. And chronic diseases. Desires for ice cold drink. And cold food. Aversion to sweet meat. Boiled milk. Salt, fish, beer, pudding. Tea and coffee.
- Many of the complaints are. Aggravated by eating. The nervous symptoms of the phosphorus drive the patient to eat and he feels better for a little while. And then he must eat again or the

nervous symptoms will come again, often He can sleep better after eating or cannot go to sleep.

- The food is eructed by mouthfuls until the stomach is emptied of the last meal. It is a great friend. Surgeon because he can always antidote the stomach affection of chloroform by phosphorus. Awful sinking gone feeling in the stomach. This sometimes comes at 11:00 like sulfur. It is a very useful medicine for cancer of the stomach. Coffee ground vomiting and burning. Coldness as if freezing in the pit of the stomach.

- It has a peculiar gurgling, which begins in the stomach and gurgles along down through the Intestine attended by involuntary stool, the Gurgling that occurs in. Arsenic is down the esophagus.

- Stitching pain from the coccyx up to the spine to the base of the brain, drawing the neck backward and this symptom occurred. During stool.

- It has cured rectal polyp.

- It is a good medicine for diabetes mellitus present. Of sugar in the urine, gradual emaciation, profuse, thirst for ice cold water. Considerable heat of the head, coldness of the extremities.

- Violent. Sexual desire driving. Him frantic. Erection. Frequent and painful day and night. Seminal emission at night. Even without. Lascivious dreams. Frequently discharge day and night of thin, slimy, colorless fluid from the urethra discharge of prosthetic fluid during a heart stool Sexual abuse with. Spinal disease. It has cured. Hydrocele following gonorrhea.

- Powell and pin in the ovaries extending. Down the inner side of the thigh during menstruation Copious hemorrhage from uterus. Bright red plotted blood after. Confinement during. Menstruation or during the activity. Climacteric period Frequent and profuse Too long casting. Copiously. Yellow leucorrhea with great weakness leucorrhea instead of menses bleeding.

- Warts Erectile. Tumors on the external genitalia.

- The general modalities of phosphorus is aggravated from motion, which is not found in Dr. Kent. (R.IJH 72-117) Due to quick perception of finer. Appreciation. They have a sense of beauty, and they become the best artist. They have long tapering fingers like artist.

- Craving for salt like all other tuberculosis remedies.

- Anxious and afraid of everything such as being alone of a crowd of death disease evil. That something will happen. Ghost robbers sudden noises. Thunder, Etcetera.

- Wants company. Of somebody. Should be touched. Like a child. Hold its mother hard.

- Nine out of 10 cases of. Infective hepatitis in children. Phosphorus is the remedy.

- The patient wants to give and receive affection. He is also over-sympathetic and cannot see others suffer.

- Feels better than before. An attack hungry. Before an attack Hungry during fever and before and during headache.

- It towards the end of whopping cough disease threatens to take an unfavorable course. Involuntary stool while coughing bronchitis fever, very high. Pulse rapid. Lies upon the back. Breathing very fast. Cough, provoked by a strong odor and the appearance of strangers. Cough from confusion. (JH.70-47)

- Violent sexual desire during pregnancy and lactation Increase secretion of milk out of season.

- Inflammation of the larynx with hoarseness in the morning. Every change of weather. From becoming overheated and cold settles in the larynx. Producing loss of voice and hoarseness, especially for public speakers and singers.

- With the cough bronchitis pneumonia. And cardiac symptoms There is more or less construction of the chest, as if bound or as bandaged as If tied with a string. Sensation of heat in the chest mounting to the head flushes of heat in the chest extending upward. Violent pain in the chest with coughing the patient is compelled to hold the chest with hand.

- In all in. all incurable cases after the fever has been receded. Phosphorus should not be given as will intensify the fever and do just what it was given to avoid. It is not. It should not be given in high potency. In last stages of thesis.
- It often suitable and. Restrains the progress of. Multiple sclerosis, where there is weakness and trembling of the extremities.
- Ulcers bleed on appearance of menses.
- Could see better when? Pupils are dilated by? Shading the eyes?

Dr. Chowdhury
- Emotiveness and. Shamelessness are the characteristics of phosphorus. She uncovers herself and wishes to go naked as if insane. She lifts her clothes and kisses hotly whoever comes near her.
- The cough. Is constant. Aggravates in the evening till midnight.
- It has no power to cure a case usually. Silicea is necessary to finish the case. (Indian H, Journal)
- Phosphorus means light and many symptoms of this medicine are connected with light. Again, light means. Knowledge and knowledge are perceived through the senses of the nervous system. So the patient's sense is acute. He. Is sensitive to noise, touch odor. Change of atmosphere. Temperature, weather, etc. He is. Aggravated at the borderland of light and twilight. And so he is. Aggravated in the morning and evening.

Phytolacca
Dr. Kent
- It resembles Mercury, and it is an antidote to Mercury. In those lingering Mercurial bone pains come on at night from the warmth of the bed. The body aches across a bruised state.

- Soreness of the Peristomium, where the flesh is thin over the tibia joints. Soreness of the muscles. Drawing and cramping. Drawing in the muscles of the back. Worse from night. < from the warmth of the bed.

- It is a glandular remedy, the glands become inflamed and hard. It produces a sore throat with inflammation of the gland of the neck, particularly the sub-auxiliary and parotid.

- The symptoms are. < at night. Cold days in a cold room and from the heat of the bed so that there is a controversy between heat and cold.

- Settles on the breast, soreness, and lumps in the breast from each cold, damp spells become chilled, and a sore breast result.

- Almost any excitement centers in the mammary glands. Fear, or an accident, lumps form in the heart. Heart swelling, tumefaction, even violent inflammation, and suppurates.

- Diphtheria with swelling of the glands of the neck parotid, submaxillary with aching of the bones, aching of the bones. fetor from the mouth. Heavily coated tongue and salivation.

- Many eruptions are squamous. Pityriasis psoriasis. Ringworms, and barber itch, are found in the body.

- Women, who were confined years before had abscesses of the breast which were pulled. Which were poulticed and lanced, a cicatrix left and is now in the present confinement. They have trouble much (Graphities).

- Parotid and submaxillary glands swollen tongue. Swollen tongue thick coated on back quoted yellow and dry. This is found in all acute complaints like Mercury.

- Paine starts from the nipple and radiates the whole body. It has stringy milk.

Dr. Chowdhury
- There is a general soreness over the whole body of the patient moans and groans every time he moves.

- It should thus be classed with remedies like Rhus tox and Bryonia.
- It further combines with pain, intense frustration, and great exhaustion.
- It has been used with remarkable success in Sciatica and hip joint disease in the symptoms of pain shooting from the sacrum down the outer aspect of thighs to knees and toes.
- The pain occurs in such quick succession. It renders the leg powerless numb and heavy.
- It has a special affinity for the muscles and the shoulder and arms.
- The pain flies from place to place, lameness, soreness, and bruised filling are felt all over the body.
- It has a peculiar headache accompanied by an increased sense of hearing.

Picric Acid

Dr. Kent

Hot patient

- Cool air and cool bathing are grateful to him. He is sensitive to wet weather, numbness of many parts, and trembling, lassitude, and heaviness. Must lie down < from list exhaustion is a marked feature. Loss of sleep, mental worry, and mental labor are the exciting causes of symptoms. Extreme indifference. He is quickly frustrated from the least mental work, and it begins with many complaints, such as soreness and lameness, diarrhea, burning along the spine, general weakness, and heaviness of the back and limbs. In young school children, we have a common use of the very valuable and neglected remedy when the child begins to leave the alphabet. Headaches come and return with every repeated effort. Often with dilated pupils. After every exam at school come these violent headaches.

- It has violent pain at the vertex, forehead, and occiput extending down the spine with much heat. The headaches often begin to increase with the day and better sleep at night Extreme prostration and extreme sexual excitement comes with this headache.

- Looking, reading fine print, and exhaustion of vision will bring on a headache and eye symptoms. The symptoms of the eye < from artificial light.

- There is evidence of liver trouble and jaundice.

- Urine contains sugar and albumin, high S PS, urine heavy with urates, uric acid phosphorus, and poor in sulfate. Dribbling after urination. Great waste of phosphate.

- Along its characteristic symptoms, where great restlessness of feet is present, the zincum Picricum acts best.

Dr. Chowdhury

- In the first stage, he suffers from violent strong, long-lasting erections They are sometimes so hard that he feels the rupture of his penis. These erections are followed by profuse, seminal emissions, auxiliary acid comes very close to picric acid in sexual debility. Oxalic acid patient has great erections, but these come on mostly in lying down without any cause. It is also a pain in the occipital region but the pains are in a limited area < by thinking of it.

Platinum

Dr. Kent
Hot Patient

- Fear is a very prominent feature of this remedy fears. That something will happen fears that a husband will not return to her, though he comes back regularly.

- Spasms will come on fixation or anger whistles. Sinks and dances. Talks constantly about fanciful things.

- Headaches come on from chagrin, fear from vexation from hemorrhage, and sexual excitement.

- Pulsating and digging through the lower jaw, especially the right side together with numbness and coolness.

- Extreme sensitiveness of the external organ not due to inflammation, but due to hyperesthesia violent sexual desire in married women with itching, tingling, and voluptuous sensation.

- After every mental exertion palpitation, trembling, numbness, quivering, and excitement in the limbs. Nash has cured a case: of a woman who had an inspiration to kill her child.

Jules Goudy

A woman who was tormented with an almost irresistible impulse to kill her husband, whom she loved passionately and with whom she was profusely happy.

Dr. Chowdhury

- It suits young girls with premature development of the sexual organs and instincts. This often leads them to nymphomania and similar vicious practices. She generally lies on the back with her arms over her head. Thigh drawn up and knees, thrown apart. There is also a tendency to kick off the clothes and keep the leg uncovered. This posture is a great pointer and will help us to prescribe this remedy for many serious complaints, such as typhoid epilepsy, hysteria, tetanus, etc.

Plantago-Major

Dr. Chowdhury

- It has great efficacy in curing odontalgia and otalgia. The simultaneous existence of toothache and earache and the presence of salivation are two very important indications.

- The toothache. Which is of a boring digging nature < by walking in the cold air and by contact. Sometimes the tooth feels elongated.

- It is also serviceable in Neuralgia, it may be. In the teeth, ear, nose, and face, but most often in the last place. It is erratic in nature and shoots into the temporal maxillary and orbital region. Dr. Dr. Kent advises external application is essential here.
- It is a good medicine for nocturnal enuresis of children. In this connection, Dr. EW Jones. quotes the following notes. Nocturnal enuresis in children depends on the laxity of the sphincter vesicle but is not due to paralysis of the sphincter (For comparison of hernial enuresis see this book-Dr. Chowdhury).
- It is very rich in skin symptoms Itches and eruption of various shorts, but the symptoms that we deem now are important. It is a tendency to produce anticipated inflammation of various parts of the body, especially in the female breast.
- Plantago vices with calendula in lacerated and incised wounds and injuries of various kinds its special indication is the presence of pain swelling and erysipelatous.
- Punctured wound in the palm of a lady from the thorn of the fins of a cod fish. Her whole hand was swollen right up to the shoulder joint. The pain was excessive and agonizing. She was completely cured by this medicine.

Plumbum Met

Tomorrow, like that's the weather.

Dr. Kent

Chilly patient

- It is a slow and long-acting medicine. There is first paresis and finally paralysis of parts first and finally of the whole body.
- The mind is impaired, perception is slow. He memorizes with difficulty comprehension, difficult. He cannot recall words and express himself. When in conversation with such a patient, he is thinking about while making up his mind to answer.

- There is sluggishness also in the skin. You may prick him and a second later, he says ouch showing the slowness in the skin.

- There is a state of hyperplasia in the acute affections, but the chronic affections are characterized by loss of sensation, and numbness of the fingers and toes, soles, and palms. And this extends toward the skin and spine.

- The patient begins to emaciate until he becomes a skeleton. The skin is wrinkled, puckered, shriveled, and drawn over the palms. The emaciation Is sometimes local, very local. It is generally associated with pain. The painful parts wither. Pain down the arm and in the shoulder. Violent pain in the bronchial plexus and the arms whither. The paralysis usually occurs in the extension, so we have wrist drop. He cannot raise or lift anything with the hand extension. Is difficult. This occurs in piano players. They cannot lift their fingers sufficiently. rapid to keep the space. Flexion is all right. Curare Is another medicine that corresponds to this state in piano players, a paralysis from overaction of extensor muscles When the muscles become fatigued from playing fixed exercises, scales, etc, for hours at a time. When the player has to do this over and over again Rhus tox comes in but it is an acute remedy. And only holds for a short time. The change state that follows. Plumbum sometimes will be indicated.

- The bladder is also paretic. Cannot expel the urine. The muscles do not cooperate to void the urine and there is retention. It has both suppression and retention of urine.

- Deep melancholy and restlessness his thought disturbs him all night and prevents sleep. Insomnia, sleeplessness from the continual effect of thinking, inability to comprehend and to remember. Now this progresses from periods of insomnia to periods of coma and this is associated with suppression. of urine. Uraemic coma urnemia.

- Violent spasmodic. Palpitation of the heart < laying on the left side with marked anxiety in cardiac reason. Hypertrophy and dilation of the heart.

- It produces an inclination to deceive, to cheat. A hysteric woman, when she thinks. no one was near, she would get up, walk about, and look in the glass to see how beautiful she was but when she heard someone's footsteps She would lie on the bed and appear to be unconscious. She would be much pricking and you could scarcely tell she was breathing.

- Apoplexy stupor, when opium is sufficiently similar to remove the cerebral congestion, which always surrounds the apoplectic clot Plumbum may follow. Plumbum Phos, Alumina are three sheet anchors. They conform to the symptoms often, When the first state has been cited by Opium. The paralysis of muscles, the paralytic weakness of one side of the body, or a single part of the body, show its relation to such cases.

- The mental symptoms, the emotional symptoms, and the heart symptoms are greatly < by any exertion, especially exercising in the open air while walking in the open air, the patient becomes hot in the head, pale in the face, and cold in the extremities. Hands and feet cold as if ice.

- The patient is cold and emaciated and needs much clothing in warm weather, not about the head, but about the body. Extremely cold, Numb, and emaciated. Sweat on the extremities and or the feet. Feet and toes withered like a washer woman's hands, toes blistered blisters between the toes, smarting, ulceration. Molecular death and even gangrene of the skin. Of the fingers and toes. Calluses about the feet. corns and burns.

- Wandering pains, toxically swelling, yellow skin.

- Burning analysis, is in keeping with the remedy everywhere.

Dr. Chowdhury

- It is a good medicine for delirium when it alternates with colic. The patient bites and strikes those around him like Belladonna. And unlike Belladonna, there is a tremor of the head, and hands and a goodly collection of yellow makers about the mouth and teeth.

- In constipation a sensation as if a string were obstructing the anus upon the rectum.

Dr. Tyler
- Boat-shaped abdomen.
- Hypeaesthesia with loss of power Hyperesthesia in acute affection, but in chronic affection there is anesthesia.
- Dr Hollands cites a case in the patient had been suffering from agonizing abdominal pain, spasms for two days, vomiting, and suppression of stool and urine Plumbum was given and in less than three minutes, the patient fell asleep, waking after many hours, free from pain and able to relieve his bowels of masses of scybala.
- The Association of colic with constipation and constipation with colic always form its special indication.
- Its cerebral symptoms are Sometimes uraemic. More commonly primary. They start with violent headaches and amaurosis then maniacal or melancholic constriction may supervene, but most frequently eclampsia. The convulsions are quite epileptic form in character and coma or delirium may fill up their intervals. It is indicated in nephritis and cirrhosis of the liver. The patient is both hypothetic and anesthetic according to Dr. T, F, Allen. The patient becomes mentally intolerant is declines to work. His intelligence and power of expression decrease and becomes slow in perception. He answers very slowly and his memory is also impaired. Mental torpedo increases and he becomes indifferent.

Psorinum

Dr. Kent
Chilly Patient

- The patient dreads to be washed. The skin over the body especially on the face looks filthy. Though it has been well washed. Many of the complaints of the skin are < from bathing, in the warmth of the bed. The skin itches when warm. Itches when wearing woolens.

- The patient himself is one of debility. He wants to go home after a short walk, he is. Aggravated in the open air cannot breathe in the open air. Cannot breathe while he is standing up. Wants to go home and lie down So that he can breathe.

- He slowed down all of his functions in a state of paretic condition. He does not rally after a fever, his digestion is slow, and the stool is normal, yet it requires great effort to expel it. The bladder is full of urine, yet it passes slowly, and feels that some remain, he can never finish stool or urination. He has to go back several times, although the stool is soft and perfectly normal. It cannot be expelled in one shot.

- A psoriatic patient comes down with typhoid. The typhoid has subsided, but the patient has no appetite. He has no convulsions. He wants to lie down and does not desire to be moved, aggravated when sitting up > by laying on his back with his hand abducted from his side.

- Sadness and hopelessness he sees no light breaking the clouds above his head. All is dark about him. He thinks his business is going to be a failure overwhelmed, sad, dejection, He takes no joy in his family and feels that these things are not for him His business is prosperous, yet he feels as if he were going to the poor house, wants to be alone, full of anxiety, even of suicide. Despair of recovery, if sick.

- Itching at night without eruption. If he throws the covers off, then he becomes chilly. If he covers up, then there is itching. Sensitive to cold. Yet the skin is < from heat.

- Vertigo as soon as they go into the open air. Becomes dizzy and wants to go home and lie down.

- Headache with hunger. Aggravated after eating. If he goes without a meal, he has a headache. Every time the air blows onto his head, it slacks off, and the catarrh and headache come on. Either headache or Coryza from catching a cold. Headaches alternate with cough or eruption in winter. Alternating with headache.

- Complaints of aggravation from getting the haircut. (Belladonna, Sepia, Hepar Sulph).

- Otorrhea, with headache. Brown is offensive, especially from the left ear. Otorrhoea is associated with diarrhea.

- When a woman has passed through an abortion and the placenta has come away, but every few days a little push of fresh, bright red blood and clots are going days and weeks with little oozing of bright red blood. No tendency for permanent recovery. (Sulphur, Psorinum) This condition occurs due to the subinvolution of the uterus. (China)

- In fever head and body hot and hot air, or steam beneath the covers {Opium} The chill is not marked but the heat is intense and the sweat copious.

- Increased growth of hair on the face, a fuzz. (Cal-carb, Sulphur, Natrum Mur)

Dr. Chowdhury

- Eruptions are noticed over the Occiput completely hiding the scalp, the exudation is very profuse Excoriating, and offensive, its absence is contraindicated by this drug.

- All its complaints are aggravated by lying down and bringing the arms close to the body.

- It is a good medicine for abdominal colic after suppression, eczema, and other skin diseases. The mental symptoms must be there. Especially despondency. Recovery.

- Suicide deal. Tendency. Everything. Looks dark.

- Dry hard tickling cough that returns every winter it is aggravated in the morning on waking and evening on laying down the sputum is solid, green, and greenish yellow. This cough is sometimes the after-effect of suppressing itch. The cough is there while drinking.

Dr. Tyler
- It has cured more cases of hay fever in my practice than any other medicine. Among the peculiar symptoms that he draws attention to are stupid in the left half of the head as if the brain would protrude, had not having enough room in the forehead. As if the head separated from the body as if heard with ears, not his own. Teeth as if glued together, hands and feet as if broken. Psorinum cannot bear the limbs to touch each other. At night or the weight of arms on chest. (Lachesis)

Prunas Spinosa

Dr. Chowdhury
- Its pains are outshooting and out pressing, commencing at an Internal spot, they shoot and radiate out. We have sharp pain beginning in the right side of the forehead, shooting like lightning through the brain and coming out at the occiput. Sometimes the pain is pressed from within outwards Sometimes the skull feels as if it would be pressed outwards by sharp plug. This type of pain is seen everywhere.

- Input toothache, the tooth feels as if it would be raised out of its socket and thrown off.

- Another characteristic is shortness of breath to which he frequently becomes a victim. He sighs constantly as if he were climbing a high or stiff hill. This tight, short, and difficult breathing, this anxious respiration led Dr. Dippe to prescribe Prunas Spinosa With remarkable success in the case of sprint ankle in a young lady who jumped from a carriage. whilst the horse had bolted.

- Strangely, caused by the pressure of the flatus in the bladder. The desire to pass urine is continuous. If the desire is not attended to immediately, violent, crampy pain ensues in the bladder. The patient is therefore afraid to hold urine long, sometimes an apparent condition is to be met with the urging and an imperative call for urination is not always successful.

- The urine seems to pass forward into the glans penis and then seems to turn back, causing violent pain in the urethra.
- It is a good medicine during the climacteric period having heart troubles.

Ptelea-Trifoliate

Dr. Chowdhury
- It causes great congestion of the liver, stomach, and bowels and it is generally indicated in people with swollen liver, bitter taste in the mouth, and a dull, confused frontal headache A result of hepatic disorders.
- Dragging sensation of the right side of the liver while laying on the left side.
- The stools are generally thin and offensive.
- The urine is highly colored yellowish red and scalding.
- We also find excessive saliva in the mouth.
- The pain from the forehead to the root of the nose is characteristic. It can be compared with Bryonia, but the characteristic thirst of Bryonia, its sticking pain, and its dry tongue are not found in Ptelea. The stool of Bryonia has an odor of old cheese.

Dr. Tyler
- It is a great stomach and liver medicine. It causes hurry and a sensation of burning heat of skin face, even breath that burns the nostrils.
- Repugnance to animal food and rich pudding, of which it is ordinarily fond of butter and fatty foods. Even a small quantity aggravates the pain. (Epigastric)
- Hepatitis and gastric symptoms aggravate after meal.

- Chronic gastritis, a constant sensation of corrosion hot and burning in the stomach with vomiting of ingesta, constipation, and afternoon fever.

- Weight and aching distress, dull pain, heaviness. Aggravated lying on the right side. Turning to the left causes a dragging sensation.

- Stomach feels empty after eating, the sensation of goneness, pulsation, and severe abdominal pain near the umbilicus.

Pulsatilla

Dr. Kent

Hot patient

- She thinks the company of the opposite sex is a dangerous thing to cultivate aversion to marriage is a strong symptom. A man takes it into his head, that it is an evil thing to have sexual intercourse with his wife and sustains it.

- The patient imagined that the milk was not good to drink, so they would not take it. They imagine that certain articles of diet are not good for the human race. Religious freaks and freaks especially tend to dwell on religious institutions.

- Many of the complaints are associated with weakness of the stomach and indigestion, or with menstrual disorders.

- Many symptoms are aggravated after eating. It is only often a lump in the stomach, the muscle and nervous systems are also aggravated after eating. Its mental symptoms are aggravated in the evening, whereas its stomach symptoms are aggravated in the morning. Aggravation from fats and rich foods > by slow walking in the open air.

- Its skin feels hot and feverish, while the temperature of the body is normal. There is aggravation from much clothing. She wants to wear a thin dress, even moderately. In cold weather often cannot wear flannel or woolen clothing because they irritate the skin causing itching and eruption like sulphur.

- There is no remedy like pulsatilla to antidote sulphur which has been used every spring to cleanse the blood. Some people use sulphur until the skin is red hot and easily irritable by clothing.

- Old cases of psoriasis with flat brownish patches about the size of the thumbnail, which itch tremendously in the case of sulphur patients are cured by Pulsatilla.

- Pulsatilla has the usual venous constitution. Considerable bloating of the face and eyes, bloating of the abdomen, feet puffed so that she cannot wear shoes feet, are red, and the menstrual period is aggravated by menstrual flow.

- With the engorgement of veins, ulcers surrounded by varicose veins are common in this remedy, as ulcer bleeds, and black blood, which coagulates easily.

- All the catarrhal discharges are. thick. blood except the vagina, which is excoriating, causing rawness of the parts.

- Vertigo from the affections of the eyes > by wearing well-adjusted glasses attended by nausea < in a warm room, lying down in cold, open air and slow-moving in open air.

- Violent headache headaches of schoolgirls who are about two menstruate, headaches accompanying menstruation, headaches associated with suppressed menses with menstrual disorders, not caused by them, but associated with them. Pains through the temples and sides of the heads are common. Headache before, during, and after menstruation, but more commonly before.

- One sided headache and one-sided complaints are peculiar to Pulsatilla. Perspiration on one side of the head, face, and body.

- Granular lids, continued formation of little pustules, isolated granules on lids grow out here and there in batches as large as pin leads. Every cold settles on the eyes and nose. Eyes are > by both warm or cold water or tepid water Recurrent styes always have styes, pustules.

- Before menstruation in young girls especially things get black before the eyes, like a gauze or veil.

- Thick yellow purulent bland offensive discharge, frequent the ear and is very fetid, sometimes bloody.

- It is a good medicine for. Otitis especially of children.

- Dr. Harbinson's diseases of children page. 345. New York. Experience in the treatment of otitis with delirium and agonizing pains with swelling and closing of the. Kilometers. Swelling of the ear and adjoining parts. Induce me to regard pulsatilla As the specific. Form remedy in this form. Of otitis.

- Dr Bernhard Bacher and. Charles J. Hempelizer. "The science of therapeutics" Page 259. It is also. Specific for otitis event. Constipation and excessive thirst may be present, which is entirely contrasted to. Pulsatilla yet pulsatilla at magically in otitis. (See also H. Herald Nov- 1973- Page 250)

- The loss of smell is present in. acute and. Acute and caterer much stuffing up of nose occurring in the evening.

- It has loose morning cough and dry evening cough, nose bleed during the menstrual period. Before the menstrual period and nose bleed with suppressed menses.

- It is a good medicine for hay fever, the patient feels better in any way when the hay fever is present.

- Moms and inflammation of the parotid glands. If a woman suffering with mums takes a decided cold the breast swells and there is an inflammation of the memory gland Metastasis from mums to breast. In. women to testes in man.

- It has wandering pains, rheumatism goes from joint to joints, jumps around here and there. Neuralgic pains fly from. Place to place. Inflammation go from gland to gland. But here is the distinguishing feature. (Abrotanum, pulsatilla) Stick to its own text.

- She talks occasionally she becomes really insane. Subject to the strangest hallucinations. The idea of going to bed. Is detestful to her. She imagined that somebody is being naked wrapped up in the same bedclothes. We have other remedies having the similar.

Symptoms. Rhus tox patient suffers from A similar. Dilution that there is somebody in bed with her, she. Thinks of driving her out of it.

- Cholaram: As if a person were standing on the. Foot of her bed, financing her all the time.

- Eruphorbinum: The patient sees somebody walking in front. Of him And as he looks behind someone. Seems to him to be following him as well.

- It is a good medicine after grief. Modification and sorrow .

- This patient has a great predilection to styes, especially in the upper lids and Acne. on the face.

- During pregnancy and labor. The best indication for the application of this remedy is difficult breathing without any disease of the lungs.

- It gives rise to complications like. Orchidis? Epidemiotics. And prostratitis After suppression. Of gonorrhea. There is a great tennis and stinging in the nose of the ----- A pressure is also. Felt in the bladder which. Gives 2N2. N infected. Desire to pass water. Sometimes we need with hematuria for troubles like this after. Suppression of gonorrhea. We may think of the following medicine.

- Argent Nitricum: The testicles become quite enlarged and. Indurated each urination is accompanied by excessive. Burning and cutting pains extending clear up to the inus. The discharge, if any, is purulent and excoriating.

- Erechthotes: Orchitis during gonorrhoea.

- Sarsaparlia: Great swelling of the. Sparnatic chord. Much sexual. Excitement eruption on skin. And history of. Absence of.-----

- Epilepsy instead of menses. (Puls, Bufo). Pulsatilla Is. Always? Fewer in groups as if seeking company. Never or only rarely as a single specimen. Copious. Is another expression of this changeability, The personality is something rather. Infertile in character and the child. Particularly wants this Then that is never satisfied. (William Gutman)

- Cases of disease: Abrotanum Has this Metastasis. But it changed the whole diagnosis The patient has diarrhea. Today, and rheumatism. Tomorrow, the suppression of diarrhea or hemorrhage, or the piles causing an. Outcropping somewhere else.

- As a rule, it is thirstless, but in high fever there may be thirst.

- Often desires things he cannot digest, lemonade, herring, cheese, pungent things, highly seasoned things, juicy things. Aversion to meat, butter, fat, pork, milk, bread, and smoking.

- It is not uncommon for the pulsatilla patient to feel through the whole month, as if she were about to mensturate.

- Troublesome. Constipation with large hearts tool. With difficulty to expel, it has frequent urging to stool without any stool.(Nux Vom) Goes many times before. He can pass. Any. Is diarrhea and bowel symptoms aggravate in the night The stomach, throat, mouth in the morning. The mental. Symptoms are in the evening.

- Most troublesome constipation with hemorrhoids. Violent pain in the hemorrhoids amolerated laying down aggravated Laying flat on the back. Invalid, painful hemorrhoids with intense burning. Think of. Arsenic and Kali carb.

- She cannot lay on back. Without having a desire to urinate.

- Involuntary urination when coughing and sneezing from. Sudden shock and surprise, or from sudden joy, or from coughing, or from noise From a pistol shot.

- It has complaints from prostrated rain. Getting. (Dulcamara)

- Sexual desire commonly strong. From lasting erections. Sexual excess resulting in headache, Back aches head. Heavy burning and aching in Menstrual colic causing her to bend double. Distended abdomen throw away all covering. testicles with or without swelling.

- It cures many cases of gonorrhea in females. The striking feature is when the menstrual flow is present, there is milk in the breast in girls in puberty. Milk in the breast, a premature establishment of milk in non pregnant women.
- Asthma of children From. Suppressed rash. Odd in women from suppressed menses.
- In curvature of the spine, it has good valve spine irritation after sexual excess pain in the. Back. As if sprained sensation. Of cold. Water. Pour down back.
- Sleeps on back with hands over head. Cannot sleep on left side. It increases. The palpitation suffocation.

Dr. Chowdhury
More the chill, more the pain. It can be compact by the following medicine.

Bovista: The chill is intense and is accompanied by. Surging of pains, the chill is so great that the patient is compelled to seek the warmth of lighted stove to keep warm.

Colocynth: The intense squeezing cutting. Gripping nauseating pains that radiates from the umbrella. To different parts of the abdomen and chest is always a guide. Its mental condition is entirely different from.

Dulcamara: The pain in this remedy almost. Always. Caused by an exposure to cold and rain. It has fever, both in morning and evening.

- It has fever both in the morning and evening but especially at 4 pm. The attack is mostly preceded by gastric disturbances such as diarrhoea, vomiting etc. In fever its morning paroxysms are always attended with thirst but its evening are thirstless.

Dr. Tyler
- In retained Placenta two remedies are to be kept in mind and when no symptoms are present may be prescribed empirically with good results. These are Sepia and Pulsatilla-Sepia to be given for retained placenta after abortion and Pulsatilla after labor. The finer indication for these remedies are follows:

- Sepia: Little sharp shooting pains in the cervix. Sometimes with burning. Hourglass contraction ------ of heat. Cold hands and feet. Lack of any pain or contraction of uterus. Every thing wide open but nothing doing. Great sensitiveness to odors. Sensation of a ball in uterus.

- Pulsatilla: Intermitting Haemorrhage. Retention of urine with heat, redness and soreness of hypogastrium externally, which is painful to touch. Hourglass contraction in mild tearful women inclined to weep because her labor is not completed. Desire fresh air, very restless. Burning in region of heart.

- Pulsatilla is always found in groups as if seeking company. Never or rarely as a single specimen. A popular English name of Pulsatilla plant is "Samefaced maiden". In measles where pulsatilla is often indicated, the rash may disappear and the symptom shift to the respiratory organ. Pulsatilla type would tend to hypofunction of the gall bladder so that the patient cannot tolerate even aversion to fat.

Sometimes we will find out some specific symptoms for example: You question the patient whether she has got burning sensation. He gives some other answer. She says her hair is falling. Every time you question her at that point he gives some other symptoms, he runs away from the question as if he is afraid to commit himself by answering that question.

Pulsatilla is associated with slow motion. It has great pain when the flow from a abscess become scanty.

Pyrogen

Dr. Kent
Chilly Patient

- Offensiveness prevails extensively, even putrid and cadaverine odors of body, breath, sweat, and discharges.

- Sensation as though he covered the whole bed.

- Knew her head was on the pillow but did not know where the rest of the body was Feels when lying on one side, she is one person and another when turning on the other side.
- Sensation as though crowded with arms and less.
- Violent congestion of the head with pressing pain, and pulsation aggravated by pressure. Copious sweat on the head.
- The mouth is foul and tastes putrid. The tongue is coated and brown. Brown streaks down the center.
- Vomits water when it becomes warm in the stomach.
- Pain in the right side of the abdomen, going through the back amerolated on every motion, talking and breathing, lying on the right side, groaning with every breath.

Dr. Chowdhury
- Dr. J.H. Hunt reports having cured many cases of varicose ulceration with Pyrogen that refused to heal under other drugs. We should think of this medicine especially in cases of ulcers, when the indicated remedy fails to act. Complaints coming on dated back from abscess.
- She is inclined to talk all the time during fever and sometimes talks so fast that it is difficult to follow her.
- As soon as the fever came on, she commenced urinating.

Dr. Tyler
- Bowels so sore he can hardly breathe. It is so sore that the patient cannot bear any pressure over the right-side abdomen.
- Bearing down pain and prolapse uteri only aggravated by holding the breath. Pain starts at the umbilicus or just about pressing down towards the uterus, but is intercepted by just the same kind of pain starting from the uterus and passing up till they meet midway and die away till another comes.
- Pyrogen resembles Ipecac very closely in uterine hemorrhage. If you have an Ipecac case that fails then you can think of Pyrogen.

- Think of the medicine when there is a history of abortion. Never well since abortion. When the mother and the child suffer from different diseases and the indicated medicine fails give this medicine in 1M to 10 M (I.J.H.73-64).

- It has the anxiety of sleeplessness and Arsenic, prostration and coldness of Carbo Veg, the bruised soreness of Arnica, and the bone pains of Eupatorium. The > from the motion of Rhus tox and the rattling of the chest in Antim tart (H.G. June-1976).

Alphabeth

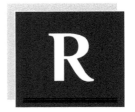

Radium Bromatum

Dr. Chowdhury

- The most important action of Radium is seen over the of this remarkable agent has been eagerly used with varying degrees of success in various lesions of the skin such as Keloids, naevi pigmented moles, urethra carbuncle, epithelioma, lupus vulgaris, papilloma, fibroma, sarcoma, and carcinoma. It increases the polymorphonuclear neutrophils.

- Severe pain over the entire body making him restless, tossing about aggravates the pain. The entire body feels as if fire with a needle pricks or electric shock. In all over the body. Anxiety, fear, apprehension feeling as if something is going to happen, fear of being alone in the home.

- Vertigo when rising, when on feet, a tendency to fall onto the left side and has to support himself. Vertigo and laying down after a warm bath, on going into open air aggravated getting up.

- P A peculiar metallic taste in the mouth with increased salivation. Perched dry sensation in the roof of the mouth, > from drinking a small quantity of cold water.

- Dysuria during the day, had to wait sometimes before the urine came, brick dust sediment in the urine. Traces of albumen in Urine. Granular and hyaline are cast in urine.

- Succession on small boils on forehead and chest. Scaly eruption on the anterior surface of the right eye. Scaly circumscribed eruption on flexure side of forearm < dry heat and open fire.

- Radiodermatitis on both hands. Eczematous eruptions, cracks, and fissures. Scaly excrescences that itch and burn most violently.

- Dreams of passing urine. Dream of committing suicide in some ridiculous way.

Ratanhia

Dr. Chowdhury

- Sometimes the straining for stool is so very great that the defecation is accompanied by protrusion of hemorrhoids. This burning for hours after stool is a characteristic symptom and is only > by application of hot weather.

- Aesculus hip: has also burning after stool and there is a sensation of fullness, dryness and heat in the rectum with severe dull pain in lumbosacral articulation.

- It is reported to have cured pterygium and itching of the eyelids.

- It has a peculiar toothache. The molar feels elongated with sensation as if ice-cold water rushes out.

- It is said to be a good remedy for pin-worms (ushing reports great success with it in such cases.)

Ranunculus Bulbosus

Dr. Kent
Cold Remedy

- It is a rheumatic remedy of great usefulness when the chest muscles are involved. It is sensitive to motion as in Bryonia and to the cold damp weather as in Dulcamara. It is extremely excitable; hence it has complaints from fright and vexation. Its complaints are < in the evening and after any change of weather especially from warm and cold. After exposure to cold air, his chest muscles are sore as if bruised. He is extremely sensitive to rainy and stormy weather.

- With the pleural effusion it is a very useful remedy. When there is extreme sensitivity along the ribs.
- It has great depression of spirits and desire to die, fear of ghosts, and very irritable even quarrelsome.
- Vertigo when going into cold air sensation of enlargement of the head.
- Violent pains over right eye < laying and > when walking and standing. All other pains are > < from motion except this.
- There is much thirst in the afternoon.
- Excoriating leucorrhea and sharp pains in the ovaries, every cold change in the weather, from motion and evening.
- Sore spots here and there on ribs.
- Sore spots in the spine. Pain along the inner margin of the left scapula, pains in the lower and inner margin of the left scapula in shoemakers, needleworkers, and knitters from sitting bent.
- Corns are very painful, sore to touch, sting, and burn.

Dr. Chowdhury

- It is equally applicable in pemphigus. The blisters are usually large. Some of them are as big as four inches in diameter. As the blister bursts, they expose raw surfaces underneath which keep on secreting a foul-smelling gluey matter. The ulcers are flat and are attended with a great deal of stinging pains.

Dr. Tyler

Differences between Bryonia and Ranunculus in Chest Troubles

- Both have stitching pains < from movement but Bryonia wants pressure on the suffering chest, to keep still while Ranunculus cannot bear the pressure to touch. Again Bryonia < in dry cold weather, Ranunculus in wet weather.

- In the evening both hypochondria and lowest ribs in the chest feel painful as if bruised.

- Violent sticking pain above left nipple near axilla, when rising in am dares not move around or raise it, dares not even raise trunk, lest he should scream with pain, has to sit or stand stooping with head or chest forward to the left.

- Sulphur does not follow Ranunculus well.

Raphanus Sativus

- It's a good medicine for the incarcerated flatus of the abdomen usually occurs after surgery. The flatus is not of extensive type. It is just like a pocket, moving hither and thither in the abdomen. It does not pass either upward or downward but continues torturing the patient (Borland).

- Great rumbling and gurgling are heard in the abdomen, particularly at night time. The pain comes in paroxysm. It is partially > by eating, hence he is obliged to eat all the time during colic. The stools are brown or yellow-brown and are extremely fluid. They are excelled with much force.

- It has a marked action on the female sexual system. We use it in hysteria, especially when associated with pain in the uterus and titillation in the genitals forcing her to orgasm. The sensation of globulus hysterics is also present. A round hot foreign body, starting or the fundus of the uterus, stops at the entrance of the throat and chokes her.

- Mentally they have a great dislike for their own sex. This is illustrated by her antipathy towards her daughter among all her children.

Rheum

Dr. Chowdhury
Chilly patient

- The milk that he vomits up becomes curdled from the excessive sourness of the stomach.

- There is a twitching of the eyelids and the corners of the mouth that gives him the appearance of frothing.

- It has constant and profuse sweat on the scalp, forehead, face, mouth, and nose (Calcarea, Sanicula, Magnesium Mur, Ammonium Mur). A sopping wet head associated with night screaming is particularly characteristic of this remedy. It has an accumulation of offensive mucus in the mouth after sleep.

- Its restlessness and irritability are as marked as in Cina and Antim crud, but it has temporary satisfaction after their whims are gratified.

- It is a capital remedy for diarrhoea and disordered stomach in children arising out of eating unripe fruit. The stools are brown, slimy, loose, thin curdled, sour-smelling, and fermented. It corrodes the anus. Sometimes it is white but turns green after remaining on the diaper. There is also cutting colic in the umbilical region and the patient is doubled up with it by uncovering arms and less.

- It has difficult micturition due to weakness of the bladder. It is invaluable in stupor of children during dentition, associated with a distended abdomen, the result of accumulation of urine in the bladder. The pale face was covered with cold sweat. The sopping wet head, twitching of lips, eyelids, and fingers and its smell never leaves us astray.

Rhododendron

Dr. Kent
Chilly Patient

- He can always foretell a storm. Chorea before a thunderstorm.

- While talking he forgets what he was talking about. Aversion to his business. Easily affected by wine.

- Violent rheumatic headaches in the morning in bed > by morning about, by wrapping of the head and external heat.

- According to Dr. Kent: There was instant relief when the Sun came out.

- Almost all their complaints are < at the onset or just before the storm. There may be > from chewing.

- Deafness due to chronic eustachian catarrh and otosclerosis. The noise complaints are various types - buzzing, rustling, loud echoes, humming, ringing, roaring, tolling of a bell, etc.

- Violent sneezing in the morning with watery discharge from the nose at times. There is a stoppage of the nose alternatively on both sides. The sense of smell and taste diminished. There is increased salivation with a sour taste.

- The stool felt to be unsatisfactory and expelled with much effort. There is no feeling. Diarrhoea < from fruit after a meal.

- Hydrocele of children since birth. Pos-gonorrheal orchitis and epididymitis have been repeatedly cured by this medicine. Metastatic orchitis from mumps (When Pulsatilla fails) Its pain is drawing and sore sensitive to touch.

- It has violent attacks of dry cough lasting hours > or ending in vomiting. At times there is involuntary urination during cough like the Sepia cough, at times it seems to originate from pressure on the epigastration-The stomach cough. Pain in the left chest or walking fast, getting chilled from standing or sitting on the damp ground. The muscles of the chest feel bruised or sprained.

- There is a feeling of sprain or dislocation in some of the joints, shoulder or wrist joints. It should take an important place by the side of Ruta and Rhustox in the treatment of sprains on the wrist especially those who play tennis or golf.

- The whole of the right arm is painful. It gives the sensation of powerlessness or dislocation, rendering holding anything difficult. This reminds us of diabetic neuritis or frozen shoulder in diabetics. The fingers and finger joints are also affected.

- The pains in the limbs seem to be felt in the bones or periosteum.

Rhus Aromatica

Dr. Chowdhury

- It is a good medicine for diabetes.

- The urine is pale and albuminous. The quantity of urine passed is very great (Acidum Phosphoricum, Natricum Acid). It is frequently characterized by great incontinence probably due to atrophy of the bladder muscles, hence it is thought of as senile incontinence.

- A lady who contracted diabetes mellitus and became extremely weak due to frequent passing of large quantities of urine, extreme thirst, backache, a slight rise of temperature, cough, night sweats, and attacks of diarrhoea, reduced her to an extreme state of debility.

- It is a good medicine for painful micturition in children (Lycopodium, Borax, Sarsaparilla).

Rhus Glabra

- It is good medicine for extreme weakness like China.

- This weakness is associated with profuse perspiration, and occipital headache when it is associated with epistaxis.

- A peculiar dream as if flying through the air.

Ricinus Communis
Dr. Chowdhury
- It is a great galactagogue. It has the effect of increasing the quantity of milk in nursing women. Its action is more noticeable in women whose breasts are well-developed.

- Lac defloratum: The diminution in the secretion of milk is due to the atrophy of the mammary gland. The breasts are usually small.

- Urtica Urens: Has always been regarded as the best remedy for the nonappearance of milk in women, when no apparent cause is noticeable.

Chandrakkhar Kali in his cholera Bromium
- It is good medicine for the diarrhoeic variety of cholera and Asiatic cholera. The symptoms come slowly and turn violent afterwards. Usually, there is a history of a disordered stomach, some hours or days before the attack. There are neither cramps nor pains but all of a sudden, the attack becomes violent with the retention of urine. It is a principal remedy when dysentery occurs during a cholera epidemic. Its most important symptom is the presence of watery blood-stained stool before the actual attack of cholera.

- It can be indicated in the stage of cholera where there is constant diarrhoea and vomiting with the absence of a pulse.

- It is the best remedy where cholera is accompanied with jaundice.

- Painless nice watery diarrhoea with frequent vomiting, and soreness of the upper abdomen by pressing it (Painful diarrhoea and vomiting, Aconite, Arsenic alb) are some of its indications.

- Retention of urine, rice water-like stool collapses, loss of voice. Slow thready pulse, cold sweat on forehead. Cold sweaty extremities, great stupper, excessive diarrhoea and vomiting with collapse. The stool becomes so enormous. There is less hope of surviving the patient's retention of urine. It is presently loaded with albumen (Dr. Lillianlbus).

Robinia Pseudacacia
Dr. Chowdhury

- Dyspepsia especially when acidity is the characteristic feature. It is excessive secretion of acid in the stomach as a result of which food soon turns sour.

- Eructation too is sour and they are accompanied by vomiting of liquid sour ingista.

- Even the water he drinks at night is vomited out in the morning in the form of a green sour ropy mucus. His body smells sour. There is constant dull heavy squeezing pain in the stomach, particularly after a meal.

- All the troubles < in the night. During the daytime, the patient is not troubled much by acid vomiting, acid eructation, rumbling, gurgling, and heartburn, which worry him all night and disturb his rest.

- It is indicated in a peculiar kind of sick headache.

- The head feels as if it were full of boiling water and the brain was constantly knocking against the skull particularly when the head was moved.

- The headache is associated with gastric symptoms caused by fat, meat, cabbage, turnips, warm bread and pastry.

- Neuralgia of the jaw bones when it spreads to the eye and forehead. The jaw bones feel as if it were disarticulated. If this neuralgia is associated with the stomach.

- There is hardly any mistake.

Rumex

Dr. Kent
Chilly patient

- The nose, eyes, chest, and trachea. The whole respiratory tract gives forth a copious flow, copious mucus discharge, copious from the nose, that it seemed a continuous flow, so copious from the trachea and bronchial tubes that the patient continually heart covered up by the mouthful thin, frothy, white mucus, so that in a little while as much as half a pint of thin mucus as thin as water would be in the cuspidor.

- It has also marked dryness of the larynx and trachea with hard dry spasmodic cough. In the latter stage, the discharge becomes thick, yellow, tough, or thick, white, and tenacious. This catarrhal state is commonly accompanied by morning diarrhoea and thinness constitutes the leading feature.

- A catarrhal headache with great irritation of the larynx and trachea, clavicular pain, and soreness behind the sternum. Extreme soreness and rawness in larynx and trachea, burning and smarting, unable to endure pressure on throat pit, tickling on the throat pit causing cough.

- A striking feature is pain under the clavicle, a sense of redness under the clavicle as if parts inside are raw.

- There is a sense of thickening, in the nasopharynx and he produces a peculiar noise in trying to get rid of it.

- Soreness, rawness, and burning especially down the trachea and under the sternum.

- Violent sneezing with fluent coryza < in the evening and night.

- Certain kinds of cough are <at 11 pm. (Lachesis), but in Lachesis, young children cough in their early sleep, but if kept awake they will not cough.

- In Rumex the cough will come on at 11 am, whether the child is asleep or not.

- Hoarse, cannot speak because the vocal cords are covered with tough mucus. Phosphorus has this hoarseness but it especially aphonia > by humming up a little mucus from the vocal cords.
- Sensation of a lump in the throat not > by hawking or swallowing it descends on degentition but immediately returns.
- Every cold settles the joint. This is a marked feature of Calcarea Phos.
- Aching pain in the pit of the stomach, gradually becoming very severe, sharp stitching pains in the stomach, becoming very severe.
- Sharp stitching pains in the stomach, extending into the chest and below a sensation of pressure like a lump in the pit of the stomach, sometimes rising under the sternum, greatly < from motion and somewhat from taking a long breath.
- Generally, < after eating > by perfectly quiet. The stomach feels sore < by talking, walking, inhaling cold air, and wanting warm things.
- Morning diarrhoea but preceded by pain in the abdomen. It is not a deep-acting medicine and is always followed by Calcarea Brown diarrhoea usually from 5 am. It is sensitive to cold baths and chilly surroundings as Rhus tox but it is < by motion like Byyonia.
- It is a valuable palliative in advanced phthisis. It will often carry a case through another winter. With Rumex, Pulsatilla, sanguine, Arsenic and Nux vom. We can patch up a phthisis Calcarea Phos.

Dr. Chowdhury

- Clavicular Pain: The patient compliments of raw pain under each clavicle while hawking mucus out of the throat.
- The objective symptoms are rawness and soreness in the trachea, extending a short distance, below the supra trachea, extending a short distance below the suprasternal fossa and laterally into the

bronchi chiefly to the left and tickling in the supra sternal fossa and behind the sternum.

- It is also very helpful in asthma of consumptives especially when the < is about at 2 am.

- Sticta Pulmonaria: Is indicated when the asthma is associated with a spating headache.

- All sorts of skin diseases < from undressing and exposure to the cold (Natrum Sulph, Oleander).

- Cough only during the day, never at night.

Ruta Graveolens

Dr. Kent
Chilly patient

- It falls under a class of complaints that resemble Rhus tox in that it is sensitive to cold < from cold damp weather and the complaints are often brought from straining the parts but principally confined to parts that often drive character aponeurotic fibers, white fibrous tissues, the flex tendons especially flexor tendons that are overstrained by exertion. Periosteal troubles where the flesh is thin over the bone over the tibia. Bruises go away slowly and leave a hardened spot, thickening of periosteum a knotty nodular condition, it remains sore slow repair. A lump on the peritoneum that has existed for months or years resulted from a fall or blow. In farmer's wooden mechanics from holding a hammer or iron instruments, hard nodules on the palm from clasping the hand over a hardened mass.

- The special location is in the wrist bursal and nodules form in this part.

- In eye troubles it is like Argentum Nitricum but Argent is > by cold whereas Ruta is < by cold.

- There is general exhaustion. The less give out on rising from the armchair. The patient totters and makes several efforts to rise from a seat. Routinists give Phosphorous and Conium for this. Ruta and Phosphorous both have a violent unquenchable thirst for cold water.

- It is a great neuralgic remedy and its pain is < by cold and lying down. The severest forms of sciatica pain commence in the back. And goes down the hips and thigh> during the day < as soon as he lies down during the night.

- Amblyopia dependent upon over-exertion of eyes or anomalies of refraction from writing by artificial light, fine needle works, etc, In Weaver could with difficulty distinguish one thread from another and could not read all mistiness of sight with complete obscuration of distance.

- Constipation with prolapses of the rectum. Protrusion of rectum after confinement. It is a useful remedy in piles and stricture of the rectum.

- It is an anti psoric but not so deep as Silecea or Sulphur.

- Regarding myopia especially where it is growing at an alarming rate in young growing children, especially girls who read a lot and are soft and lazy, give Pulsatilla 6 daily with Ruta 30 or 200 twice a week or more frequently. If there is high eye strain, tiredness gives Ruta (I.J.H. 69-153).

Alphabet

Sabina

Dr. Kent
Hot patient

- The use of this remedy is generally confined to symptoms of the kidneys, bladder, uterus, rectum, and anus inflammatory and hemorrhagic symptoms of principally of these parts. It establishes turmoil in the circulatory system with violent pulsation all over the body. The patient is disturbed by heat, is < in a warm room, or from too much clothing. It has a decided effect in diminishing knots, enlargements, or varices in veins. The principal action is on the lower tumors which bleed copiously. Great burning and throbbing in the region of the kidneys.

- Inflammation of the urethra with gonorrheal discharge or catarrhal discharge in the male.

- In the menstrual symptoms, the women suffer from bearing down, labor-like pains. Most distressing in dysmenorrhea. The manses last too long and too copious and at times in some subjects the flow does not stop before the next period begins. It suits many cases in which this flow slackens up and remains away for a while and then labor pains come on and an enormous partially decomposed blood clot is passed and this is followed by bright red blood. Such a state comes after labor and in dysmenorrhea.

- Usually its pains extend from the sacrum to the pubis or uterus. Another striking feature is itching and shooting pains, causing the patient to scream out. Stroking up the vagina to the uterus or up as far as the umbilicus. These two features, shooting pain from the back to the front and from below upwards with hemorrhages are striking corroboration.

- Bellodona and Sabina are the two most important remedies in abortion of three months, Bellodona has the same bearing down pains which expel a clot followed by copious bright red blood but in Belladona it is hyperesthesia, over sensitiveness to touch and jar.

- Chronic catarrh of the vagina with granulation, copious leucorrhea. Bloody leucorrhea, old prolonged psoric cases. This medicine especially suits gonorrhea in women. It cures warty excrescences, gonorrheal warts about the vulva and the male genital.

- In old troublesome lingering hemorrhages, starting up fresh on the slightest provocation, Sabina will stop the gush. The acute stage, but an anti psoric remedy especially Sulphur or Psorinum require to finish up the case.

- Much rheumatism and gout. Gouty nodosites in the joints. They burn so and are so hot that the patient is compelled to put the hands or feet out of bed. Gout alternates with hemorrhage.

Dr. Chowdhury

- The characteristic point of Sabina is the intermittent and paroxysmal nature of all its symptoms.

- It is an excellent remedy for rheumatic affections of the heels. The pain suddenly increases and slowly disappears. The pain is > by cold application.

Sabadilla
Dr. Kent
Chilly patient

- The Sabadilla patient is a shivering patient, sensitive to cold air, cold rooms, and cold food. It is difficult to swallow cold things.

- Coryza with discharge of thin mucus at first and then thick mucus. It has all the appearance of coryza > by inhaling hot air especially useful when the catarrhal state of the nose is prolonged, a prolonged coryza which does not yield to ordinary remedies, a lingering coryza, and the discharge is exaggerated by the odor of flowers. Even thinking of the odor of flowers makes him sneeze and increases the flow from the nose. So, thinking of various things < his complaints.

- Many hay fever patients are sensitive. To the odor of Flowers, the order of the hay field to dying vegetables matters So sensitive to the odor of fruit that the apple has to be removed from the house. They cannot bear the beautiful orders.

- Imagines that the body is withering that the. Limbs are crooked, and the chin is elongated. And larger on one side than the other. Imagines himself sick. Imagine parts are shrunken. That she is pregnant when she is merely swollen from flatus. Then she will have some horrible uh throat disease that ends fatally. The imaginations. are groundless. Nothing visible. And the suffering is greater than if something is seen.

- Mental exhaustion in the headache and produces sleep. Comes from thinking, meditating, and reading for a while. Mediating in a chair. He falls asleep like. Nux Muscata and phosphoric acid.

- Dizziness, Vertigo. He wakes up at night with Vertigo. Vertigo in the open air. All sorts of. Circumstances, headaches in school girls, feeble children who have to be taken from school. Because of the headache come home with a strange imagination. Concerning school and themselves. Attend schools to be fine and associated with coryza in the frontal sinuses and above the eyes

- Up in the morning with headache increases during the full noon. Head covered with cold sweat.
- A peculiar kind of itching coming on in some hay fever is an itching in the roof of the mouth on the soft palate with the coryza. Sneezing Etc. Weethia will cut the attack short.
- When the eating extends to the larynx and trachea with great irritability and sensitivity to cold- Nux Vom.
- It takes the midway between Allium cepa and. Euphrasia, Sometimes the national discharge is bland, and sometimes it is acrid. Sometimes the acrimal discharge is bland, and sometimes it is acrid.
- Great thirst for hot drinks. A pregnant woman does not want to take her milk, but when sits for her, dishes take a full meal. Disgust for all foods to meet, sour things for coffee, for garlic.
- A routine remedy for pinworms seat worms, and all sorts of worms, Sabadilla, and Synapis Niagra are well adapted to cases in which pinworms are present.
- Nymphomania from ascarides.

Dr. Chowdhury
- It brings on fluent coryza and violent spasmodic Sneezing. So violent. Once the sneezing commences, there is no knowing as to when it will end. The sneezing is followed by profuse lacrimation and a copious discharge from the nose.
- It is a good medicine for students and scientists when it is due to too close an application of concentrated attention.

Salicylic Acid
Dr. Chowdhury
- It acts upon the Bony tissue of the body, the bone to which it is particularly destructive, is the tibia.

- It is a great remedy for articular rheumatism attacking. One or more joints, particularly the elbow or knee joints. It causes great swelling, redness, and high fever, and excessive sensitivity to touch motion or jerks is also to be noticed.

- Intense pain, profuse sour smelling sweat, heavy sediment in urine, great swelling, sleeplessness, and great emaciation with anemia. The pain is > by application of any heat.

- It is extremely useful in dyspepsia. The particularly characteristic symptoms are putrid eructation, excessive accumulation of flatus, the acidity of the stomach, great belching of gas, anemia, and despondency. It is even recommended in gastritis and gastric ulceration with a great deal of pain in the epigastric region. Nausea, gagging, vomiting, and waterbrash are frequent. The stools are loose, green, acid and putrid-smelling.

- Its action on the mouth is considerable. The mouth feels hot and dry and the tongue is covered with burning vesicles. The whole mouth becomes dotted with white patches of scalding sores and emits foul breath.

- Big bulging lips express people who are very greedy for eating, good eating. Also for love because you kiss with the lips.

Sanguinaria Canadensis

Dr. Kent

- Headache < by vomiting and the vomited matter is bile, slime bitter substance. Headache > by passing flatus. Usually, the patient suffers from hot palms and soles, so he must put them out of bed. Take an individual who has missed his chronic headaches by some means for a considerable time, but since then he has become increasingly sensitive to cold and cold settle in the nose, throat, and bronchial tubes, and these parts feel as if on fire with rawness and burning. The expectoration is thick, tenacious mucus, disturbance of the belly with much belching, and the belching is especially noticed after a violent attack of coughing.

- **It is not a very long-acting remedy. When a periodic sick headache is interrupted by** sanguinaria, if a deeper drug, an antipsoric is not given, the headache will return, or something worse will come on as sanguinaria does not go deep into the nature of the case. If a chronic sick headache is interrupted the patient will tend to phthisis. Its ability to palliate phthisis is very well known.

- **There is a class of remedies that suits these phthisical patients better than Sulphur, Silicea, and Graphities. Remedies such as Pulsatilla,** sanguinaria, and Senecio Aureus which palliate and mitigate his suffering.

- The patient has a rare cold in June, sensitive to flowers and odors. Subjects with hay fever.

- Thickening of the skin of the palms and soles.

- Headache as if stomach would burst with chilly and burning in stomach.

- Rheumatic pains in the right shoulder joint, so that he cannot raise the arm, and all the muscles of the neck and back of the neck become involved, stiff neck. If the pain comes on in the day it increases as the day advances at night. Complaints < at night. When the patient comes after exposure to cold and cannot raise his arm it hangs by his side. Pain < at night.

- In the chest complaints it has a circumscribed red spot over the malar bones, such as seen in hectic patients.

- Headaches from stomach disturbances, overeating rich food, drinking wine. Almost as useful as Nux vom in old drinkers. Those who disorder their stomachs and weaken their digestion by beer drinking, cannot eat. Vomiting at even a teaspoonful of water, no food or drink stays in the stomach. Headache, vomiting, and diarrhoea are associated with such troubles.

- Acridity of its all discharges, copious loud empty eructations present after cough, no other remedy has this.

- Nausea with burning in the stomach with much spitting, nausea not > by vomiting. Keeps on vomiting and retching Arsenic is given by mistake because of its burning.

- Vomiting of bitter water sour, acrid fluids of ingesta of worms preceded by anxiety with headache and burning in stomach. Such symptoms occur in headache disorder stomach and sour stomach.

- Belching up of acrid fluid in asthma. Asthma with a stomach disorder.

- If you watch a chronic sanguinaria, patient you will notice that the stomach will be disordered for a week. Spitting up of bile, mush flatulence. Sour hot eructation, then all at once this will disappear and a diarrhoea which fairly floods him comes on suddenly, a bilious liquid gushing stool (Natrum sulph, Pulsatilla, Lycopodium).

- Cough < at night with diarrhoea.

- When the asthmatic attack comes on by burning incense (IJH. 67-62).

Dr. Chowdhury

- The patient feels a sensation of rapid movement as if in a car or vehicle and a peculiar vibratory sensation throughout the body. A great desire to be held as in Gelsemium is noticed.

- Offensive nature and acidity of all the discharges of the body. Sensitiveness comes in next. She is painfully sensitive to certain sounds. The sense of smell is equally acute. The least odor produces a tendency towards fainting. The patient cannot stand light, odor, noise, and jar.

- Headache often brought about by the foregoing of an accustomed meal.

- In pneumonia, it is a good medicine for red hepatization. The symptoms are an unwanted amount of dyspnea. The patient finds comfort in no position and practically gasps for breath, his lungs inside his chest weighing like lead. The cough is at first dry and is excited by a tickling and crawling sensation in the trachea and upper portion of the chest. The sputa looks rust-colored. A great accumulation of blood in the lungs also gives a sensation of heat ebullitions. Sharp stitching pains are complained of in the region of the nipple, and offensiveness of the sputa is present. The patient usually prefers lying on his back.

- It is a good medicine for polypus. It is reported to have dissolved many such cases in various parts of the body such as the ear, nose, larynx, and womb.
- It is full of rheumatic pains. Acute muscular rheumatism is when the pains are sharp and erratic in nature. Particularly affects the muscles of the back and neck and sometimes in the deltoid region. The pain vanishes from the painful parts of being touched and appears in some other parts of the body.

Dr. Tyler

Flushes of heat extend from head to stomach as if hot water were pouring from the breast into the abdomen.

- Asthma worse from strong odors- Sanguinaria.
- Fear of darkness and downward motion, obstinate, violent anger, dirty. More or less skin affection, cold sweaty palms, and soles, sweat in head, burning soles. Does not want to cover even in the coldest weather (Sanicula).

Sanicula

Dr. Tyler

Hot Patient

- Sensation of bursting in perineum bowels, bladder, vertex, chest.
- Falls asleep after vomiting (Aethusa, Ipecac).
- Vomits large tough curds, like white at hard-boiled eggs. Vomits after drinking cold water.
- Stomach sensitive to pressure and jar. Cannot laugh without holding stomach and bowel, when stomach is empty.

- Rumbling and gurgling like distant thunder along the course of large intestine bowels bloated as if they would burst.
- Feels as if a hard body like a lead pencil were forced up and back from the bladder to the kidney.
- Child cries before urinating, urine stains diaper red (Lycopodium).
- Odor-like fish brine about genitalia. The child's parts smell like fish brine even after bathing.
- During pregnancy, swelling of stiffness of hands and feet. The sensation that os. uteri are opening and dilating.
- On swallowing sensation of hard substance in trachea.
- Bursting feeling on a vertex on coughing.
- Sharp pain from least during. Most hold themselves stiff and turn their whole body to look down.
- On putting hands together, they sweat until it drops from them.

Dr. Nash mentions it has the combination of the following medicines:

- No two stools alike-Pulsatilla.
- The crying infants after which the sand appears on diaper red-Lycopodium.
- The bashful stools-Silicea, Thuja.
- The immense stool, long retained painful and receding when partly expelled of-Silicea.
- The thin neck-Natrum Mur.
- The emaciation while eating well-Iodum.
- The terror of downward motion-Gelsemium and Borax.
- Every time the child feeds it passes stool (Sanicula, Aloe).

- Rickety child with bed wetting, fishy smell (Sanicula, Medorrhinum).

- When stools are too large, a diameter, appears in the constipation of infants, a dose of Sanicula 50M cures (Dr. C.M. Bogyay).

Santoninum

Dr. Chowdhury

- It is a powerful parasiticide. It is inimical to lumbricious oxyuris and other varieties of intestinal worms. Two or three grains of the 1st or 2nd trituration in a spoonful of sweetened milk on an empty stomach is sure to kill all intestinal worms.

- It has specific action over the eyes. It is found to be curative in amaurosis and blindness. This blindness is due to nervous failure of sight. As Dr. Hole calls it, it is due to paralysis of the optic nerve. It has also been found to be curative in cataracts.

- It is very effective in chronic cystitis. It causes an immediate relief of many of the worst symptoms, such as sensitiveness and soreness of the bladder, incontinence of urine, and dysuria. There ia urine that brings great relief to the patient.

- I fevers in children who are troubled with worms and where on account of worms, it frequently takes on a remittent form, a few doses of Santoninum will remove irritation and cause the fever to come down and also allow other remedies to act more satisfactorily.

Sarsaparilla

Dr. Kent

Chilly patient

- It is suitable in low forms of chronic diseases, especially in complex states, resulting from mixed maism, especially in cases of sychosis, and syphilis, where the tissues become flabby, and refuse to heal when injured. Ulcerate from slight cause. After An

- injury, open sore remains. Or is indolent or become phagedenic and spreads like (Arsenic or Lachesis).

- All the organs are slowed down, weak, sluggish, becomes congested, with weakness and dilation of Veins, and tendency from Varicus in the limbs. Varicose ulcers, hemorrhoids, varicose veins of the face and body. The face is often red and discolored in patches. Useful in old ages when black and blue spots appear on the backs of the hands and elsewhere.

- The skin of the backs and palms of the hands become thick and indurated with barn-like scurf resembling psoriasis intermingled with blue spots.

- Warm food and drink < the complaints. Wants cold food, but heat applied externally is grateful.

- Suitable in old syphilitics, whose complaints have been suppressed by Mercury.

- Marasmus of children from hereditary syphilis. Emaciation about the neck dry purple, copper-like eruption. No assimilation.

- The child is always Passing stool in its diaper yellowish or whitish like chalk.

- Eruptions appeared in the spring. All the various remedies are brought up by winter and go down in the spring. (Lachesis)

- Jerking sensation along the male urethra. Each time he makes water air it passes out of the urethra with a gurgling noise. This symptom is common in catarrh of bladder.

- The medicine has many times dissolved the stone in the bladder. It changes the character of urine and it is no longer possible for the stone to build up.

- Old dry sychotic warts are. Remaining after mercurial treatment for gouty pains.

Dr. Chowdhury

- The urinary complaints are at abeyance during the menstrual period. The bladder does not have trouble during that period of flow, but as soon as the flow seizes, the trouble restarts and lasts the next monthly function.

- Chronic obstinate constipation sometimes calls for this an attempt to pass stool is accompanied by an intense desire to urinate. The patient goes to the closet, sits there for a long time, and strains hard till he breaks out into profuse perspiration and faints (Aloe, Sulphur).

- Sad, discouraged, idiot type.

- Coppery colour eruption which comes and goes with itching.

- Its discharge is offensive eruption and ulcer on both thighs before menses.

Secale Cor

Dr. Kent

Hot patient

- Purplish sports on Withered, skin, purplish, bluish Skin, especially where the circulation is feeble, as on the back of the hands and feet and the tibia, the extremities prickle, burn, and tingle, creeping and crawling as of insects under the skin, as if between the skin and flesh numb. Dead, wooden sensation in the fingers, and especially in the toes.

- Oozing of black liquid blood oozing when there is an inflammation, nose bleed of dark venous offensive fluid, blood bleeding from the throat, lungs, bladder, and rectum of dark blood, urine-like ink, prolonged uterine hemorrhage so that one menstrual sinus runs to another, considerable flow on the first-day fluidly and blackish. This goes on for a couple of weeks and then a dark, watery flow comes on, which lasts until the next. Then comes the thick fluid, horribly offensive flow, again, such as state is found in women who have taken ergot To produce abortion, she says, "I have had no health since I aborted."

- A patient with an ulcer wants to be uncovered. In inflammatory conditions of the stomach and bowels, wants the abdomen to be uncovered.

- Active mania with great excitement exposes her body and tears the genitals put her finger in the vagina and scratches until the lips bleed All idea of modesty is lost.

- Those poisoned by Argot become victims of the opacity of the lenses in. senile debility cataracts of old persons.

- Paralysis of the lower extremities of one side of one arm or one leg. Paralysis of the upper extremities with tingling, numbness, and pricking numbness and burning down the whole length of the spine. General emaciation only of diseased parts.

- Establishes sterility so weak is the uterus that it can never hold the fetus. Hence the value is sterility and repeated abortions.

Dr. Chowdhury

- It is a good medicine for afterpains (Cimicifuga, Gossypium, Sabina). It is similarly used in cases of retained placenta, where the patient complains of strong and constant bearing down in the abdomen.

- In some women, the uterus is in such a state of irritability that the slightest violence, as that caused by an act of coitus, a misstep tripping over a carpet, or a ride over a rough road, will bring about an abortion.

- The miscarriage in this remedy generally takes place about the 3rd month, with a copious flow of black, bad-smelling liquid blood, she gets cramps in her fingers, and she holds them asunder. This distressed her more than the hemorrhage.

- **Viburnum opulus:** The abortion takes place in the first month. The pains are very great, almost labor-like, and of extraordinary severity. The spasmodic pains shoot from the uterus into the legs.

- **Apis:** Abortion of the second month, the stinging and burning pains first start in the ovaries. They get more and more severe till the labor pain starts. Finally ending in miscarriage. The urine is scanty. Absence of thirst and prolonged and obstinate constipation are two other important conditions.

- **Kali carb:** Abortion takes place in the second month. The pains are more of teaching character. The patient complained of very severe backache when walking. So that she must sit or lie down.

- **Crocus Sativus:** Miscarriage in the third month. As soon as blood flows from the vulva it forms Into black string masses. The patient is in a fickle hysteric temperament. She cries and laughs alternatively. This changeability of mood is one of the guiding symptoms.

- **Sabina:** Abortion at third month, the patient generally has a dirty appearance with brown or brownish white spots all over her face and body. Large speedy pedunculated warts are in general abundance. She sweats much, and the sweat is fetid. She has many funny ideas, and very often she's insane.

- **Sepia:** Abortion at 7th month is sepia symptoms.

Selenium

Dr. Kent

Hot patient

- All his nervous symptoms are < after coition, pulsation on all the limbs and in the abdomen after eating.

- Irresistible desire for alcoholic stimulants symptoms < after sleep, especially on a hot day.

- He is excitable and talkative in the evening. Dreads of company.

- His mind dwells on lascivious thoughts, yet he sometimes is impotent All mental symptoms < after coition.

- Headaches from strong odors. Increased flow of urine in headaches.

- The ear is stopped and ear wax becomes hard from which he has a hardness of hearing.

- Aversation To food much salted < from sugar, salt food, tea, and lemonade.

- Soreness in the liver from pressure and inspiration with a rash over the right hypochondrium, stitching pain in the liver from motion and pressure.

- Involuntary urination while walking after urination and after stool Twinge pain outward along the urethra sensation as though drops were pouring out. Sensation as it biting drops where. Forcing itself out.

- Pulsating in the abdomen during pregnancy < after eating.

- It has cured syphilitic psoriasis in palms, itching palms, hands withered, and tearing pains in hands at night.

- He is sleepless until midnight sleeps in short naps, awakens early, and always at the same hours symptoms < after sleep.

- Burning heat in spots, sweat perfuse on chest arm speed, and genitalia, staining yellow sweat from exertion.

- Eating about finger joints and between fingers.

Dr. Chowdhury

- The most characteristic feature of this remedy is debility.

- It is indicated in the headache of nervous origin. It is associated with profound melancholy and profuse flow of urine. This headache is brought on by drinking wine. Tea or lemonade or debauchery. Headache is located over the left eye. < from exposure to strong odors.

- It has strong action over the lever. It is especially used in the enlargement of the liver when such enlargement is associated with loss of sleep, white coated tongue, absence of thirst, sharp stitching pain in the region of the liver, and the onset of a peculiar rash over the hepatic region.

- Hoarseness due to nodes in vocal cords (I.J.H.M-71-78).

Sepia

Dr. Kent
Chilly Patient

- It is suited to tall slim women with narrow pelvis and. Lax fibers of muscles. Such a woman is not well-built.

- A woman who has the hips of a well-built man and is not built for childbearing. She cannot perform the function of a woman without becoming relaxed in the pelvic organ and tissues.

- It abolished the ability to feel natural love. To be affectionate, this state often comes on when nursing an over-vigorous child or twins, who require much lactate fluid and drag her down. It may be brought out in a woman who has an over-vigorous husband, excessive sexual excitement, and overindulgence brings on coldness and she becomes a cold woman.

- She is worse in company, yet dreads to be alone. The Sepia woman permits no opposition to her opinions.

- The whole face is covered with numerous fickles, and great brown patches, as in pregnancy, brown spots on the cheeks, brown warts, and warts that have been red or pink, become pigmented. Lever spots on the face, chest, and abdomen.

- The face is generally puffed, often smooth and rounded, and marked by an absence of intellectual lines and angles. This patient is anemic, with pale lips and ears, a Shallow face fingers, and hands that become shriveled, yellow bloodless. It establishes a progressing emaciation of the body. Premature old age. A woman of 35 years of age looks as if she were 50.

- All gone sensation in feet in the abdomen not > by eating or > for a moment.

- It has a marked catarrhal tendency to milk discharge from the mucus membrane long after digestion has ceased, and the stomach is empty, comes nausea and sometimes vomiting. It is a catarrhal state of this stomach. It persists with milky vomiting.

- Cough during 1st sleep (Lachesis, irritable children).

- Spasmodic dry cough in the evening until mid-night holds the chest during cough (Byonia, Natrum Sulph, Phosphorus).

- It has cured epithelioma of the lips, wing of the nose, and eyelids.

- Never happy unless annoying anyone.

- The headache that particularly affects the occiput < In the morning. Great pain through the eyes and temples > by. Sweat.< or going to move. I'm going upstairs jaundice is often set in with a headache. At the close of the headache, vomiting, and in a few days, jaundice which passes away and returns with the next headache.

- Craves spicy punch and bitter things and beer.

- Pain in the stomach < vomiting.

- Chronic dry stools jelly-like lumpy alternating diarrhea and constipation. A great amount of mucus in the stools. Whether constipated hard stool is covered with a great quantity of jelly-like mucus. Goes for days without a stool and then sits and strains until a copious sweat breaks out and yet no stool but after assistance with finger and prolonger straining, a little stool is passed followed by a cupful of jelly-like mucus, yellow. yellow white is very offensive. The acute diarrhoea and dysentery with jelly-like stools are more in keeping with Kali Bichromicum but it is meant for chronic diarrhoea and dysentery.

- It has much offensiveness. The stool urine and sweat all are offensive. The stool has a putrid, sourish, and fetid smell that expels suddenly, and the whole of it at once.

- In voluntary urination, when coughing, sneezing. The slam of a door and shock. Or when the mind is diverted, sudden desire to urinate and cut. Like knives. And chilly all over the body, if unable to pass it.

- Cypriot patients abort in the 3rd month. Metrorrhagia during the. Climacteric or during pregnancy, especially 5th and 7th months.
- Both males and females have an aversion to the opposite sex.
- A wife has been normal in her relationship with her husband. Brings forth a child. And then the thought of sexual relations causes nausea and irritability.
- In prolapses of the uterus, it has symptoms like Murex but Murex can be differentiated by the following points:

1) Copious menstrual flow violence sexual desire Murex has great soreness and congestion of the uterus and She is constantly reminded of the uterus, acute pain in the sight of the uterus, which crosses the body diagonally upward to the left side of the chest.

2) Its back symptoms are > By heart pressure. (Natrum Mur). The patient commonly puts a book down. On the chair and presses the back against it.

3) The sleep is full of distress and dreams. Cannot sleep on the left side because of palpitation of the heart.

Dr. Chowdhury

- It acts particularly on the portal system and causes a great deal of Venus congestion. We find flushes of heat in various parts of the body, finally breaking out in pools of perspiration. The engorged uterus of Sepia, The sensation of heaviness in the hepatic region. The burning of the palms and soles frequent attacks, and headaches are all to be. ascribed to the same pathological cause.
- When the legs become cold, hands become warm.

- The lower lip is usually swollen, giving the patient. Almost a vulgar appearance. She sweats profusely, but especially in and about the genitals, back, and axilla.

- Its headache is usually hemicrania in nature and mostly reflects her uterine trouble and neuralgic inc character. It begins in the occiput and hence spreads over the whole head to the eyes. It commences in the morning and lasts till noon or evening. It is accompanied by. Nausea, vomiting, and contractions of the pupil > from rest and dark room.

- Profuse sweat around the genitals as in Thuja. It further resembles Thuja in the preponderance of work and condylomata growths around the penis. Numerous cures such as growth ascribed to Sepia even after Thuja failed.

- Slightest injury tends to ulceration, Sepia is particularly our remedy for ulceration about joints especially on the bends of the knees and elbow joints and the tip of the finger. In this respect, it is similar to Borax.

- It is a good medicine for Urticaria, especially when it appears on the bend of joints < from cold baths but when a patient has a particular desire for a warm bath takes a warm bath for a long time.

- Sensation as if a ball moving in the abdomen (Aurum, Silecea, Sepia).

- Sensation as if the Sepia fetus in the uterus, stopped moving (Sepia 1M) (Dr.Knerr).

- The author has used Sepia in ringworms with great satisfaction especially. When they are isolated and cover a small area. In Tellurium large surface of the body is involved and the multiple rings intersect one another.

- Worry (Shock) on arrival of guest.

Senecio Aureus

Dr. Kent

- It is to be studied about young girls with menstrual irregularities. Those who have suppression of menstrual flow from getting wet, from getting the feet wet. Those who have menorrhagia and also who suffer from dysmenorrhoea. In this remedy, with these general features, the young girls gradually tend toward catarrhal phthisis. The menstrual l flow is sometimes suppressed for many months. She begins to look pale. Has dry hacking cough with bleeding from the lungs instead of the menstrual flow. A vicarious spitting of blood. There is a catarrhal state throughout the chest. They are pale and weak girls. They tell you they have lost their menstrual flow and have a chronic cough or are sensitive to every draft of air and are always taking cold and finally expectorate profusely. The phthisis may go on as caterer of the chest for years, but at least. Sets in, especially in this condition, associated with this order of menstrual flow and a general catarrhal state.

- Phthisis with obstructed menstruation. When the symptoms agree in this kind of case, it is the most useful medicine for establishing the menstrual flow.

- These waxy, anemic chloritic girls who have lost their menstrual flow become dropsical after slow hemorrhage from the uterus, kidney, and bladder. Dropsy from anemia. It is the medicine of the highest order for hemorrhage in catarrhal conditions.

- It has many distressing symptoms in the urinary organ. Painful micturition, uncomfortable heat in the neck of the bladder, renal colic, the pain's being so great that it produces nausea, renal dropsy, intense pain over the kidneys. The whole urinary tract is painful and subject to bleeding, but bleeding especially in the absence of menstrual flow, is the feature of this remedy.

Dr. Chowdhury
- It has all the disturbances between the non-appearance of menstruation and a host of other ailments, sore throat, headache, leucorrhoea,, bronchitis, hoarseness, cough, and dyspnea.
- Show decided improvement as soon as menstruation commences.

Senega

Dr. Kent
- It is an old lung tonic. Its chief use has been in chest complaints, asthmatic complaints in various forms of dyspnea, cardiac and asthmatic. There are violent pains in the chest, especially pleurisy. It has also symptoms like pneumonia.
- A violent attack of pleurisy associated with pneumonia. Too deep and too vicious for Bryonia. Often finds its remedy in Senega. Senega is sort of a cross between Bryonia and Rhus tox, the violent symptoms are those of Bryonia, yet are worse from rest. Unlike Bryonia, the symptoms of Senega are not so much like Rhus tox, but it has a similarity to that of Rhus tox> from motion. The pain being < from rest.
- The chest pains, rheumatic pains, and inflammatory pains are <during rest but the cough is < from motion, the asthmatic troubles are <Slightest motion. The patient cannot walk uphill. He cannot walk against the wind because it brings on chest symptoms and dyspnoea.
- The rattling in the chest is as marked as Antim Tar. The tenacious mucus is as copious as gluey and stringy, as in Kali-Bich.
- It is a remedy of deep action as well as an acute remedy, suffering that comes on rapidly from taking a cold or from a cold that involves the whole chest.
- It has cured the opacity of the vitreous humor.
- Aphonia from severe cold or excessive use of voice, causing tickling and burning in the larynx. Leaving the patient not a

moment of rest and preventing him from lying down. Fear of suffocation when Senega is indicated there is dryness of the mouth and throat. And the cough is incessant. There is a constantly metallic taste in the mouth and throat.

- Grippe with stitches in the right eye when coughing.

- Sensation as if chest were too narrow Most violent suffocation with asthma.

- Dry cough with aphonia < From cold air and from walking like Rhus tox and Rumex. Those two remedies cause a cough, which commences when it first goes into the air. Senega has another feature, like phosphorus, in that the cough is so violent it makes him shake from head to foot. It brings on a. tremorous feeling all over the body.

- He breaks out in cold sweat, especially on the upper part of the body. The chest is full of coarse rales from the mucus which he cannot expectorate.

- The concussion from the cough causes the discharge of urine involuntarily and causes violent pain in the head and eyes. The pains are increased, and it seems as if the chest would be torn on coughing. Walls of the chest are sensitive or painful when touched.

- Senega is one of the leading remedies for the tough. Mucus and coarse rales in old people. Without any other symptoms, the profuse secretion of mucus in the lungs of old people.

- In the advanced case of phthisis it acts as a palliative. It is not so deep acting like sulphur and silicea.

- The pains of the chest are < during rest and on inspiring. Stitching pain in the chest when laying on the right side, pain under right scapula when coughing, the chest pains are > in the open air.

Silicea

Dr. Kent
Chilly patient

- The action of Silicea is slow. In the proving it takes a long time to develop the symptoms. It is therefore suited to complaints that develop slowly. At certain times of the year and under certain circumstances, peculiar symptoms will come out. They may stay with the poor throughout their lives. Such is the long-acting, deep-acting remedies. They are capable of going so thoroughly into the vital order that hereditary disturbances are rooted out. Symptoms come on cold damp weather and after baths.

- If he has any mental work to perform, he fears he will make a failure of it. Yet he does it well.

- An old ulcer heels with indurations.

- It suppurates old wounds and indurated tumors. It has cured recurrent fibroids and old indurated tumors.

- Complaints from the suppression of discharges, suppressed sweat, thick yellow catarrhal discharges for a long time.

- Sweat on the upper part of the body and head. Rus tox sweats on the body. The head is dry.

- It will remove blood tumors.

- Pairatoids enlarged from every cold and get hard.

- All sorts of abnormalities in hearing even deafness and roaring in years associated with many diseases and hardness of hearing, hissing, roaring like a stream, like a train of cars, many times from mechanical causes and other times from a condition of the nerves. It is commonly the beginning of a dry cataract of the middle ear.

- Especially with ear troubles, there will be associated, indurated, parotid glands.

- Baby suffers from bloody nasal discharge.

- It has rough leaves cracks and Peel. Fissures in the corners of the mouth indurate.

- It competes with Natrum Mur in inveterate sore throat.

- Decided abortion to warm food wants cool things wants his tea moderately cold. It is sometimes impossible for him to drink hot fluids. They cause sweat on the face and head and cause hot flashes (Baryta Carb).

- The patient is disturbed by extremes of hot and cold. Easily affected by changes even of a few degrees. He complains of being overheated. He gets overheated easily, sweats easily from the slightest change in the temperature, and comes down with a cold. The acute complaints of Silicea often < from warm rooms and heat.

- Cannot bear mother milk diarrhea from it. (Natrun Carb)

- The abdominal symptoms are.> By taking cold food and cold drinks, but the chest complaints and the general symptoms are.<From cold. Abdominal paints> From external heat and last abdomen in children (Baryta Carb). Disturbed by the pressure of clothes.

- Great straining at stool (Alumina, China, Natrum Mur, Nux vom, Nux Moch).

- Patients, who tend to phthisis, are subject to abscesses about the region of the rectum that break inside or out and from complete. Or incomplete opening. If healed by operation or other external means, the tendency is to end in. chest trouble either in the form of a fixed catarrh or tubercular infiltration. Silicea is one of the remedies that turn the constitution into the order In 1 to 5 years the opening ceases to be necessary, and it will heal Silicea here follows Thuja well.

- Involuntary discharge of urine at night. Enuresis in little boys and girls.

- It cures hydrosalpinx and pyosalpinyx with copious watery discharge from the uterus. Sometimes a woman lumps one or the other side of the uterus, which. Steadily increases and all at once there is a flooding of watery, bloody, purulent fluid and the lump disappears. This process repeats again and again.

- Humid asthma coarse rattling the chest seems filled with mucus. Seema as if he would suffocate. Especially the asthma of an old sycotica patient it competes with Natrum Sulph in such cases. The patient is pale, waxy, and anemic with great prostration and thirst. Chronic tendency for colds to settle in the chest and bring asthmatic symptoms. Slow recovery after pneumonia.

- Corns: Ingrowing toenails. Rheumatism of the soles of the feet (Antim Crud, Ruta, Medorrhinum).

- Begins to sweat as soon as he falls asleep (Pulsatilla).

Dr. Chowdhury

- There is a sense of coldness in the ulcers.

- Sense of weakness and debility is constantly on him and he wants to lie down all the time.

- The long list of skin diseases, where Silicea is curative clearly shows that it is useful in psoric and scrofulous diathesis. The patient is as a rule emaciated, pale, and light complexion. There is a marked sensibility to touch, particularly of the scalp and the objects even to the pressure of having to brush the head is also out of questions owing to the same tenderness. Despite this great tenderness a desire to wrap the head warmly to get >.

- Mentally he is feeble, in reading, writing, and thinking bring on fatigue. He experiences great difficulty in fixing his attention on any subject and as a consequence, he makes many mistakes and becomes quite confused. The other aspect of Silicea is irritability. He also suffers from certain fixed ideas for instance, he feels as if pins are scattered all over the place and he is in constant dread of stepping in them.

- In this respect he is similar to Spigelia. He believes as if he were divided into halves. That something alive was in the ears, that his eyes were dragged into the head by a string that a hair was on the tip of his tongue, that a pin was lodged in his throat.

- This patient is also subject to a peculiar type of vertigo. It may be the effect of suppressed foot sweat.

- In diarrhoea the stools are pasty, offensive, and painless. It contains particles of undigested food and is attended with great exhaustion. It suits tiny pot-bellied children during dentition who sweat profusely in the heat. Persistent diarrhoea appears after vaccination.

- Sharp pain either in the breast or uterus of a nursing mother.

- It moderates the too-violent action of the fetus in the gravid uterus.

- It applies to all kinds of fevers, intermittent, hectic, and typhoid. The curative factor always is suppressing foot sweat. The shaking chill begins at 6 pm and obliges the patient to lie down. The foot legs as far as the knees are ice cold. Violent chilly and strong thirst, There is usually a loss of taste and appetite with a marked aversion to warm food. In hectic fever, the sweat starts mostly at midnight and wets the pillow far and wide.

- The convulsion always starts from the solar plexus in or is dragged in or his mothers < at the new moon and full moon.

Dr. Tyler

- Typical Silicea crawls nervously in or is dragged in his mother's hand and you can hardly miss him.

- Rough and yellow nails and feeling as if he had got a splinter in his finger or gets red, swollen fingers that throb and feel like a felon.

- He is an awful boy for knocking, bits off of himself or falling and scratching his knees, and every little hurt or scratch faster and ulcerates and they would never heal and is very sore, he gets burning and sticking pain. Such is the case with a boy with boils, which you would never see. A boil on his chin, neck, pustules, or boils anywhere in the body. He has never been right ever since vaccination.

- One nipple seems to be swollen and painful and shooting pain on the other.

- Abdomen hard tense.

- Bruised feeling over the whole body after coition.

- Dreams of his youth.

- For Molleseum Contagiosum: both Silicea and Sulphur are good remedies. Give it according to hot and chilly (I.J.H- 67.206).

- The soft parts become hard in glands, muscles, etc. Hard parts become soft in teeth, cold abscesses, etc.

- The patient is timid (Lack of courage) but obstinate. The patient is quite nervous and exhibited in various ways, cold, perspiration in palms, soles, etc, A boy was appearing for his Law exam, and he would start vomiting violently,m every time 3 days before his final exam, Silicea cured him.

Sinapsis Alba

- Sinapsis alba cured a woman 8 months into the pregnancy, who was constantly suffering from burning in her stomach extending from the esophagus to throat and mouth. Her mouth was full of canker sore and it was with great difficulty that she could either eat or drink.

- The cough which is barking in nature is > by lying down. The breath of the mouth is very offensive. Sweat on the upper lip and forehead.

Sinapsis Nigra

Dr. Chowdhury

- Dryness of the anterior nares. The left nostril stopped up all day. Scanty acrid discharge from the nose, mucus membrane of nose dry and hot. No discharge. Symptoms. < at afternoon and evening, feeling as if the nostrils were stopped up, although they discharged profusely.

- Hacking cough < during day and > from lying down.

Solanum Nigrum

- It is very similar in its action to Belladonna Its pains too are throbbing, and they come and go quickly. The differentiating points, however, are to be found in its action over the skin, where it tends to produce blackness. The affected parts become swollen and gradually become darker and darker till they look almost black as if dyed. It is a good medicine for gangrene when. Lachesis and Arsenic fail.

- Its application in convulsions and spasms. Is based on a peculiar movement of the hand during an attack. The patient stretches his hands as if to grip something, and then carries them eagerly to his mouth and goes through the motion of mastication and swallowing.

Spigelia

- The patient is easily irritated or offended.

- Vertigo may develop due to digestive upset with a lot of flatulence passing upwards or maybe even due to labyrinthitis.

- It is indicated in eustachian and catarrh. Stopped feeling in the ear and partial loss of hearing.

- It is usually preceded and accompanied by infection of the frontal sinuses.

- It is indicated when any complaints are associated with left frontal sinusitis or affection of the left maxillary.

- Most of the complaints are associated with palpitation.

- Most of the heat complaints are associated with troublesome constipation.

- Fear of pain and sharp pointed instruments.

- Sensitive both physically and mentally.
- Left-sided complaint.
- Slight touch brings on shuddering but > from hard pressure.
- < from slight movement and noise.
- Vomiting and sweating during neuralgic pain.
- Indication for worms: Increases appetite, neuralgic or pressing pain in the stomach.
- There is at times sour regurgitation after eating.
- Pain is pressing upwards both in the stomach and abdomen.
- There are pains and she always has a headache whenever she rides a train.

Dr. Kent
Chilly patient

- Pain in the neck and shoulders are > from heat. Those about the eyes are > from cold, causing a feeling of oppressive in the heart > passing of flatus.
- Shooting and tearing pains in the extremities like a hot wire. Sometimes the pains are < from laying down, but in commonly > from laying still < light, motion, ear jarring.
- There is intercostal neuralgia, tearing pains, shooting into shoulders and neck, especially the left side and down, arms, and pains shooting hither and thither.
- It is full of visual symptoms, visual symptoms bring on complaints. At times he can do nothing but look straight ahead for he has vertigo, even when there is no pain, from looking downward and everything goes round in a whirl.

Dr. Chowdhury
- The Spigelia patients are generally of rheumatic diathesis with Ascaridae and Lumbria. These patients are like Kali, Stannum

Metallicum- very sensitive to youch, the least touch sends shudders to the whole frame. They are pale, sickly, and bloated in appearance.

- Yellow Discoloration around eyes.
- A marked presence of sweat on face and general < of all symptoms from Sunrise.
- Fear of pointed things.
- Dr. Hering cites a case of a man, suffering from extreme pain over the temple and forehead, the effect of injury caused by a brick striking over the eyes, sustained years ago. The symptoms were at irregular intervals, extreme pain came over the site of the wound, It was at times so severe that he feared he would lose his reason. The pain came at about 10 am and reached its height at about 3 pm.

Spongia Tosta

Dr. Kent
Hot patient

- In this drug we find without any cerebral symptoms, marked anxiety, fear of death, and suffocation, associated with palpitation and uneasiness in the region of the heart. It is especially related to cases where there is pain and a sense of stuffiness and fullness in the cardiac region, in the chest with dyspnoea, anxiety, fear of death, fear of the future, fear that something dreadful is going to happen.
- It is just like Aconite, which also excites the heart, brings on anxiety, fear and restlessness, fear of death, and Predicts the hour of death, but Spongia has febrile excitement in a minimum degree. It is much deeper in its action than Aconite. Spongia is a deep-acting medicine though its complaints, sometimes come suddenly.

- When there is rattling of the chest and if the patient wants to be covered (Hepar Sulphur). If the patient does not want to be covered and gets < from it (Causticum).

- Spongia patient < from warm room from heat but > from warm drinks.

- Hypertrophy of the thyroid, goiter, when the heart is affected and the eyes protrude.

- Cardiac dyspnoea and the most severe forms of asthma. Dryness of the air passages with whistling and wheezing, seldom rattling, must sit up and bend forward at times after great dyspnoea. White tough mucus forms in the air passages, difficult to expectorate, it comes up and often has to be swallowed.

- Violent basilar headaches force him to sit up in bed and keep still. This headache is associated with goiter cardiac affections and asthma.

- Dyspnoea and cough are > by warm food and drink.

- Laryngeal troubles with great hoarseness in individual tendons towards phthisis with tubercular heredity, cachectic aspect, weak lungs but no deposit at the trachea. But all at once hoarseness sets in. There is a tendency for the larynx to become involved in phthisical patients, that need Spongia. This patient takes an acute cold and it settles in the larynx with hoarseness.

- In cardiac troubles, the patient, lies without a pillow.

- At times an adult takes cold and rawness of the larynx and trachea is the result. On going to bed she is taken with a spasmodic constriction of the larynx. Laryngismus stridulus is commonly found in women. 1 g Gelseminium will cure 8 out of 10 cases.

- In cardiac and asthamatic troubles it resembles Lachesis in the rising from sleep in suffocation. The Phosphorous, dyspnoea is often < after sleep.

- In phthisis, when the patient is going to die, there is sweat on going to sleep, dyspnoea on going to sleep, and on walking- Lachesis palliate and must be repeated.

- Cardiac affection accompanied by thick, yellow, or green expectoration like pus and dyspnoea on falling asleep, so that he must keep awake for as long as he fears to sleep in advanced chest troubles. Grindelia robusta will palliate that case.

- In acute endocarditis, the principal remedies are Spongia, Abrotanum, Sepia, and Kali.

Squilla Maritima
Dr. Kent
Chilly patient

- It has a loose morning cough and a dry evening cough. (Aluminium, Carboveg, Phosphoric acid, Sepia, Pulsatilla). Pulsatilla He is also strong here, but Squilla has hard cough, gags, and sneezes. Urine escapes and quite frequently feces. The patient coughs. Until he is covered with sweat, he gags and coughs and finally succeeds in raising two or three little lumps of white tenacious mucus. It is a spasmodic cough caused by mucus in the trachea or tickling, creeping sensation in the chest. The loose morning cough is worse than the dry evening cough. The patient is a chilly one and wants a lot of clothing. Urine is generally copious, watery, and colorless. It is one of the important and associated symptoms with cough of chest troubles.

- About 11:00 AM to 12 or 1:00 PM. There is the most common dyspnea for filling of the chest with mucus.

- Copious colorless urine in diabetes when this seems to disappear, chest symptoms appear. The troubles disappear and kidney troubles appear These would disappear and dropsy comes up when the urine would get copious. Again, these dropsy symptoms would disappear.

- Respiration difficult with stiches in the chest when breathing and coughing, great dyspnea. The child cannot drink, seizes the cup eagerly, but can drink only in sips, frequently obliged to take a deep breath, which provokes a cough, and shortness of breath. On exertion pains in the chest < in the morning. Dull rheumatic pains < when exercising > from rest. Evening dry cough with sweetish expectorations. Follows well after Bryonia, absolute lack of sweat is the great characteristic.

Dr. Chowdhury

- Acrid corrosive, fluent coryza, sneezing, soreness of the nostrils as in Allium-Cepa.
- The cough is caused by a tickling sensation in the chest, sometimes tickling is felt as low down as region of the spleen. Hence it is recommended very highly for splenic cough. Stitches are felt during cough under the free ribs of the left side.
- Dr. Boger brought great relief to a patient suffering from angina pectoris on the principal indication of profuse urination accompanying severe chest pains and much loose mucus in the throat and trachea.

Stannum

Dr. Kent
Chilly Patient

- Some deep-seated constitutional state must be present. There is a sensitiveness to pain and an increasing aversion to doing anything.
- The countenance becomes increasingly sallow, even to a waxy cachectic aspect.
- The pain sometimes begins with sunrise, increases until noon, and gradually diminishes and ceases with sunset. On the other hand, it may begin at any time, as often at 10 am, and increase for 10 or 20 minutes, then gradually decrease until gone.

- If the Stannum neuralgia is suppressed. we will see phthisis making its appearance. If the neuralgia is not permitted to have its way, the patient becomes over-sensitive to cold and takes cold easily.

- Headache every morning over one or other eye, mostly the left, gradually extending over the whole forehead and increasing and decreasing gradually after vomiting.Intermittent supraorbital neuralgia.

- If you ever meet with a case, who has suffered with violent neuralgia and she says since the obliteration of the pains, she has copious thick, yellow, green leucorrhoea, think of Stannum. This leucorrhoea may save her otherwise he may be developing phthisis.

- Paralytic symptoms, winter cramps. Women cannot let go of the broom (Droserea cures most cases).

Dr. Chowdhury

- Most of the time the patient lies on her back with one leg stretched and the other drawn up.

- Pain in the molar lone and its great sensitivity to touch also of < occurring before and during menses.

- It is essentially a voluptuous remedy. The slightest irritation and least approach of thoughts brooding on sexual subjects bring on emission. Hence it is frequently used in nocturnal emissions, spermatorrhoea, and neurasthenia, especially when such sexual sensitiveness is great. Emission takes place without the least sexual dreams. Scratches arms produce an intolerable sensation of pleasure in the genital organs, which extends to the uterus and produces sexual orgasm.

- There is a marked hectic fever towards the evening with profuse sweat at night.

- Nausea and vomiting from the odors of cooking food.

- Diarrhoea and Monday constipation or constipation appearing particularly on the day following rest.
- Stannum: is a good medicine for chronic amoebiasis. If there is a lump of mucus gushing out during stool.
- Cina: Every stool contains mucus and sometimes blood.
- Teucrium: Irritability is not so marked as Cina. The tongue is somewhat coated, and every stool does not contain mucus. Usually changeable stool.
- Santoninum: Tongue usually coated, the ulcer-like appearance of the tongue.

Staphisagria

Dr. Kent
Chilly patient

- First the impression made upon the mind, and thereupon on the body. The person becomes speechless from suppressed indignation, anger with indignation.
- Irritable bladder with frequent urging to urinate, lasting many days after suppressed wrath, after insults.
- Person having blue lips, trembling hands, pains about the heart, and all over.
- He thinks he is going to die. This is a great indication of Staphisgaria and it is caused by suppressed wrath or anger.
- The senses are in an irritable state so the tips of the fingers are sensitive. The ears are sensitive to sound. The tongue is sensitive to taste and the nose to odors. Every little inflamed spot will have its center-sensitive points. Little nerve spots, and ulcers when touched cause the patient to go all to pieces and a convulsion threatens. Little nerve tumors form in the skin, and little polypoid growths, the size of a wheat grain, when touched will throw the patient into convulsion and suffer for days and

nights. A hyper-sensitive new growth will come out on the hand or the back sometimes it turns black.

- The Staphisgaria headache is a numb, dull pain in the occiput and forehead especially in this nervous constriction headache from vexation and indignations.

- Scrofulous glands, glands of the neck enlarged, enlarged and indurated ovaries and testes, stitching, tearing pins in the gland everywhere. Hardness and chronic indurations. Hardness of tonsils. Pains come on after eating.

- Chronic diarrhoea or dysentery of weakly, sickly children, After anger, after being punished, after emotions.

- Stitching in the region of the heart, and trembling of the body with nervous excitement is an excellent indication of Staphisagria.

- A patient has an eruption on his legs as high up as the knees, that looks like a pair of trousers with arthritic nodosides on the fingers, which was cured by this remedy.

- It has nightly bone pains.

- It is a good medicine when the insomnia of a patient comes suddenly. The sy, symptoms are either suppressed wrath anger, or due to sexual excess.

Dr. Chowdhury

- It is regarded as a great germicide and the allopaths still use it to destroy lice and itch mites.

- These patients look abashed. They cannot look you straight in the face. The nose is pointed and the eyes are sunken.

- The diarrhoea or dysentery is always < after a meal or after drinking cold water.

- It is a very good medicine for eczema. The erumption may be dry and scary, or moist, with yellow crust discharging a very offensive secretion. The usual site is the head, especially the obsequent and the region behind the ears. The whole hair is skull becomes covered with a dark, scaly eruption, a scratching causes bleeding and a discharge of clear. Nonloutinous fluid, which dries quickly, leaving the whole head covered with yellow offensive crust.

Dr. Tyler

- Pressive, boring stitch left forehead from within outwards. Its violence wakes him up from sleep in the morning.
- Inflammation of white off-eye with pains.
- Gum's bleed when pressed or when brushing teeth.
- Hard painful pressure in the right abdomen below the navel.
- Call to urinate, Scarcely a spoonful passes, mostly reddish or dark yellow in thin stream or by drops, and after he has passed it, always feels as if the bladder were not empty for some urine continues to dribble away on waking from sleep, pressure in the bladder.
- Every time water is passed, burning in the whole urethra.
- Frequent sneezing with or without coryza.
- Correca at first blows only thick mucus from Lowe's. Afterwards, thin discharge.
- Tightness in the chest at the end of coitus.
- Violent yawning, so that tears come into the eyes.

Stramonium

Dr. Kent
Chilly patient

- Fever with hot head and cold extremities, high fever, big delirium. The heat is so intense that it may be mistaken for Belladonna. But it is usually continued fever only at times, remittent, while the intense fever of Belladona is remittent always.

- Crushing tearing the cloth, erotomania (exposing the person). The symptoms are found in continued fevers, insanity, and cerebral congestion. It is useful in violent typhoid.

- When the delirium is not on. The patient has the appearance of great suffering, forehead wrinkled, face pale, sticky haggard in headache. This anxious look is indicative of intense suffering from meningeal involvement.

- Screams until he is hoarse or loses his voice.

- Screeches and screams day and night with fever with forms of mania. Violent laughter with sardonic expression of his face.

- In cerebral congestion, the delirium subsides into unconsciousness. The patient has the appearance of profound intoxications, pupil dilated or contracted, Marked stuper, stertorous breathing, lower jaw dropped. In typhoid and other low forms of fever, Using a blood from the mouth and other passages through the mouth, dry, tongue dry, swollen so that it feels the mouth pointed red like a piece of meat, bleeding from the mouth, sordes on the teeth, lips dry and cracked at times, violent thirst, yet dread of water, diarrhea, copious involuntary abdomen, lymphanitic involuntary urination.

- Maningitis from suppressed ear discharges, forehead, eyes glassy, staring, dilated pupils. Awful pain through the base of the skull.

- Violent headache from walking in the sun and from the heat of the sun < All day and at night, the patient must sit up because of increasing pain of laying down < From every motion.

- It cures troubles of irritation of the brain from overstudy in students who are much obliged to do networks to keep up with day literature.

Dr. Chowdhury

- The beseeching and the brain attitude is often marked within young women with suppressed menses, girls who are naturally form a religious bent of mind, turns pious on such occasion. They sing pious songs, solemnly utter words of wisdom and even delivers sermons of great virtue. They lie on their back with their knees flared and their hands join together. These patients in their unconscious delirium jolts up their heads from the pillow and then drop them back again. They think they are very tall, and other. Objects around them are dwarfish. The patient had a great desire to hide themselves.

- In cholera hiccup with very frequent black almost jet black and offensive stool is found,

- The secretion of urine becomes either suppressed or scanty, as this condition is often to be met within cholera, eclampsia and nephritis. The urination is accompanied with. Vigor and rumbling in the abdomen and with symptoms of cerebral hyperaemia.

Dr. Tyler

- Seen more at the sides than in front curiously.

- Sexual irritation hands constantly on genitals.

- The glass of water, which ready for drinking, looked black, and her face was black.

- Fever at noon.

Sticta-Pulmonaria

Dr. Chowdhury

- The whole of the buccal cavity of the throat is so dry, parched, and leather-like that our patient finds it hard to sleep. He sits up all night. Unfortunate man, sneezing and coughing. It is towards the later part of the morning when the palette and throat get a bit moistened that he can sleep.

- It is almost specific for hay fever. Dr Herring says at night, discharges almost cease, and air passages become dry. Paroxysms of sneezing are more frequent, as explosions seem to number more at each paroxysm until sneezing and coughing almost incessantly, and very little sleep until morning when hyperemia gradually subsides. Air passages become more moistened at sunrise. There is again a profuse discharge from the eyes and nose, which is hot and excoriating, causing rawness and soreness of the cheeks border of the nose and upper lip.

- Its cough is rather dry, incessant, and titillating. It has proved very successful in that distressing teasing cough that follows in the wake of measles and influenza. It also gives relief in the distressing and treating cough of phthisis.

- It is a good medicine for the rheumatism of the right shoulder. Wrist knee and ankle joint.

Dr. Nash

- Heavy full feeling and pain and pressure in forehead and root of the nose > by discharge.

- Secretion in the nose dries up and from crusts Constant inclination to blow the nose without result on account of the excessive dryness.

- Dry night cough cannot sleep or lie down. Must sit up. Cough after measles.

- It is meant for inflammatory rheumatism of the knee joint. It is very sudden in its attacks and unless promptly relieved by Sticta will go on to the exudative stage and become chronic in character.

Stilliangia- Sylvatica
Dr. Chowdhury
- It produces symptoms very similar to those seen in secondary syphilis such as bone pains, modular growths, or forehead and tibia, caries of nasal bones, chronic rheumatism, etc.
- Where Merc Sol, Aurum, and Thuja failed, think of this medicine.

Strophanthus Hispidus
Dr. Chowdhury
- It is an important heart remedy. Weak heart due to great debility of the heart muscles.
- Quite a lot of dyspnea is experienced due probably to the edema of the lungs.
- Mentally these patients are irritable.
- A certain amount of loquacity is well marked as Lachesis.
- Nausea without actual vomiting is an important symptom. There is great loathing of food if however he eats any food, it is vomited out.
- The patient experiences great burning in the esophagus and stomach.
- It is good medicine for hypertension and the indications are as follows: irritable heart of tobacco smokers with urinary troubles. Use Q. (1970, H. Gleanings).
- Spartium: Hypertension of heavy smokers who grow weak with albuminuria and dyspnea, Calcarea symptoms (H. Gleanings, 1970, Hypertension).

Strontiiana Carb

Dr. Chowdhury

- < of its congestion from least movement, there are people whose face becomes livid and flushed every time they move about. These patients are great subject to appoplexy. It is a valuable medicine for congestive headaches and climaxes. The flushes are frequent and continuous. The symptoms that help Strontiana to differentiate the symptoms of Lachesis is great desire on the part of the patient to have the head wrapped up in spite of the fever and warmth.

- The author himself has written as follows "I'm ever grateful to Strontina for the relief it gave me, while still a medical student at. Chicago from an attack of persistent nocturnal diarrhoea, to which, unfortunately, I became a subject. It used to come at every night with a peculiar urging that made me sick to the closet for hours. I would Scarcely be off the vessels before I had to return. It used to leave me. Particularly. After 3:00 AM" H. C. Allen prescribed Strontiana. It is equally great for constipation. The stools are large, hard and expelled with great effort. Defecation is followed by pain in anus and burning lasting for hours and compelling the patient to lie down.

- Chronic spins of ankle joints when other remedies such as Arnica, Ruta and Rhus tox fail, there is almost always a certain amount of edema associated with this. Dr. Borger Cured with Strontiana a case of sciatica with inciation of its being associated with edema of ankle joint of the same side. It is a great drug for anginal pain. The angina is accompanied with high BP pain in cardiac region with frequent startling (I.J.H. 91-110).

- The acute case corroborating to that of.Strontiana, Is always found to be thoroughly responding to Syphillium (I J H M 71-55).

- If there is severe pain in White low. Give this medicine to relieve the pain. Dr. Rue said. It would relieve the pain of white low instantly.

Strychinium

Dr. Chowdhury

- Great hyperaesthdesia of pharynx and esophagus.

- A great feeling of stiffness and a marked visibility of the cervical muscles.

- Spasmodic twitching and jerking and a general tremor of. Almost all muscles of the body.

- Great relief by laying on back and continued hard massage and rubbing.

- < From slightest touch and the constant presence of consciousness from the beginning to the end.

- There is a great sensation of eating of the roof of the mouth.

- Sensation as if head and face were enlarged.

Sulphur

Dr. Kent

Hot patient

- The child is subject to catarrhal discharges from the nose, the eyes, and other parts. And he offered. And he often eats the discharge from the nose. The sulphur patients are very selfish in nature.

- The patient is always imagining and hunting for offensive odors. He commonly has such a strong imagination that he smells the things that he has only in memory.

- Filthy discharge is characteristic of sulphur. He has filthy-smelling genitals, which can be smelled in the room despite his clothing, and he smells them.

- They have all sorts of eruptions, there are vesicular, pustular, and scaly eruptions. The skin even without any eruptions itch as much itch from the warmth of the bed and from wearing woolen clothing. Many times the sulphur patient cannot wear anything except silk or cotton.

- Nightly. < Other feature headaches beginning after the evening meal and increasing into the night. He cannot get to sleep because of the pain. Intermittent periodic neuralgia. < Every 12 am and 12 pm. Midday is another time off. < It has a chill at noon, fever, increase at noon, an increase of mental symptoms, and headache at noon.

- Thirsty patient always drinking water. He also speaks of hunger feeling a desire for food. But when he comes to the table, he loathes food, aversion to milk and meat.

- The skin will not heal easily small wound continues to suppurate.

- The tissues seem to take on weakness so that every little pressure causes soreness, sometimes inflammation and suppuration. Old sores come on easily. Induration from pressure is a strong feature.

- If a shoe presses anywhere on the skin, a great corn develops. Where the teeth come in contact with the tongue and other parts of the buckle cavity nodules and these little nodules over time commence to ulcerate.

- Feeling as if hot steam were inside the body and gradually rising. And then she breaks out in a sweat. When the flushes begin in the chest about the heart It is more like sulphur But when in the back or in the stomach, it is more like phosphorus.

- < after sleep, especially mind and sensorium. Most of the complaints are < after eating.

- Is full of excitement. Is easily startled by the noise. Much trouble sleeping, he's very sleepy in the. 4th part of the nighttime. Sleeping till 3:00 AM. But from that time on, he has restlessly or does not sleep at all. He dreads daylight. Want to go to sleep again and then when he does not sleep. He can hardly be roused and wants to sleep late in the morning.

- Sulphur like silicea is a dangerous medicine to give where there are structural diseases.

- In suppressed gonorrhea, it is often the remedy to start up the discharge and. establish the condition that have been positive disappear.

- Person to work in the coal mine or handle the coal.

- Measles when they are out with a purplish color very often requires sulphur.

- The dreadful effects of vaccination are often cured by Sulphur. In this, it competes with Thuja and Malandrium.

- It has an aversion to following up things in an orderly fashion, an aversion to real work and systematic work. The patient is a sort of inventive genius, with an aversion to business.

- Foolsh happiness and pride, thinks himself in possession of beautiful things, even rags seem beautiful.

- He is slow in gathering himself to gather after sleep < from sleep.

- Most headaches are coming on Sunday in working men who are cured by Sulphur. Sunday is the only day he does not work and he sleeps late in the morning and gets up with a headache that involves the whole head with dullness and congestion, being busy and active prevents the headache during the week. Headache by stooping, headache t times in those who suffer constantly from drinking.

- Left ankle sprain (Sulphur, Natrum Carb). When Natrum Carb fails give Sulphur.

- Sulphur patients are curious like a scientists and go on questioning about everything.

- Extreme craving for milk, bat milk <.

- Useful in persons who get up in the morning with a headache, dizziness, and red face. Before the headache comes on there is flickering before the eyes and flickering of colour. Scintillations strart. Saw teeth zig zag are forewarning of headache. Whenever he disorders his stomach, he has this peculiar vision. It comes also when he is hungry in the evening and delays in eating. This state is also found in Natrum Mur and Psorinum. The zig zag flickering sparks stars and irregular shapes appear before the eyes periodically and may last an hour or so.

- Much dandruff in the hair and less of hair. There is a slow closing of fontanelles.

- There is a tendency for every cold to settle in the eyes. Ulceration of thickening of the eyelids rolled out and inwards loss of eyelashes.

- Thickening of the mucus membrane and the drum of ears, All sorts of strange noises in the ear until the hearing is lost. Frequent stoppage of ears, especially when eating or blowing the nose.

- Smell before the nose as of an old catarrh and so troublesome is the Sulphur nose, catarrhal states that with odors he is made sick. He thinks he smells his catarrh and thinks others also smell it.

- Periodical neuralgias in those that live in a malaria eliminate especially on the right side of the face.

- Erysipelas begins on the right side of the face and about the right ear and there is considerable swelling of the right ear it spreads slowly, and moves with sluggish and unusually purple. In erysipelas, Arsenic and Apis burn like fire. Rhustox has blisters upon the erysipelatous patches.

- Scabby lips, chapped lips, cracks about the lips and corners of the mouth.

- White patches in the mouth very useful remedy in the sore mouth of nursing infants.

- These patients are commonly dyspeptic and digest almost nothing.

- Every cold, every bath, and every change of weather < his liver symptoms.

- He cannot stand because the abdominal viscera hang down so they seem to be falling.

- He has spells of colic without being flatulent. The winds are confined, dreadful spells of colic, cutting, tearing pain and > In no position, burning and smarting in the whole abdomen and soreness of the intestine.

- Morning is the typical time for diarrhea, but diarrhea comes on after midnight.

- It is a wonderful remedy in cholera and in these cases of diarrhea that occur in cholera times. It is also great medicine in dysentery when the stool is bloody mucus with constant strain sulphur often cures. This case after Natrum Sulph fails.

- Every cold settles in the bladder like sulphur, and when Dulcamara fails, gives sulphur.

- Sulphur and Sepia are suitable in most violent cases of dysmenorrhoea in girls and even in those of advanced age. Most violent cases have existed for a long time since the beginning of menstruation in women who always needed Sulphur.

- Septicaemic condition with purulent lochia on suppression of lochia, on that day there has been a chill, and the lochia was suppressed. The woman has a high temperature and is covered head to foot from sweat. If you put your hand under the covers you feel steam come up from the body. She is dazed and sensitive over her whole abdomen. Give sulphur in this case instead of giving other medicine. Now, on the other hand, if in such a case with hot sweat and other general features, you have one rigor following another in rapid succession and no end to them. You cannot get out of that case with lycopodium. When there is a continuous intermingling of little chillness and little quiverings throughout the body and the pulse has lost its proper relationship to the temperature, Pyrogen must be administered. If there is a purplish appearance of the body, cold sweat all over, if there are remittent or intermittent chills with thirst during the chill and at no other time and the face is red during the chill. Give Ferrum.

- Full of difficulty breathing, and shortness of breath from very little exertion. Every time he gets cold, it settles in the chest or on the nose. In both these instances, the catarrhal state hangs on and holds for a long time. Every cold ends in asthma. The patient is never well, since the attack of pneumonia. He has had a chronic cough ever since the attack.

- It has the most violent cough that rakes the whole frame. It seems that the head will fly off pain in the heart when coughing. The head is jarred by the cough.

- Pain in the back or rising from the seat, compelling him to walk bent. And he can only straighten up slowly after moving. The pain is principally in the lumbosacral region.

- Tightness in the hollow of the knees. Tightness in the tendons. Rheumatic and gouty character. Cramps in the soles of the feet.

- After childbirth give a dose of Sulphur 1M to both child and mother (I.J.H.72-7).

- For bed wetting always give a dose of Sulphur, when it fails try Sepia.

- Sulphur children may be playing all the time in water.

Dr. Chowdhury

- In Laryngitis, the prominent symptoms are hoarseness and aphonia< in the morning. The more chronic the case, the better indicated.

- Sharp stitching pain through the left lung to back.<When laying on back and least movement.

- The cough is accompanied by pain in the chest, as if. It would burst to pieces. Sometimes there is a peculiar sensation of coldness in the chest, as from a lump of ice.

- In dysentery, there is tenusmus after school and as in Colchicum, the patient falls asleep as soon as the tenusmus ceases.

- The patient sweats very much on the head, especially during sleep.

- During fever, ice coldness of the genital is a great indication of this remedy.

- There is an involuntary discharge of cement with burning in the urethra.

- In epilepsy, the aura seems to proceed from the extremities up to the back as a creeping sensation, or up the leg to the right side of the abdomen. The patient is apt to fall on the left side.

Sulphuric Acid

Dr. Kent
Chilly patient

- The sensation of quivering All over the body and in the limbs, without visible trembling, is a very strong symptom of sulfuric acid. It is especially associated with long-standing weakness. Black fluid blood from all the orifices of the body. Blue-black spots on the skin from a slight injury. It has many of the complaints found in old people. The morning < of symptoms And general sweat after eating are the guiding symptoms. The symptoms are The brain seems loose and seems to fall to sight. predominant on the right side.

- Prostration of mind and body with extreme sadness. Weeps continuously. Nothing can be done to please him. All things must be done at once Unwilling to answer.

- The brain seems loose and seems to fall to the side < walking. The blood flows strongly from the. Head and feet become cold. The hair falls out or turns gray. Lacrimation when reading.

- Slowly oozing dark thin blood from the nose in the evening.

- Violent neurologic pains of the face coming on gradually and ceasing suddenly > By warmth and laying on a painful side.

- Craves brandy and fruit. Aversion to the smell of coffee.

- Diarrhoea with a great general sinking sensation in the abdomen after stool. Diarrhoea is brought on from the least indiscretion in eating fruits especially if unripe and after oysters.

- Pain in the bladder if the desire to pass urine is postponed.

- Menses too frequently and copious and the flow is dark and thin and has nightmares at the close of menses.

- Oppression of the chest and suffocation unless he lets the leg hang down. It has been a very useful remedy in the first stage of phthisis, with profuse sweat and great weakness. But when given in the last stage, it appears to bring on hemorrhage and increase the inflammation condition of the lungs. Soreness between the shoulder blade and coughing, stitching pain in the shoulder joint on lifting the arm.

- Late falling asleep and wakens, too early. Nightmare before menses.

- Copious sweat mostly on the upper part of the body.

Dr. Chowdhury

- It is needed in the coughs of drunkards and women in their climacteric years. It is a short of hacking, dry, constant cough, very frequently they complain of sudden violent pain in the upper left chest, passing through the supra on that side.

- It is indicated in hernia scrotalis when there is a great tendency for the hernia to come down. Dr Guernsey recommends it for Hernia in profoundly weak infants.

Syphilinum
Dr. Kent
Hot patient

- Whenever the symptoms that are representative of the patient himself have been suppressed, in any case of syphilis and nothing remains but weakness is present.

- When a syphilitic patient has suffered from a course of typhoid, he may be very slow in convulsing. Hereby a single dose in high will restore the case.

- When there. Is violent neuralgia of the head in the sides of the head over the eyes, great soreness in the bones of the legs and head, and a multitude of symptoms of nerve Syphilis.

- There is great prostration in the morning on walking.

- Sleeplessness. Sometimes only one half of the night. Again, the whole night's complaints.

- Aggravates in both cold weather of winter and summer.

- Dwarfish children, curvature of the spine and other bones and last glance offensive order of the body, soreness to touch in many parts, especially bones.

- Sulphur often produces prolonged aggravation when there are many tissue changes in advanced cases of syphilis. Such changes are most likely gummata. It often causes the suspension of latent syphilis. When such aggravations are very severe after a sulphur high dose.

- It is a very good medicine for skull injury. Both Ruta and Symphytum are effective in bone injury, but in Symphytum pricking pain is felt on the affected part. During the treatment pf duodenal ulcer for intermittent pain give Symphytum 6 (Dr. Kent).

- Asthma appears in warm weather.

- The patients are liars or cheats and are full of vices. These patients want to remain in a neat and clean position. (I.J.H.M-72-62)
- Laughing and weeping without cause cannot remember face, names, dates, events, books, or places, fears he is going insane Imbecile, indifferent to his friends, and feels no delight in anything.
- Analysis of the eye muscles is a common chronic recurrent phlyctenular conjunctivitis, interstitial keratitis.
- Carries off the mastoid bone, Paralysis of the auditory nerve.
- Offensive green or yellow discharge from the nose in children with a specific history. Dryness in nose obstructed at night. Frequent attack of coryza. Always taking cold in the nose.
- Ulceration of soft palate carries of hard palate.
- Longing for strong drinks, thirst aversion to food. No desire to eat. All food disagrees.
- Nodular formation in testes, spermatic cord, and scrotum induration of testes and spermatic cord.
- Leucorrhoea of little girls with a specific history.
- Ulceration of the larynx and loss of voice, asphonia before menses.
- Dry cough from laying on the right side.
- Aching in whole spine pain in reason of kidneys.< after urinating. Pain in sacrum < while sitting. Caries of cervical and dorsal vertebra.
- Rheumatism muscles are cracked in hard knots or lumps. Pain in lower extremities, preventing sleep < from hot application > from pouring cold water. Pain in back of foot and toes at night.

Dr. Chowdhury

- Constant stream of boils, which breaks out in endless succession, one after the other.

- Foetidity of all the discharges and secretions.

- Excruciating headache that. Cause sleeplessness at night. It makes him restless and keeps him constantly on the move. This tendency to move and walk during severe headaches is a keynote indication.

- Desires to wash her hands constantly.

- It has chronic constipation and is due to a kind of stricture high up in the rectum The breath of the patient is very offensive.

- Fistulous opening exostosis, fissures, tubercles, and warts have been cured promptly (Dr. Kent).

- Abdominal colic < night, if Syphilinum fails, give pituitaria.

- It is a very good medicine for any kind of fever. When the fever does not abate, despite giving the best-indicated medicine, give a dose of.Syphilinum High dose. Usually, there is a history of abortion of the mother history of Blood pressure erosion of the cervix or heavy leucorrheal discharge. 4 to 8:00 PM.< (Lycopodium, Helonias). When these medicine fails think of Syphilinum. It has also an itching eruption > from the warm application.

- DR. Wheeler in his book "Introduction to the Principles and Practice of Homeopathy" writes that whenever there is a Syphilitic miasm that patient has a low resisting power and as a result, children of syphilitic parents succumb to diseases like pneumonia, typhoid, etc.

- Constant desire to wash hands. The patient does not allow anybody to touch, thinking that she may be polluted by touching others. So she washes the parts quickly which are being touched or used. (KI.J.H.N, 71-61)

Alphabet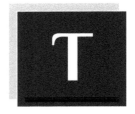

Tabacum

Dr. Chowdhury

- Intense nausea with incessant vomiting like Ipecac but Ipecac is wanting in great prostration. The tremor the cold, clammy sweat, and the palar of the skin.

- Dr. Hering Reports of a case of a lady aged about 70 ailing upwards for a year. Her complaints were nausea, vomiting, and constant pain in the stomach. She often threw up mucus and blood together with the food taken. But what ailed her most was the incessant pain in the stomach and the intense and constant feeling of sickness.

- Its symptoms are > From exposure to a draught of open fresh air and from uncovering <From slightest movement even that of opening the eyes.

Dr. Chandra Sekhar Kali : Cholera

- It is a very good medicine in the stage of collapse coldness of the extremities, heat of the abdomen and chest, constant nausea (Ipecac) I am vomiting with pain in the abdomen. The whole body covered with cold sweat wants to. Uncovered the abdomen, which > the symptoms < from motion cramping of the extremities.

- Difficulty in breathing.

Taraxacum Officinale

Dr. Chowdhury

- Mapped tongue. This is caused by little patches of white coating, off from different places, exposing the red, tender, sensitive, surface of the tongue. Bitter taste in the mouth.

- The liver becomes enlarged and indurated.

- Billious diarrhoea.

- Another important symptoms is chilliness.

- It is a good medicine for thphoid and its symptoms like Rhus tox.

- We have the same muttering delirium, the same intolerable pain in the lower extremities during rest as great prostration, but in Taraxacum violent tearing pain in the occiput, great chilliness after eating and drinking.

- The mapped toungue and the coldness of the finger tips makes this remedy successful.

- It is a right sided medicine.

Tarentula Hispanica

Dr. Kent

- Anxiety and restlessness prevail all through its condition. It is much like Arsenic, when Arsenic fails we should think of this medicine Cardiac anxiety is a strong feature. A strong aversion to colors, such as green, red, and black. Desire to run about, to dance, to jump up and down. Sometimes music > all the symptoms and sometimes it < the symptoms. Emaciation is so marked, that it may be said, sometimes that the flesh falls off him.

- Creeping and crawling in the skin all over the body.

- It has an appearance like " St. Vitus's dance" and has cured Chorea when > from music. Sometimes it is also < from music.

- It is full of pains in the body and limbs and pains in the bones, arms, and joints.

- Periodicity is so well marked, it has been marked as a curative remedy in intermittent fevers with restlessness in limbs., aching of the bones with stitching pains and anxiety, especially when these come in the evening followed by fever without sweat is a marked feature.

- Susceptible to cold and the pains in the limbs < from cold air and becoming cold < in cold damp weather.

- Walking in the open air, when not cold > its symptoms > from rubbing.

- Violent pains in the rectum and bladder.

- Burning is a strong symptom in many parts but especially in the rectum, in the palms, and soles and the uterus.

- Excessive hyperaesthesia, all the symptoms are < from grief and excitement.

- They not only imagine themselves sick, but they pretend to be sick when they are not.

- She pulls her hair and presses her hands upon her head constantly complaining and threatening. Threatens her nurse and her attendants. She strikes her head with her hands and tears her clothing. Consolation causes weeping. Mental symptoms are < in the evening after eating. She wants to hide because she imagines that she will be assaulted.

- Frequent attacks of dizziness, even so great that she falls to the ground.

- Constantly rubs the head against something. Sometimes it is the pillow, when in bed. Pains are pressing and often wander around from place to place in the head. Violent pains in the temples and occiput at the same time.

- Dim vision < in the right eye. The sensation of sand or splinter in the eyes. Itching in the eyes. Many symptoms of the body are confined to the right side.

- Aversion to food and meat but craving for raw food.

- Diarrhoea has been brought on after washing the hair attended with dark fetid stool.

- Oppression in the chest when raising the arms and when laying on the left side.

- Constant want of air and desire for fresh air and sensation as if the heart turned over, A sensation as if the heart were squeezed and compressed. It has cured angina pectoris.

- Upon the back, there are boils, abscesses, and carbuncles, especially on the back of the neck and between the shoulder blade, and violent pain in the lumbar region.

- Weakness, numbness, and restlessness are always present. The pains of the limbs are so great that he cannot stand the weight of clothing. Numbness of the left upper and right lower extremity.

- Sleeplessness before midnight is very marked.

- It has cured dry itching eczema of the extremities and other parts of the skin after Arsenic and Sulphur failed. It is a very deep-acting and long-lasting medicine and very useful for the skin.

Tarentula Hispanica & Tarentula Cubensis

Dr. Tyler

- Sudden violent or sly (cunning), destructive movements are characteristic and unique to this drug.

- The urinary symptoms suggest (cantharis). The skin < septic troubles, abscess (Anthrax), etc reminds me of Tarentula Cubensis.

- Has a reputation for cancer of the tongue etc,

- Laughs, runs, dances, gesticulates, sings till hoarse and exhausted.

- Attacks of hysteron mania daily about the same hour, first quarrelsome and despondent, suddenly a state of great exaltation, hits, and abuses everyone. Destroys whatever she can lay her hand on, tears her clothes, laughs and sings, mocks aged people, if restrained becomes violent, and ends in a comatose sleep.

- Rolling from side to side to relieve the distress is a characteristic symptom of this remedy.

Tarentula Cubensis
Dr. Chowdhury

- It is useful in various affections like chorea, hysteria, and paralysis. The constant movement of the arms and legs and various muscles of the body.

- There is hyper irritation of the terminal points of the nerves. Hence constant movement of friction is necessary with these patients. They rub their hands and legs and even their heads against something. They must roll something between their fingers and put their fingers in their mouth. This extra irritability of the entire body is the red-strand symptom of the remedy.

- Troubles occur at the same time every year.

- Extreme sensitiveness, particularly marked in the spine.

- It causes great hyperemia and hyperesthesia of the female sexual system which leads to extreme sexual excitement. It is a leading remedy for Nymphomania. In the male, it leads to orgasm and inability ending ultimately in insanity.

- It is a good medicine for intense unbearable painful vulvae extending into vagina. The itchness is indeed great at night time with dryness, heat of the parts, burning and frequently, expulsion of gas from the vagina.

- The patient is almost driven made every night. The urine generally is thick, hot and full of sediments.

- It is a good medicine for cystitis with high fever, Great difficulty in passing even a few drops of urine.

- Cough > by smoking. Stool followed immediately on washing the head. Pain in the ear associated with hiccough.

- Tarentula Hip: Weeping, causeless in sleep. Light L, wants tom scream, noise <. Averasion to any kind of colour.

- The patient is a 1st class lier, thief, deceiver and disguisher. The patient pretends himself in a different way (I. J.H 69-20).

Tellurium

Dr. Chowdhury

- Ring worms affect the face, body, and the hair roots. The lesions are round shaped just like rings, from exude a watery excoriating fluid, that smells like fish-brine.

- Useful in otorrhoea and its indication here is a fish-brine smell.

- It is used with benifit in case of injury. DR. Dr. Kent has cured a case by the following indication. An extreme hyperesthesia of the back. The sensitiveness is so great that the least tactile impression sends vibration of pains to remote parts of the body.

- Sweats profusely and the odor of the sweat is offensive and garlic-like.

- Suppose the root of the nerve is crushed and the pain shoots downwards and is < by coughing and sneezing etc. Tellurium helps much better than Hypericum. IN hypericum the pain shoots upwards towards the root of the nerves. 80% case of slipped disc cases may need Tellurium as well as cervical Spondylosis. In cases where the pain shoots up without any history of injury, it is Palladium.

- Natrum Sulph: It is a good medicine for after effects of Lumber puncture such as headaches, lumber pains, etc. When there is oozing out of C.S.F. after fracturing at the skull (IJHM-January-March,75), and prolapse disc think of Rhus tox.

Terebinthinae Oleum

Dr. Chowdhury

- It is a first-grade remedy for Bright's disease. In the 1st stage when blood and albumen are more abundant than casts and epithelium. When the urine is scanty and surcharged with albumen, casts, and blood discharge, edema of the legs sets in. When the urine becomes dark-colored due to the decomposition of blood capsules. Violent burning in the urethra, great tenesmus of the bladder, dyspnoea, and peculiar sweetish odor of the urine, resembling the odor of violets. No remedy can take the place of Terebinthinae.

- Violent burning and cutting pain < at rest and > from walking.

- Uraemia and ureamic coma. It removes the stupefaction and deep sleep that follow uraemic poisoning.

- It is a great hemorrhagic remedy. It checks hemorrhage from the bowels, kidneys, bladder, lungs, uterus, and anus especially when the ejected blood shows signs of degeneration.

Dr. Tyler

- Burning in the umbilicus, the umbilical region seems retracted, cold, just as though a cold round plate were pressed against him.

- It has the credit of inducing stupefaction and deep sleep.

- Toungue remains dry with abdominal tension after cleansing becomes dry again.

- As if the intestine were being drawn towards the spine.

- It is said, it prevents and dissolves renal calculus.

- Constant colic of the whole abdomen, extending into the leg.

- Movement in the inguinal region as if a hernia would protrude.

- Very drowsy, difficult to awake, cold and clammy perspiration all over the body.

Teucrium Marum
Dr. Chowdhury
- In excluding its worm symptoms it is a first-class remedy in the treatment of polyps- nasal, vaginal, and rectal. Mucus polyp of the nose, as well as flushy polypus, springing from nostrils or elsewhere accompanied by a crawling sensation in the nose, stoppage of the nose and sensation of formication and shooting at the root of the nose finds Teucrium a ready help.
- It cured hard fibrous growths on the inward side of the eyelids which prevented him from properly closing.

Theridion
Dr. Kent
Chilly patient

- Emaciation, enlargement of glands, constant hunger and thirst > by warmth and during rest. So restless that she must keep busy though she accomplishes nothing.
- Joyousness and singing with a headache.
- Awakens at 11 pm with vertigo. Vertigo and nausea from closing the eyes and when kneeling in church.
- Headache is almost violent < on motion, talking, hot drinks with nausea and vomiting, sensitive to light and noise. Pain in forehead extending to occiput, Sensation as if vertex did not belong to her. Complaints from sunstroke.
- Flickering even when eyes are closed.
- It has cured most obstinate catarrh of the nose with offensive thick-yellow or greenish-yellow discharge. Pressing pain of root of nose. Paroxysms of violent sneezing.

- Lock jaw in the morning on waking. Foam at the mouth with a chill. Salty taste in the mouth, and the tongue feels as if burnt. The mouth feels numb. Taste impaired.

- Liver condition with burning pain < from touch motion and noise and bilious vomiting.

- Pain in the groin in man after coitus or motion and on drawing up the limbs.

- Enlarged prostrate gland with a sensation of a lump in the perineum. Must arise several times during the night to pass urine. Copious urine during the night. Seminal emission during sleep in the afternoon.

- Singing and short breath on ascending stairs.

- Spinal anaemia. Itching of back and nape. Violent itching of calf.

- While coughing he jerks his head forward and draws his knees up to abdomen while coughing (Dr. Dr. Chowdhury).

- Craves oranges, bananas, wine, brandy, tobacco, acid fruits and drinks (Dr. Tyler).

Tilia Europaea

Dr. Chowdhury

- An intense sore feeling about the abdomen. The whole abdomen feels painful when touched, especially about navel.

- This symptom leads to its successful application in peritonitis.

- The next important indication is hot sweat.

- A peculiar burning sensation was felt in the genital urinary and rectal region.

- Sensation of a veil before the eyes. She feels as if there is a veil or gauze spread before the field of vision.

Trombidium
Dr. Chowdhury

- It is prepared from a parasite found in the common house fly.
- It is an invaluable remedy for the treatment of diarrhoea and dysentery.
- Its grand key note < after eating and dinning.
- The stools are generally thin brown and facial.
- Crampy pain before during and after stool.
- Great tenesmus, prolapses on and burning in the anus.
- Stools are generally expelled with great force.
- They occur generally after dinner and supper and hardly any evacuation after breakfast.
- Stool after eating and drinking it can be compared with the following medicine:
- Aloes: Want of confidence in sphincter, early morning diarrhoea, during out of bed < in hot weather and jelly-like mucus, rumbling in the abdomen.
- Desires for juicy things.
- Passing of much flatus during stool can make it differentiate from Trombidium.
- Argent Nitricum: Usually greenish diarrhoea and nocturnal aggravation.
- Diarrhoea after taking sweets and candy.
- Nervous diarrhoea: Greenish, slimy diarrhoea.
- Arsenic: It is serious, the rapid sinking of the vital force, anguish, restlessness, putrid blackish stool.
- Thirst at midnight.

- China: Diarrhea after meals. It is painless and mostly nocturnal. Diarrhoea is caused by taking fruit. Distension of the abdomen and the stool contains undigested food particles.

- Colocynth: Intense colic and > by hard pressure.

- Croton Tig: The stools are copious, yellow, watery and they come out forcibly. Though < from eating and drinking but > from warm water is a characteristic. The slightest movement of bony renew and fresh desire for stool.

- Ferrum sulphuricum: the patient can hardly wait till the meal is finished. It is almost simultaneous with eating and drinking. The stools are undigested and mostly nocturnal. It is generally indicated in chronic cases where the evaluations are mostly painless.

- Gambugia: Particularly indicated in diarrhoea of old people. The urging is excessive and the stools are expelled all at once with considerable force followed by a feeling of general relief.

- Kali Phos: White putrid diarrhoea with great weakness. The breath is extremely offensive.

- Trombodium: It is a good medicine for ulcerative colitis.

- In ulcerative colitis even when there is no history of T.B. in this case either T.B. or bacillus, gives in good result. Sometimes Thuja interposed +- helps these cases.

- Chaparro Amargoso and Trombodium: Both are good medicine for ulcerative colitis as well as chronic diarrhoea,

- Cortisone: If you take cortisone, it produces a peptic ulcer. It should be tried in duodenal ulcer, where the indicated medicine fails, It should be tried in ulcerative colitis (IJHM-71-70 pages).

Thuja Occidentalis

Dr. Kent

Hot patient

- It has a waxy, shiny face, it looks as if it had been smeared with grease and is often transparent. HE is sickly looking individual, looking as if entering after some cachexia.

- The perspiration is peculiar. It is sweet in odor and swells like honey. Sometimes like garlic. A pungent odor emanates from the genitals. He smells his genitals.

- Arsenic is the acute of Thuja and Natrum Sulph. In most cases usually, these two medicines are required to finish the case. But in Syphilis and Psoriasis. Arsenic acts for a long time and eradicates the complaints when similar to them, but it is not similar to sycosis.

- It throws out wart-like excrescences which are soft and pulpy and very sensitive. They burn, burn, itch, and bleed easily when rubbed by clothing. Horny excrescences more upon the skin, warts of a brownish color, especially if upon the abdomen. Great brown spots like liver spots, from upon the abdomen. Zona around the chest. Herpetic eruptions everywhere and there like Sepia.

- When warts have been suppressed in a non-homeopathic way, we get symptoms of Thuja and Staphysgharia, but Thuja leads all medicine from symptoms coming from suppressed warts.

- There are probably several varieties of urethra discharges, but there is one that is sycotic and when that has been suppressed, it has produced maism with soreness in the bottom of the feet and in the knees and particularly through the back and loins and sciatic nerve, in the knees and ankle joints. Sometimes it affects the upper extremities, particularly the lower.

- Most violent < from keeping still like Rhus tox, great aching that increases so long as he keeps still, he is very often compelled to keep in bed and then he constantly moves and turns. This symptom is cured by Rhus tox when it is not sycotic, but when it comes from suppressed gonorrhea. Medorrhinum and thuja will cure.

- It is preeminently a strong medicine when we get the history of animal poisoning, snake bites, vaccination, and smallpox.

- Sometimes the pain is so severe in the left ovary that the right one suffers apparently from sympathy. When the ovaries have been affected sometimes there will be measle symptoms, most violent irritability, jealousy, quarrelsomeness, and ugliness. She wants to be alone and takes upon herself fixed ideas. Associated with this condition, we have violent intense headaches, and tearing in the eyes > by heat. Pain localized in a small spot. A nail is driven in the head sides of the head and forehead.

- Rheumatic head symptoms are < in damp air from sour things and also from stimulating and exciting.

- In the urethrae discharges and sycotic character. Thuja leads all other remedies. In non sycotic variety Cannabis Sativa is sufficient but in those cases that have proved to be sycotic Cannabis Sativa is left uncured.

Dr. Chowdhury

- It is also called Abor vital which means tree of life.

- Its action upon the human constitution is that of at unlimited cell proliferation and on this account we meet with a lot of pathological vegetative growths, spongy tumors, and many other varieties, and manifestations. It is said to have a strong action over the lymphatic secretion.

- He is constantly in a hurry. When he talks he talks in a rash. His movements are hurried and impatient. The merest approach of a stranger sets him on his edge. When spoken to he answers with tears and sobs. These patients are extremely quarrelsome and they get angry easily about trifles, loathing of life, depression of spirits, sleeplessness, and dissatisfaction are distinctly marked.

- The headache is always < from sexual excessed and at night > by exercise in the open air looking upward and turning the head backward.
- Neuralgic pain in different parts of the body accompanied by frequent micturition.
- It is not only a remedy for smallpox but also a preventive applied during the suppurative stage it prevents pitting.
- It is a very useful remedy in cases of persistent indigestion and loose bowels. There is distension of the abdomen with flatus and great rumbling, cracking, and grumbling noise in the abdomen. The abdomen protrudes here and there from the flatus as though something live were moving inside.
- The anus smarts and burns all day after the morning diarrhoea.
- The urine spurts out while laughing, coughing, and sneezing. Suddeness of the desire for urination, cannot retain the flow of urine. He runs to the vessel, grasping at his penis, and even then fails in retaining it.
- Its cough comes on during the day. Ait hardly troubles at the night time. It is excited by a choking sensation and followed by an expectoration of yellow or green lumps. Sometimes this cough is < after eating.

Dr. Tyler
According to Hahnemann
- On exposure of the body to warm air, shivering all over. Rigor with much yawning, the warm air feels cold to him, and the Sun seems to have no power to warm him.
- Eruptions only on covered parts, burn after scratching.
- Yinglings Accoucheur, 's Emergency Manual- a small discharge starts with pain, gradually becomes worse, and ultimately ends in abortion (200 or 1M Thuja) is the remedy here.
- The remedy here:<

Piles with pain sitting (Thuja)

Baby: Sad, depressed, sensitive to music and people, riding carriage, usually faulty dentition. Hesitate to speak, because they do not find the proper words to speak Weeping easily Homeopathic Herald-June 73.

- Palpitation insomnia > Headache from excessive tea drinking.
- It is a good medicine for the history of old animal poisoning.
- < From taking onion. (Lycopodium).
- Weeping and trembling of feet from music.
- A dazed and confused stage is marked especially after sleep(Arsenic, Antim tart, Lycopodium).
- The heart must beat violently on ascending stairs (Calcarea carb, iodium).
- With the coryza, there is nocturnal and morning cough and shooting pains on the left side. Of trachea. < By swallowing and Inspiring.
- Urine is frequent and copious and the clear urine becomes cloudy with break due to sediment after standing. Jerky urination, the stream stops, and stairs.
- Pain and cracking in the shoulder joints It is a good medicine for newborn babies when complication arises after primary vaccination or when we get a history of repeated vaccination of parents. It tends to wild hair all over the body.
- Hair on unwanted parts as on the face Of a woman on the upper. On the upper lip At times, the movement Is felt in the abdomen, just like a child. The mother feels the knee or the elbow. This is more like a spurious pregnancy. These symptoms are found in women where there is a great desire for a child. Inquire into the dream where Thuja seems a remedy. Its dreams are very important and often a guide for the selection of this remedy. Dreams are falling from a height and dreams of dead people are very prominent indications.

- Recurrent cystitis or a history of bladder complaints.
- Fear of Touch she never let anybody handle or touch her. She hated being fondled or kissed. She cried and struggled even while she was dressing.

Tuberculinum

Dr. Kent
Hot patient

- One of the prominent remedies in intermittent fever is when the best-selected remedy like Silicea and Calcarea fails to bring a cure when the well-selected remedy has acted and the constitution shows a tendency to break down, we should think of this medicine.
- 10 M, 50 M, and CM, potencies, Two doses of each potency at long intervals. All children and young people who have inherited tuberculosis may be immune from their inheritance and their resilience will be restored. It cures most cases of adenoids and tuberculosis glands of the neck.
- Hopelessness in many complaints, anxiety, evening until midnight, loquacity during fever, cosmopolitan. The intellectual symptoms and lung symptoms are interchangeable.
- When chronic constitutional headaches have been broken up, sometimes the patient tends to lose flesh and becomes feeble. The headache has been resolved, but the patient has become feeble. A new manifestation comes a new organ is affected.
- Sore bruised Feeling all over the body. Acting on the bones. Sore bruised condition of the eyeball. Sensitive to touch on turning the sideways. Persons who have long felt the weakness of tuberculosis. Tubercular conditions are subject to cold sweat on the head.
- The relationship between the tuberculinum and. Calcarea is very close. Tuberculinum and silicea are also well-related.

- Craving cold milk and all gone hungry feeling that drives him to eat. This has been cured by Tuberculinum after sulphur failed.

- Stool large and hard or constipation alternating with diarrhoea. Constipation is a strong feature of the Tuberculinum. Itching of the anus. Excessive sweat in chronic diarrhoea. A drum belly. Diarrhea driven out early in the morning. This is a common feature of pthisis or patients going into pthisis..

- Dry hacking cough before the evening chill. The patient says "I know my old chills are coming back again because of the cough I have".

- Burnett thought that ringworms commonly formed upon those who have inherited phthisis. He thought it was a sign of approaching phthisis, and he used Bacillinium 200. He used it somewhat as a routine remedy for every child with ringworm.

- Patients who suffer from weakness in the evening rapid pulse in the evening. Palpitation after the evening meal.

- Aking drawing pain in the limbs during rest > by walking (Rhus tox) In acute cases when Rhus tox fails. Give this medicine. Pains all over the body, but mostly in the lower limbs.

- Complaints aggravated from standing. (Sulphur)

- Red purple eruptions that are nodular in character. The patient wants to sit all the time by the fire, etching in cold air > By going to the fire < From scratching. Always< before a storm.

Dr. Chowdhury

- Tall slim stoop shouldered and flat-chested. Mental precocious, very weak physically.

- It has three characteristic symptoms:

    1) Changeability of symptoms.

    2) Great sensitivity Crops of boils intensely painful. to cold.

    3) Profound and rapid emaciations.

- Crops of boils intensely painful. Keep appearing successively in different parts of the body, especially on the nose. The puss discharge is generally greenish-fetid.

- Morning diarrhea, where the attacks are sudden and imperative after the failure of sulphur.

- According to Dr Dr. Kent, it is almost specific for ulceration of cornea in children. Give Bacillinum instead of Tuberculinum.

- According to Ghatak, we should always think of Bacillinum instead of tuberculinum, where there is a history of ringworm.

Tubercular patients are over-intelligent over enthusiastic and over agile. They are particularly sick before a thunderstorm or cloudy weather due to electrical changes in the atmosphere.

Aversion to meat, desire for cold milk feels > in the open air.

Alphabet

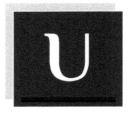

Uranium Nitricum
Dr. Chowdhury
- It is a good medicine for both diabetes mellitus and diabetes insipidus. It is meant for. Heptagonic diabetes. These symptoms generally are great languor debility, Cold feeling Vertigo profuse urination, complete loss of sexual power, dryness of the mouth, tenacious salivation, coated tongue, and great thirst.
- Dr. Dr. Kent: Consider this medicine for excessive thirst polyuria and dry tongue. He used. 30.
- It is also used in gastric and duodenal ulcers. Boring pain in the pyloric region, sinking at epigastrium, irritations, gnawing, sinking feeling of the cardiac end of the stomach. A short while after dinner and recurring hematemesis.

Urtica Urens
Dr. Chowdhury
- Dr. Burnett used Urtica Urens in acute gout associated with fever.
- He however used it in five drop doses of the Q in a glass of warm water every 2/3 hours. Under this influence, urine became free and plentiful and the patient made steady progress until complete recovery ensued.
- It is an excellent remedy for. Nettle rash. It causes intense itching and burning of the skin with a sensation as the part is scorched, red and red raised blotches appear in different parts of the body,

and they are characterized by a constant desire to scratch these. Blotches generally precede an attack on rheumatism. They are also periodical. They affect the patient every year at the same time. Both the eruption and etching disappear as soon as the patient lies down and reappears immediately on rising.

- The Association of rheumatic pain and continued fever with nettle rash is an important keynote symptom.
- It has a special affinity for the deltoid of muscles. We use it for the rheumatism of the arms when the deltoid muscles are affected.
- It is one of our best remedies for causing the free flow of milk. When that has been impeded, it was used repeatedly in insufficient or entire want of milk sensation, with almost astounding results.
- Dr Dr. Kent reports a case of a woman with a lump in her left breast of many years' duration, who, after childbirth altogether, lacked in milk secretion She had severe pain on the whole of her right lower limb, breast chest sacrum, and in the muscles of her neck. Urtica Uranus was given and after three doses, the breast was full of milk together with a general relief.
- It is a good medicine for bee stings.
- It is usually meant for the right deltoid rheumatism.
- Uraemia with highly urinus odor of the patient.

Ustilago
Dr. Chowdhury
Hot patient

- This is a fungus, that grows in Indian corn, hence it is similar to Secale-Cor. The affinity between these two remedies is more marked in their action on the female sexual system. It is noted as abortifacient. Dr. Burt administered two drachmas of Ustilago to two pregnant bitch dogs and in both it caused abortion.

- Passive hemorrhage from retention of placenta after miscarriage. The blood that keeps oozing for days and weeks is darkish and coagulated. The patient complains of constant bearing down sensation. There is a profuse discharge of blood from the enlarged uterus and the flow is accompanied by cache and sharp pains across the lower abdomen from the hip to hip. This flow of blood is sometimes intermittent. It stops and then on slightest excitement reappears.

- The patient complains of constant aching, and distress in the testicles, more especially in the right Hemamelis has similar symptoms. The pain is severe and it shifts suddenly to the bowels. The pain is accompanied by nausea and cold sweat on the scrotum. It is particularly useful in. orchitis after gonorrhea when the disease becomes chronic.

- Oxalic acid: It is also a good medicine for neuralgia of the spermatic chord, where the pain is almost unbearable. The patient avoids all movements. as much as the pains aggravated by the slightest motion.

- Frequent attacks of tonsillitis. They are congested and enlarged. The left tonsil is especially affected. It looks large and dusky, and the pain on swallowing is intense. It is a lancinating character and it extends from the tonsil to the ear. The throat is dry, and there is a feeling of lump behind the larynx which makes her swallow constantly.

- Alopecia: We find a complete loss of hair under this remedy Dr. Hurandall relates a case of Alopecia in a bitch dog that he cured with. Ustilago. The symptoms which led to the prescription were her tendency to abort. He used 3x in five drop doses three times daily.

- Carboveg: It is good medicine for falling hair during parturition, especially from occiput.

Urva- Ursi

- It has a selected action upon bladder, Very frequent urination, and this hardly leaves the patient for rest. At night time he had to get up three to four times every hour to pass urine and each time it took 10 to 15 minutes to finish Although the quantity of urine was passed very meager.

- Its greatest indication is that the patient can only pass urine by lying posture.

Alphabet

Valeriana

Dr. Kent
Chilly patient

- Sensation of something warm rising from the stomach, causing paroxysmal suffocation.
- All these general symptoms come on during rest> by motion and moving about.
- Complaints change and pains wander from place to place.
- Erroneous ideas thinking she is more than one, moves to the edge of the bed to make room. She again thinks of an animal lying near her, which she fears. She may not fear in the evening in the dark. Vertigo when stooping.
- Headache from exposure to the light of sun and heat.
- Flashes of light before the eyes in the dark.
- Voracious hunger with nausea symptoms. < when the stomach is empty > After breakfast complaints from fasting child vomit as soon as nurses after the mother became angry.

Dr. Chowdhury
- All the senses of organs are in a state of excitement. The vision becomes extremely acute. He seems to see even in darkness. His hearing is true in a state. Hyperesthesia.
- It has a strong affinity for Achilles tendinitis when other remedies fail Valeriana cures. The pain in the heels. The pain is

< from, standing and letting the foot rest on the floor. A certain amount of relief is obtained by resting the foot on a chair or lying down. This pain comes and goes quickly in Belladona.

Veratrum-Alb

Dr. Kent

- Coldness running through this remedy, coldness of discharge. Coldness of the body with. Complete relaxation and exhaustion.

- Full of cramps looks as if he would die.

- Always wants to be busy to carry on his daily work in insanity. He would pile up chairs on top of one another when asked what he was doing. He replies that he was piling up stoves. When not occupied with this, he was tearing his clothes or praying for hours on his knees an exalted state of religion, and frenzy, believing that he is the risen Christ. Screams and screeches until he is blue in the face. Head cold as ice. Exhorts to repent, preaches, howls, sings obscene songs, exposes the person, fear of death, imagines the world is on fire, is full of despair and hopelessness, with approaching insanity, despair of his recovery, and attempts suicide.

- Young girls go on for years with menstrual difficulties and preceding each menstrual sinus is a state of despair, never smiles. The world seems blue. Everything is dark. These are preparing for a marked state of insanity. It is a remedy that keeps many women out of the insane asylum, especially those with uterine troubles. Girls at puberty suffered from dysmenorrhoea. Historical mental state diarrhea and vomiting.

- He has a strange sensation when he drinks water as if it ran down the outside and did not go down the esophagus.

- All fruits cause painful distention of the abdomen.

- Gnawing hunger despite nausea and vomiting, empty and all gone sensation in the abdomen after stool.

Dr. Chowdhury

- Chronic constipation the first portion of which is large and the later parts consist of thin strings. He has to urge and strain so hard each time that he breaks out with cold sweat on his forehead, and he feels quite weak and exhausted.

- He believes himself to be a man of very great importance and enormous wealth and wealth and he squanders his money.

- They kiss everybody they come in contact with from an affectionate nature they may merge into an amorous and lascivious state. They talk about indecent things makes. Impudent gestures and gesticulation, phenomena like this are caused by the suppression of the catamenia.

- It is particularly efficacious in all varieties of pernicious fevers, accompanied by general exhaustion, rapid synching of strength, and profuse diarrhoea on this indication it is useful in quotidian, tertian, and quaten fevers. The time of paroxysm is generally 6 am. The stage of chill is very prominent. It starts with great severity, with the ice coldness of the entire body, despite great chilliness. The patient craves for cold and refreshing drinks.

- It has epistaxis during sleep, but only from. Right nostril. It can be compared with the following medicines in Epistaxis during sleep:

1) **Merc Sol:** The blood discharges from the nose is black, and it hangs down the nose like black. Icicles are just exactly what we find in Kali Bichronicum.

2) **Nitric acid:** Very exhausting hemorrhage of Venous blood. The gums are swollen and dark red and bleed easily. The patient complained of splinter-like pain in the nose.

Dr. Tyler
- Cutting pains. Flatulent colleague, which? Attacks the lower bowels here and there, and the whole abdomen.

- The longer the flatus is retained, the more difficult it is to be expelled.

Veratrum Viride

Dr. Chowdhury
- There is great cerebral congestion, the feeling in the head as if it would burst open. This congestion may be due to extreme plethora, vascular irritation, alcoholism, teething or suppression, and some natural discharge. one. A unique feature of this congestion is the Concomitance of nausea and vomiting with the congestion. The patient complains of feeling sick and vomits often during the attack.

- Suddenness is another feature of this medicine. The patient is at her best, but all of a sudden there comes an attack of fainting, headache, prostration, nausea, and vomiting. These symptoms are all prominent by the suddenness of their onset.

- Red streak down the middle of the tongue. And sensation as if scalded, were the guiding symptoms for the selection of this remedy.

- Stupefaction, confusion, loss of memory, and depression of spirit are prominently marked. It has been highly advocated in puerperal mania of the symptoms of silence and suspicion. The patient is mortally afraid of being poisoned. She refuses to see her physician, whom she thinks has come to terrify her. This antipathy and aversion towards the medical man to whom she was accustomed is almost a guiding symptom.

- It is used in metritis, ovaritis, cellulitis, and inflammation of other appendages, Provided we have a high fever accompanying such inflammation. It is an important remedy for dysmenorrhea and menstrual colic in purothic women. Prone to cerebral congestion.

- When the fever is accompanied by drowsiness and throbbing of the temporal arteries. A frequent fall in pulse. Vomiting of mucus and bile and showing a tendency to spasm, it ought to be a good remedy.

- Pulmonary congestion is apprehended during the emotive stage of measles is manifested by. Dyspnea, cough, and pain in the chest So in scarlet fever variola and other exanthematous ailments attention should be particularly directed to Veratrum Viride by the intensity of the arterial excitement. Hardness and fullness of pulse, restlessness, dyspnea, sensation of constriction of chest, and high temperature are sure indications of this remedy.

- No remedy is prompted and more liable in checking convulsion whether. Epilepticform or puerperal. Then Veratum Viride when given in a big dose to a healthy individual causes contractions of the muscular system, particularly of the muscles of the face, neck, fingers, and toes. The head is drawn to one side, the mouth is drawn at one corner, and facial muscles get affected with violent convulsive twitching.

Dr. Tyler

- The patient has an aversion to sweets and may complain that water tastes sweet.

- In one case, clothes would not fit him seemed as if they were scratching him somewhere, constantly. Twitching of the different parts of the body.

- Sensation as if head would burst, as if stomach tightly drawn against spine.

Viburnum Opulus

Dr. Chowdhury

- It is a good medicine for spasmodic dysmenorrhea, a great sickening feeling. Severe pain in the back, going around to the loins and across to the pubic bones, a bearing down sensation with a feeling as if the body from the west downwards would collapse. Severe aching in the rectum and great depression of spirits > from laying down and < from motion.

- Before the onset of menstrual flow, the patient complains of a severe bearing down sensation and drawing pain in the anterior muscles of thighs, both the sacral and pubic region have a heavy aching feeling.

- Dr. Hale says it is especially indicated in spasmodic dysmenorrhea for false labor pains, A dose after every pain. He says that cramps in the abdomen and legs of pregnant women are. controlled very quickly by it. It will prevent miscarriage if given before the membranes are injured. And when the pains are spasmodic and threatening it prevents abortions, especially. In the 8th month when children so delivered die soon after birth. Pain and cramps in the abdomen and legs during pregnancy.

Dr. Tyler

- Pains begin in the back and go around to loins and cross pubic bones like labor pains.

- Cramp-like pains and spasms of the stomach, bowel bladder, or other organs when reflex from uterine irritation.

- Opening and shutting in the left parietal region in occiput (Coccus and cannabis indica).

- Pelvic organs, turning upside down.

- As if she would collapse from the waist to the lower pelvis.

- In sleep sensation of falling wakes with a start.

- Dr. Boger: Frequent profuse urination during headache, menses hemorrhage, etc.

Vinca Minor

Dr. Chowdhury

- Various skin diseases are marked with this remedy and its special affinity is found on the scalp. It has been used with great success in. crusta lactea, flatus, plica polonica, eczema, and alopecia. Humid eruptions with intense burning and itching are numerous on the head. There is an oozing of moisture that mates the hair together. Sometimes the whole gets full of vermin. It is just like Graphities and Mezereum.

- The slightest mental excitement or emotion throws a quantity of blood into the nose and it looks almost purple.

- Excessive hemorrhage during menstruation either from fibroid or climacteric, hair falls out in patches when renewed and becomes grey.

Viola Odorata

Dr. Chowdhury

- Obstinate cases of Otorrhoea and deafness that after resisting every sort of treatment had, at last, given in to Viola odorata (infertile eczema of the face).

- The most characteristic symptom is a sensation of tension felt by the patient everywhere. He complains of tension in the forehead, oxycodone, and scalp. This feeling of tension originally begins in the scalp. From there, it extends to the upper half of the face, forehead, and temples as far as the ears alternate with a similar sensation in the occiput and cervical muscles.

- The patient constantly knits his brows and if asked As to the cause, he will tell you that this inclination is due to an uneasy sensation of tightness on the forehead. A peculiar burning sensation in the forehead is equally characteristic. Great weakness in feet in the muscles of the nape of the neck. The head feels too heavy to be carried straight. It frequently sinks forward.

- It is a very useful remedy for eye, particularly in choroiditis particularly for the eye, particularly in chloroids. LIT S, sensitiveness to light, painful, forcible drawing together of lids are from irresistible sleep. The illusion of vision. The vision of fiery, serpentine circles, intense headache, and tension beneath the eyes.

- It is an important rheumatic remedy, especially of the right deltoid muscles and the right, carpal and metacarpal joints. It is also indicated in the rheumatism of the wrist.< by slightest motion.

- Unusual discomfort of breathing quite disproportionate to the height of uterus turning pregnancy. It is a good medicine for chyluria whether the urine is milky and smells like cat's urine. Very offensive or where the urine is milky and thick like condensed milk.

Viola Tricolor
Dr. Chowdhury

- It is a great remedy for eczema and impetigo with urinary disturbance. The urine is too copious or sudden arrest of urinary secretion accompanies most of its skin symptoms.

- It causes involuntary seminal discharges with lewd dreams. The dreams are very vivid and the loss of seminal fluid causes a certain amount of exhaustion and weariness of mind. The urine passed is cloudy and has a strong smell resembling cat's urine.

- It is an anti-syphilitic and deep-acting remedy.

Vipera-Torva
Dr. Chowdhury

- Its modality is very important for the application of this remedy in any sort of complaint.

- A bursting sensation of the affected limbs when hanging down is the characteristic indication of this remedy.

- Other modalities are: < from warm and night > by cold application.
- Exposure of the affected parts to cold air.

Viscum Album
Dr. Chowdhury

- It is a good remedy for rheumatism and its modalities are like Rhus tox. We should think of this medicine when the Rhus tox fails.
- It is a good medicine for epilepsy. The aura felt like a glow of fire rising from the feet to the head. He also feels a large spider, crawling over his hands.

Alphabet

Xanthoxylum
Dr. Chowdhury

- It is an excellent remedy for dysmenorrhea of nervous women. The pain is almost agonizing along the course of the genitocrural nerve. It almost drives the patient's distraction. It shoots down as low as the knee and no position relieves. The desire to take deep breaths during pain is the greatest indication of this remedy.

- Another important symptom is the sensation of weakness of the lower limbs. The patient wants to sit or lie most of the time. The menstrual flow is too early, and it is always accompanied by pain down thighs. Ovarian pain with scanty and retracted menses, extending to genito crural nerves and associated with great backache also call for this medicine. Leucorrhoea coming on when it is time for menses to appear is another important indication of this remedy. The menstrual blood is almost black, coming in springs and clothes and intermittent every other day, and generally lasting two weeks.

- It has been used with success in chlorosis, particularly in these cases in severe oedema. Swelling had appeared in the face and leg and all symptoms pointed to a fatal end. The indication here is sharp, severe neuralgic pains that radiate downwards from the scitic cfrest rest to the knees.

Alphabet

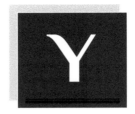

Yucca Fillamentosa

Dr. Chowdhury

- Its symptoms are very much like the symptoms of Chelidonium. The patient complains of sharp, cramping pain in the liver, which. penetrates straight through the back. There is also a bad taste in the mouth and an excess of bile in the stools which becomes loose and diarrhoic.

- The tongue, which is coated yellow, takes the imprioned of teeth like. Chelidonium. In Yucca filamentosa the tongue is rather bluish-white, then yellow.

- The patient passes many flatus by rectum while having stool, and complains of frontal or temporal headache most of the time.

- It is used in Gonorrhea and urethritis. The patient complained of a sensation of burning while urinating.

Alphabet

Zincum Metallicum

Dr. Kent

Chilly patient

- Oversensitive in one part and lack of feeling in another. This extreme sensitiveness is like Nux vom, which is inimical. The overwork and excitable persons belong to Nux vom.

- Difficult expulsion of urine paralysis of the bladder and tedious constipation associated with spinal symptoms. Urine slow in starting can pass it only when sitting and in some cases, only when sitting, leaning back against the seat with hard pressure.

- Aching in the dorsal lumber. And sacral region > when walking < from rising from a seat. Calcarea, Rhus tox, Phosphorous, Suphur, and Sepia, have this in the highest degree. Zinc occupies a lower grade.

- Always chilly sensitive to cold, full of neurologic pains, and tearing pains, in all parts of the body, when exposed to draft. When it comes to rest, the limbs want to draw up. Hence, historical contractures draw the fingers all out of shape.

- When you put a question to him? And he stares at you in perfect amazement, then says, Oh and answers.

- Some deep-seated brain troubles that will go slowly and gradually into unconsciousness. Rolling of the head for days, eyes listless, body emaciated, involuntary discharges of feces and urines in the bed. Tongue dry and parts so shriveled that it looks like leather, lips also. Face withered each day. older paralysis of one hand or one foot, or it seems that the whole muscular system is paralyzed. Screaming out in pain, but not so shrilly like Apis. A dose of zincum will sometimes bring this patient back to life in a few days after the remedy, there will be jerking and quivering in the past that were motionless, or its action will be shown in copious sweat and much vomiting. Sudden arousing that is alarming for it looks like a threatened sinking, but this. Is the beginning of the reaction. Now, for days and nights, while this little one is coming back to consciousness, the restoration of sensation in the parts is accompanied by the most tormenting formication, tickling, pricking, creeping, and crawling. The parents and neighbors will want something done for it. But if you antidote the case will return where it was before. It will go in this way for a week or two and then will begin to show signs of falling back. It needs another dose of zincum. You will find this. Spinal meningitis after the relief from Gelsemium, Belladonna, and Bryonia, give Zincum.

- It is good medicine for pterygium of the eyes, itching, and stinging pain in the inner angles of eyes with cloudiness of sight. Much burning of the eyes and lids in the morning and the evening with a feeling of dryness and pressure in them. It has cured distressing thickening of the lids, ectropion, and entropion. Granular thickening of the lids, zincum, and Euphrasia are closely related to eye troubles.

- Strabismus after brain troubles.

Dr. Chowdhury

- It causes a sensation of formication as of ants walking over the body, a sensation of tremulousness gradually comes on, developing later, or into a regular tremor, vertigo, fainting, and even convulsions may supervene till death ensues.

- Dentition of children who are very weak and badly developed. The teeth fail to appear in spite of the hardening of the gums. The child shows the great weakness and prostration. The pulse usually is slow and the child soporous and drowsy. It lies with the back of the head pressed deep into the pillow and eyes half closed and squinting rolls the head from side to side.

- It is useful in headaches, a great symptom is the pressure of the root of the nose. This headache is brought on by indulgence in wine or is < by it. It also increases after dinner. Cannot tolerate liquor. This is considered an important indication of this remedy.

- He forgets even those things that have been done. In the course of the day, he finds it difficult to grasp ideas and coordinate thoughts. Evening is usually the time of aggravation wants to get out of bed and run away like Belladonna.

- Aversion to meat fish, and sweet things, particularly to Veal. The taste in the mouth is bitter, and there is intolerance of water.

- It is an invaluable remedy in serious types of diarrhea accompanying typhus, typhoid, meningitis, hydrocephalus, and other varieties of adynamic disease. The stool is foamy, profuse, soft, papescent, and thin. At times it is almost pitch-like and expelled involuntarily. This diarrhoea is mostly accompanied by stupor (Opium) It is usually present with a deficiency of nerve power and an absence of high temperature.

- In Chorea, Zincum finds application in the later stages when symptoms of hydrocephalus Superveins.

- It is a great remedy for constipation as it is with diarrhoiea. The stool are generally large in size and are evacuated with great effort of abdominal muscles. They crumble to pieces due to great dryness. After stool, this patient complains of a pressure and a chewing sensation in the anus. The dryness of stool is like Bryonia and Graphities. Like Sulphur there is great burning in rectum after stool due to dryness. There is often discharge of blood from the anus. It is almost a specific for constipation in newborn babies.

- It has important action over the circulation of blood. It produces great stagnation of blood in the veins of the legs, particularly during pregnancy.

- Heartburn in pregnant women after taking sweet things.

- Its cough is spasmodic and accompanied by severe pain in the chest. The patient during a violent coughing puts his hand to his genitals. It is.<By taking wine and during menstruation. The cough is excited by a tickling sensation in larynx and trachea, as far down as middle of the chest. The sputum is yellow, purulent, tenacious, bloodtinged, sweetish, putrid and metallic.

Zingiber Off

Dr. Chowdhury

- It is reputed to be a good remedy for diarrhoea, when caused by drinking impure water, melons, and bread.

- It is also indicated in humid asthma. The patient feels the great difficulty of respiration. He sits up till night, but the peculiarity lies in the absence of all anxiety, even in the face of threatened suffocation. He seems to be quite cool and collected.

- When the condition in smallpox, measles, or typhoid leads to coma, despite the treatment or abruptly after the onset, the background should immediately be investigated. It is always the syphilo mercurial background, which remains responsible in this condition. A few doses of Merc Sol high solve the problem.

- When a simple cold develops into pneumonia and leads to coma, the background is also syphilis mercurial and Merc is the remedy. The indication here is Merc tongue and a history of dysentery or stomatis is sufficient indication.

- When Encephalitis is wrongly treated the sequel gives serious nervous complications, leading to paralysis of various types, brain disorders leading to idiocy, Insanity cerebral palsy, or muscular atrophy of the affected parts. These conditions are covered up by a list of indicated medicines, but it must be remembered that either. Syphillium, Aurum met, and Merc Sol should be prescribed for a day to loosen the grip of this background, which is always syphilitic (I J H M-71-50).

Zincum Metallicum- Baby (Borland)

- Delayed in everything, slow understanding, and slow grasping.
- Tired from both physical and mental exhaustion, especially pain in the cervical region and sometimes burning along the spinal cord.
- Very sensitive to talking to others.

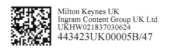
Milton Keynes UK
Ingram Content Group UK Ltd.
UKHW021837030624
443423UK00005B/47